A
CONSUMER'S
GUIDE
to
"ALTERNATIVE
MEDICINE"

A Close Look at Homeopathy, Acupuncture, Faith-Healing, and Other Unconventional Treatments

KURT BUTLER

edited by Stephen Barrett, M.D.

PROMETHEUS BOOKS

Buffalo, New York

Published in 1992 by Prometheus Books.

A Consumer's Guide to "Alternative Medicine": A Close Look at Homeopathy, Acupuncture, Faith-Healing, and Other Unconventional Treatments. Copyright © 1992 by Kurt Butler. All rights reserved. No part of this publication may be reproduced, stored in a retrieval system, or transmitted in any form by any means, electronic, mechanical, photocopying, recording, or otherwise, without prior permission of the publisher, except in the case of brief quotations embodied in critical articles or reviews. Inquiries should be addressed to Prometheus Books, 59 John Glenn Drive, Amherst, NY 14228-2197, 716-691-0133 (FAX: 716-691-0137).

96   95   94   93   5   4   3   2

Library of Congress Cataloging-in-Publication Data

Butler, Kurt.
A consumer's guide to "alternative medicine": a close look at homeopathy, acupuncture, faith-healing, and other unconventional treatments / by Kurt Butler.
        p.   cm.
Includes bibliographical references and index.
        ISBN 0-87975-733-7
        1. Alternative medicine. 2. Quacks and quackery. I. Title.
        [DNLM: 1. Alternative medicine—popular works. 2. Quackery—
        popular works. 3. Therapeutic cults—popular works. WB 890 B985c]
R733.B956 1992
615.5—dc20
DNLM/DLC
for Library of Congress   92-19859
                                                                         CIP

Printed in Canada on acid-free paper.

A
CONSUMER'S
GUIDE *to*
"ALTERNATIVE MEDICINE"

The Smoke-free Workplace
William Weis and Bruce Miller   Paper $17.95

Toxic Terror: The Truth behind the Cancer Scares
Elizabeth M. Whelan, Sc.D., M.P.H.   Cloth $26.95

Vitamin Politics
John Fried   Paper $18.95

Your Guide to Good Nutrition
Fredrick J. Stare, M.D., Ph.D., Virginia Aronson, MS., R.D.,
and Stephen Barrett, M.D.   Paper $13.95

The books listed can be obtained from your book dealer or directly from
Prometheus Books. Please indicate the appropriate titles. Remittance must ac-
company all orders from individuals. Please include $3.50 postage and handling
for the first book and $1.75 for each additional title (maximum $12.00, NYS
residents please add applicable sales tax). Books will be shipped fourth-class
book post. **Prices subject to change without notice.**

Send to _____
                          (Please type or print clearly)
Address _____
City _____ State _____ Zip _____
                                          Amount enclosed _____

Charge my   □ **VISA**   □ **MasterCard**

Account # [ ][ ][ ][ ][ ][ ][ ][ ][ ][ ][ ][ ][ ][ ][ ][ ][ ]

Exp. Date _____/_____ Tel.# _____
Signature _____

Prometheus Books Editorial Offices
700 E. Amherst St., Buffalo, New York 14215

Distribution Facilities
59 John Glenn Drive, Buffalo, New York 14228

Phone Orders call toll free: (800) 421-0351
FAX: (716) 691-0137
Please allow 3-6 weeks for delivery

**This book is to be returned on or before
the last date stamped below.**

About the Author

Kurt Butler, a nutritionist and former science teacher, is a free-lance science and health writer based in Hawaii. He holds a Bachelor of Science degree in physiology from the University of California, Berkeley, and a Master of Science degree in nutrition from the University of Hawaii in Honolulu. He founded and served for two years as president of the Quackery Action Council, a consumer-protection group. He has written many articles on health and nutrition and is coauthor of *The Best Medicine* and *The New Handbook of Health and Preventive Medicine.*

About the Editor

Stephen Barrett, M.D., who practices psychiatry in Allentown, Pennsylvania, is a nationally renowned author, editor, and consumer advocate. An expert in medical communications, he edits *Nutrition Forum Newsletter* and is medical editor of Prometheus Books. He is a board member of the National Council Against Health Fraud and chairs the council's Task Force on Victim Redress. His thirty books include: *The Health Robbers; Vitamins and "Health" Foods: The Great American Hustle; Health Schemes, Scams, and Frauds;* and the college textbook *Consumer Health: A Guide to Intelligent Decisions.* In 1984 he won the FDA Commissioner's Special Citation Award for Public Service in fighting nutrition quackery. In 1987 he began teaching health education at The Pennsylvania State University.

Contents

Acknowledgments

The author is grateful to the following individuals for their many helpful
suggestions during the preparation of the manuscript:

Project manager	Jeanne O'Day, Associate Editor, Prometheus Books
Legal advisor	Michael Botts, Esq., Kansas City, Missouri
Technical editor	Manfred Kroger, Ph.D., Professor of Food Science, The Pennsylvania State University

Introduction

Everyone knows that "the world's oldest profession" is the selling of fake passion. We learn about this as kids, and we read and hear about it throughout our lives. But few people give much thought to the equally widespread and lucrative second-oldest profession—quackery. This entails the selling of fake medicines, miracle diets, worthless supplements, bogus youth potions, and phony cures of all kinds. Like prostitutes, quacks make the "right" noises at the right times. Unlike most prostitutes, however, quacks often become prominent in their community, and many achieve national acclaim.

Health fraud, especially nutrition fraud, seems to enjoy a privileged status in our society. Americans are generally well protected from such scams as counterfeit money, stock swindles, and fake jewelry. But there is almost no protection from fake cancer cures, bogus arthritis remedies, miracle diets, and scores of other snake oils that are worthless, dangerous, or both. These items aren't sold in dark alleys but in modern shops, elegant malls, and professional offices.

The health-fraud industry is large, entrenched, and institutionalized. Large and growing guilds of fringe practitioners are pressuring legislators for more recognition and privileges. Pyramid-style organizations are creating armies of zealots intent on getting rich by selling herbs, vitamins, and weight-loss products to their friends and neighbors. Legions of "experts"—many with diploma-mill degrees—crowd the tabloid talk shows to peddle their books and supplements. Almost anyone with an "alternative" health-related product, procedure, pill, diet, or book is free to market it with little or no social opposition or government regulation. Moreover, the kookier the product, the more irresponsible and ridiculous it is, the better chance the promoter has of being booked on major talk shows and receiving enormous amounts of free publicity.

There's gold in them thar' hills! And the rush is on. Pandering publishers, manufacturers, drugstores, "health food" stores, pharmaceutical firms, and bookstores all profit from the misinformation and mythology. But quacks are not content to peddle their nostrums and leave it at that. They also work tirelessly to undermine confidence in scientific health care—including public-health measures that can save lives. Attacking doctors enables the "health food" and "alternative medicine" industries to increase the market for their wares.

Unfortunately for the general public, an army of true believers accepts the logic of the quacks and demands, in the name of "health freedom," the right to be lied to, cheated, sickened, and killed by all manner of fringe practitioners and snake-oil peddlers. The quackery industry and many of its clients comprise a large and aggressive lobby capable of blocking legislation that would treat health fraud for what it is: theft by deception, combined with assault, battery, and an occasional murder.

The late Congressman Claude Pepper took special interest in the problem of health fraud. The investigations he led threw floodlights on the darkest corners of the industry. As Chairman of the Subcommittee on Health and Long-term Care of the Select Committee on Aging, he worked for years to expose and combat quackery. His landmark report, *Quackery: A $10 Billion Scandal*, and subsequent Congressional hearings were greeted with a yawn from the media. The talk shows were too busy with their usual promotion of fad diets and miscellaneous snake oils to interview Pepper or any of the experts who had contributed to his project. Moreover, Pepper's attempt to gain passage of three antiquackery bills was unsuccessful, however, because the quackery lobby bombarded Congress with letters opposing these bills. Not surprisingly, the problems he described have become worse.

As the twenty-first century approaches, the ancient art of quackery is one of the growth industries of the industrialized world. The American public has wasted countless billions of dollars on worthless health products and services during the past decade and seems hellbent on wasting even more in coming years.

In the areas of nutrition and health care, you can follow the flock and repeatedly get fleeced. Or you can learn to see through the schemes and scams, and to stay healthy without all the paranoia, pills, potions, and paraphernalia now in vogue. The first five chapters of this book throw light on diet quackery, "alternative" practitioners, and a long list of other scams. The final two chapters show how the media promote quackery and how consumers, health profession-als, educators, journalists, legislators, and others can fight back. Throughout the book, the word "alternative" appears in quotation marks because the methods it characterizes are not true alternatives. A true alternative to an effective health-care method is another method that has been proven effective. The methods described herein are ineffective, unproven, or both.

1

The Great American Diet Hoax: An Assortment of Hogwash, Hype, and Half-Baked Baloney

The American public is being swindled by the extremely lucrative diet and diet-book industries. As the public's clamor for weight-loss miracles has reached new highs, peddlers and publishers have reached new ethical lows.

Almost anyone who can put pen to paper or call himself a "nutritionist" can play the game. No education or certification is needed, just a new or recycled gimmick and facility with words like "revolutionary," "miraculous," and "breakthrough." It helps to collect celebrity endorsements and drop their names at every opportunity or to obtain a mail-order "Ph.D." degree in order to use the title "Doctor," but many diet phonies do well without these trappings. Some of the worst offenders don't need a phony doctorate because they already have a genuine medical degree.

In most scientific fields, experts have a dominant influence on society's attitudes and applications of the science. For example, physicists and chemists working in industry, education, and research all have one or more degrees from an accredited college or university. As far as I know, no renegade chemists are claiming that the Periodic Table is all wrong or that the chemical formula for water is not H_2O. And when a bridge or highway is built, engineers with appropriate training are utilized. No "alternative" engineers are earning their living by denouncing academic engineers and claiming to have discovered new principles of stress and strain that enable highways to be suspended from clouds.

In nutrition, however, the situation is quite different. Scientifically trained nutritionists are fighting an uphill battle against the quackery that dominates the marketplace. Large pharmaceutical companies, publishing conglomerates, and armies of pseudonutritionists mislead the public at will, while real nutritionists often are ignored. Most bestselling books on nutrition and diet are written by self-anointed "experts." Trade publishers rarely ask genuine nutrition experts to write books for the general public or to help decide whether manuscripts promoting "miracle" diets are valid. Fad diets dominate the tabloids and women's magazines, while live phonies dominate the radio and TV talk shows. Preposterous and potentially hazardous claims seem to be magnets for publicity and financial success.

A good lifetime diet consists of a wide variety of foods with a reasonable balance of proteins, fats, and carbohydrates. Valid weight-loss diets have the same balance but fewer calories. Most diet books are based on a gimmick of imbalance, as though there is magic in eliminating or emphasizing one or two of the major food categories. However, some "classics" are objectionable because they involve unnecessary supplements, pseudonutrients, and/or bizarre theories that lead to irrational food choices. In this chapter we take an irreverent look at recent bestsellers and old favorites that still are widely available in bookstores, "health-food" stores, and public libraries.

Body-Type Hype

Dr. Abravanel's Body Type Diet & Lifetime Nutrition Plan [Bantam, 1983], by Elliot D. Abravanel, M.D., and his wife Elizabeth A. King, claims that "body type" depends on the dominant endocrine gland and that each type is prone to craving and overeating certain foods in an effort to stimulate that gland. This, they say, is the fundamental cause of obesity. Their solution is to determine body type, to avoid foods that stimulate the dominant gland, and to eat "nonstimulating" foods that strengthen the other glands, overcome the cravings, and cause weight loss.

The book contains a lengthy questionnaire for determining body type. The questions involve appearance, fat distribution, food preferences, and personality traits. For each body type there is a diet-and-exercise plan that includes an herbal tea for soothing the dominant gland and reducing cravings and hunger. Here's what the authors teach about body types:

"Pituitary-type" individuals tend to have a big head, a round, childlike face, and baby fat evenly distributed all over the body. They invariably crave dairy products (which stimulate the pituitary) and should therefore avoid them and eat more meat (to stimulate the adrenal glands and the gonads) and drink fenugreek tea.

"Thyroid-type" individuals crave sweets, starches, and caffeine, which eventually exhaust the thyroid gland, leading to sluggishness and obesity. They should let the thyroid rest, eat more meat and dairy products (to stimulate the other glands), and drink raspberry leaf tea.

"Adrenal-type" individuals crave cholesterol-rich meats and salty foods, which stimulate the adrenals, the most powerful of the glands. Adrenal-type men are solid, strong, broad-shouldered, and steady. Adrenal-type women tend to gain weight around the waist and breasts. A vegetarian diet and parsley tea is best.

"Gonadal-type" individuals are women who tend to gain weight in their legs and buttocks and are susceptible to "cellulite." They crave fats and spicy foods, which stimulate the sex organs. They should eat more plant foods and leaner meat and should drink red clover tea. There are no "gonadal-type" men.

Responsible physicians who observe correlations between body build, glandular activity, behavior, food preferences, and weight problems would do careful studies before jumping to conclusions. They would weigh and measure their patients, determine their hormonal levels, monitor their eating habits— and then do statistical analyses to look for patterns. The Abravanels, however, present no evidence to support their claims that specific foods stimulate specific glands and eventually exhaust them, that each individual has a "dominant gland" at the root of any weight problem, or that herbal teas help control weight by soothing the errant gland and moderating its cravings. All this is nonsense dressed in scientific-sounding terminology.

People who actually attempt to take the book seriously may wind up quite befuddled. Because most individuals do not fall clearly into one of the body-type categories, the questionnaire will give ambiguous results. I assume, however, that some readers manage to fit themselves into a category and follow the recommended plan. They might just as well base their eating habits on astrology.

The cover of *Dr. Abravanel's Body Type Diet & Lifetime Nutrition Plan* calls the book "revolutionary" and "based on the latest scientific discoveries." But in 1991 Bantam followed with *Dr. Abravanel's Anti-Craving Weight-loss Diet* —"based on the revolutionary 8-week Skinny School Program." And guess what? "Now there's a revolutionary new way to lose weight and end your cravings forever." Like Marxists of the Trotskyite and Maoist varieties, the American diet-book industry believes in "perpetual revolution."

Every so often they proclaim a new and improved "revolution" similar to the old one—or worse. The Abravanels' sequel merely adds "pop" psychology and mystical appetite-control methods to his body-type nonsense.

The High-Fat Revolution

Robert C. Atkins, M.D., says thousands of his patients have lost weight without counting calories and without a single hunger pang. He says that his followers can eat as much as they want as often as they want, including such rich foods as heavy cream, butter, eggs, bacon, seafoods, mayonnaise, cheeses, and meats. On his diet, he assures us, you can eat 5,000 calories a day, be sedentary, and still lose weight, feel better than ever, and have more energy.

If this sounds miraculous, it is. In fact, Atkins calls it a "biochemical miracle." He has made these claims in *Dr. Atkins' Diet Revolution* [Bantam, 1971], *Dr. Atkins' Superenergy Diet* [Bantam, 1977], and on his nationally broadcast radio show.

The key to it all is a zero- or near-zero-carbohydrate diet. In the first week, during which no carbohydrate foods are allowed, ketone bodies will appear in the urine as a by-product of fat metabolism. Carbohydrates are gradually added until ketone excretion stops, then the dieter keeps the carbohydrate intake just below this level and eats as much fat and protein as desired. According to Atkins, ketosis causes "hundreds of calories to be sneaked out of the body every day in the form of ketones and a host of other incompletely broken down molecules of fat" in the urine and in the breath.

Atkins has never published scientific studies to support the above claims—which is not surprising, because they are false. The caloric value of ketones is about 4.5 calories per gram. People who fast or eat only fats and proteins excrete only a few grams of ketones in their breath and urine. So the maximum loss would be less than 15 calories a day, the equivalent of about a third of a teaspoon of butter. This is much less than the "hundreds of calories" Atkins claims are "sneaked out of the body" and certainly not enough to account for his alleged weight losses.

While a near-zero-carbohydrate diet will not cause excretion of calories from the body, it will cause excretion of water. It is well known that carbohydrates in the diet help retain water and that high-fat, high-protein diets cause water loss. This can produce rapid weight loss in the first week or two and the illusion of success. But obese people need to lose fat, not water. More important than these theoretical objections to Atkins's "diet revolution" is the hazard involved for people prone to atherosclerosis and coronary artery disease.

Atkins encourages a high intake of cholesterol and saturated fats, which can dangerously increase blood cholesterol. Despite this, he claims that his diet is appropriate for most people with diabetes and high cholesterol levels.

Long before Atkins's "Diet Revolution" produces a heart attack, it is likely to cause fatigue and hypotension (abnormally low blood pressure). In one study, ten healthy, normal adults were placed on diets of 1,500 or 2,000 calories and zero carbohydrate. After two days, all complained of fatigue that was brought on by physical activity. Taking glucose quickly relieved the fatigue.[1]

A diet rich in red meat can also increase blood levels of uric acid, which can be hazardous to those with gout. The excess amino acids and ketones in the blood can harm the kidneys. Moreover, experts suspect that a high-fat diet promotes certain cancers.

In recent years Atkins has widened his claims considerably. In *Dr. Atkins' Nutrition Breakthrough* [William Morrow, 1981] and *Dr. Atkins' Health Revolution* [Houghton Mifflin, 1988], he states that reactive hypoglycemia is extremely common and causes a host of symptoms. He advocates six-hour glucose tolerance tests for everyone. Endocrinologists insist that hypoglycemia is very rare, but Atkins doesn't listen to the experts. Instead he espouses the notions of Carlton Fredericks, Ph.D., a chain-smoking, self-anointed nutritionist whose doctoral degree was based on a study of responses to Fredericks's own radio broadcasts. Atkins calls him "my mentor and the mentor of many of the great minds of complementary medicine." Fredericks died in 1987 of a heart attack at the age of 73. Prior to his death he performed "nutritional consultations" costing $200 in Atkins's office.

Besides hawking his diet plan as a panacea for scores of health problems, Atkins has embraced many forms of "alternative medicine" now huckstered to the American public. In addition to his unbalanced diet, he has touted laetrile, chelation therapy, so-called "vitamin B_{15}," cytotoxic testing for food allergies, hair analysis to determine nutrient requirements, high-colonic enemas, applied kinesiology, homeopathy, acupuncture, dubious herbs, an "anti-yeast diet," and megavitamins. On his radio show, he has claimed that a machine called an Electro-Acuscope focuses healing energies and makes chiropractic adjustments hold longer. He has suggested taking 200,000 International Units of vitamin A (forty times the RDA) at the first sign of a cold and said that AIDS should be treated with thymus gland extracts to build up the immune system. Even years after it was firmly established that high doses of vitamin B_6 can cause severe nerve damage, Atkins continued to advocate megadoses of the vitamin. And he says that orthodox medicine has made no progress in treating cancer, while alternative medicine has made much progress. As an example he cites German physician Hans Neiper, who uses laetrile and other types of cancer snake oils. I wonder how many cancer patients Atkins may have led astray.

Atkins claims to be highly successful in treating diabetes, atherosclerosis, coronary artery disease, hypertension, rheumatoid arthritis, multiple sclerosis, cancer, and many other serious diseases. His treatment typically includes avoidance of almost all carbohydrates; avoidance of foods claimed to produce adverse reactions; prescriptions for dozens of nutrients and pseudonutrients, some in potentially toxic doses; and prescriptions for various drugs that the scientific community considers worthless. He has developed and markets his own line of supplement products, including Heart Rhythm Formula, Anti-Arthritic Formula, Hypoglycemia Formula, Urinary Frequency Formula, and more than a dozen others. In *Dr. Atkins' Health Revolution* he claims that food intolerances can be discovered through (1) cytotoxic testing, (2) muscle-testing (applied kinesiology), (3) making observations after placing suspected foods under the tongue, (4) interpreting blood sugar elevations, and (5) using an "electroacupuncture" device that measures "differences in electrical potential transmitted through acupuncture meridians." None of these approaches has the slightest validity.

Rather than publishing his results in scientific journals so fellow physicians can evaluate his claims, Atkins tells stories for the lay public through his books and radio shows. He provides lots of dubious "case histories" of miraculous cures. Given all this, it may not be surprising that he failed the oral examination for certification by the American Board of Internal Medicine.[2] The test measures skill in diagnosis and treatment.

Appeals for Sympathy

Promoters of quackery would like you to believe that they are underdogs being picked on by Big Brother and that the critics of quackery are part of a self-serving "Medical Gestapo." The truth is quite the opposite. During the last two decades, quackery has so dominated the media that the public has been duped into wasting billions of dollars on worthless (and sometimes hazardous) health products. Atkins's own radio show is a perfect example. For years he has used it to promote practically every snake oil on the market without opposition or fair discussion.

In the introduction to *Dr. Atkins' Health Revolution: How Complementary Medicine Can Extend Your Life*, Atkins states:

> The War Against Quackery is a carefully orchestrated, heavily endowed campaign sponsored by extremists holding positions of power

in the orthodox hierarchy. They work through organizations with names like the National Council Against Health Fraud, American Council on Science and Health, and the Quackery Action Council. They even have nonprofit status, which gives their adherents, often the officers and stockholders of major pharmaceutical firms, a chance to pay less taxes than do hardworking stiffs like you and me.

As cofounder and ex-president of the Quackery Action Council, I can assure you that Atkins's statements about it are 100 percent false. The Council's annual budget has never been more than $3,000, almost all of it from the pockets of its officers, none of whom are officers or stockholders of any drug companies, and none of whom ever got paid or got a tax break for serving as an officer or director. The National Council Against Health Fraud has only one employee, a part-time secretary. Its annual budget is about $50,000, almost all of which comes from dues from its 1,200+ members, most of whom are dietitians, physicians, and health educators. Atkins could have learned these facts with a little research. I wonder whether the "case histories" that supposedly prove his diets and remedies work are equally unfounded.

Houghton Mifflin is a major publisher of textbooks in a variety of fields. These are written by responsible experts and carefully fact-checked. However, some of its mass-marketed titles are fiction masquerading as fact. Those in charge of Houghton Mifflin's trade division apparently have little sense of responsibility and don't believe in checking far-fetched claims even when correct information is easily obtainable.

The Quackery Action Council was formed primarily to combat the absolute domination of the media by people like Atkins and Carlton Fredericks. Years of listening to TV and radio talk shows and perusing bestselling diet books had convinced us that the public needs an alternative to the flood of misinformation that saturates the airwaves. We still believe that the media have little interest in presenting a factual picture of controversial health issues, that they tend to favor quackery and exclude responsible professionals who oppose quackery. Unlike Atkins, we and similar consumer advocacy groups have no vested interest in any industry. The motivation for our whistleblowing is like that of good citizens who witness a mugging or burglary.

"Immune Power"

In 1981 psychiatrist Stuart Berger, M.D., issued *The Southampton Diet* [Simon and Schuster], which, the public was told, unveiled a biochemical miracle that keeps the "beautiful people" beautiful, thin, and superactive. The cover proclaimed the diet the most revolutionary weight-loss system ever devised, one that would allow people to lose a pound a day safely, without hunger or fatigue. *American Health* magazine reported that Berger received a $200,000 advance for writing the book.

The diet's key feature is to eat only "happy foods," which contain amino acids that produce "positive neurotransmitters" in the brain. These include dairy products, poultry, fish, eggs, whole grains, leafy greens, and various fruits. The no-nos are "sad foods," which produce "negative neurotransmitters" in the brain. Examples are sugar, chocolate, lobster, lentils, chick peas, and foods containing choline and lecithin.

Dr. Berger supplied no evidence to support these notions. The brain has a complex balance of chemicals that work together to produce feelings, moods, and behavior. Neurotransmitters are chemicals that transmit impulses between brain and nerve cells. The concept that some are "positive" and others are "negative" is nonsense. Berger's meal plans supply about 1,000 calories per day, so weight loss is assured if you follow them. But this does not mean there is anything to his theory.

Berger's next book was quite different from his first. *Dr. Berger's Immune Power Diet* [New American Library, 1985] offers to provide lasting weight loss; increased resistance to infections, heart disease, and a host of other ailments; enhanced sense of happiness and stress-free well-being; heightened sexual energy and interest; a more youthful appearance; and greater longevity. "These are no empty promises," the book's jacket assures. *American Health* even reported Berger's claims to be treating "pre-AIDS syndrome" (whatever that is) with "remarkable" results.

The book's gimmick is its notion that people are fat and sick because they binge on foods to which they are unknowingly allergic and because they don't get enough vitamins and minerals. He says the immune system regulates the digestion, absorption, and storage of nutrients, as well as the amount of fat we burn or carry around. The solution is to determine what foods we are allergic to, eliminate them from the diet, and supplement with lots of vitamins and minerals. Poor science, but trendy marketing; the book sold hundreds of thousands of copies.

Berger's offices are located on Fifth Avenue in New York City, where, he tells us, he treats beautiful and famous people. When the book was published, he used cytotoxic testing as the basis for determining that patients were allergic to foods. This test—which cost several hundred dollars—was regarded as worthless by real allergists and immunologists as well as by the FDA. It was performed by inspecting white blood cells under a microscope after blood samples were added to special slides containing dried foods. About two years after *Dr. Berger's Immune Power Diet* was published, the test was driven from the marketplace by government enforcement actions.

The book advised readers who did not have access to cytotoxic testing to determine their own allergies by observing the effects that foods seem to have on their body. Did your low-back pain flare up within four days of eating bell pepper or eggplant? Did your hay fever get worse hours after an orange? It's a hypochondriac's delight.

Berger claims that everyone has hidden food allergies, but real immunologists say only 5 percent of us have any significant ones. If you have good reason to think you are in this small minority, you should consult a board-certified allergist with experience in food allergies. Berger's claims that the immune system determines body weight and that people binge on food to which they are allergic are absurd.

Equally ridiculous is Berger's Immune Quotient (IQ) Quiz, which is supposed to determine the reader's exact requirements for supplements. Berger claims you can determine exactly how much of each nutrient is needed by answering multiple-choice questions and adding up your score. If your score is high, your immune system is supposedly strong, and you should take a regimen of supplements that ranges up to 50 times the RDA. If your score is low, you should take up to 150 times the RDA.

The questions on the IQ Quiz include the following. How regular are your bowel movements? Do you remember your dreams? And how much TV do you watch? None of these has any bearing on immunity. Moreover, while gross malnutrition can decrease an individual's resistance to infections, there is no evidence whatsoever that large doses of supplements can boost resistance. In fact, excessive doses of vitamins and minerals might decrease immune response by damaging the bone marrow, liver, and spleen. And, as noted in Chapter 5, megavitamins can cause a host of other problems.

Berger repeatedly mentions that he was educated at Harvard and Tufts. But he doesn't mention that the nutrition and medical experts at these schools say his theories are full of baloney. The *Tufts University Diet and Nutrition Letter* (September 1985) says, "Berger's book is filled with unscientific claims and unwarranted advice." The *Harvard Medical School Health Letter* (September 1985) says the book should be listed in the fiction category because it is "a collection of quack ideas . . . a rich collection of errors of fact and interpretation."

Much of Berger's first book contradicts his second. In the first book, for example, he promotes whole grains, dairy products, and eggs as "happy foods" that should be eaten frequently. In the second, he includes them among the "sinister seven," which "create immune damage in the overwhelming majority of patients" and are closely linked to food binges and excess weight. Moreover, he no longer regards the amino acid phenylalanine as a villain; in fact, he recommends taking it as a supplement. He provided no evidence to support either his earlier dogmas or his flip-flops. In sequels titled *How to be Your Own Nutritionist* [William Morrow, 1987] and *What Your Doctor Didn't Learn in Medical School* [Morrow, 1988], Berger provides more misinformation and recommends potentially toxic doses of several vitamin supplements.

In January 1990, the television magazine "Inside Edition" aired a devastating undercover investigation of Berger's practice. A former employee said that Berger had ordered him to fake the results of blood tests and would tell practically all of his patients that they were suffering from chronic fatigue syndrome and candidiasis and were allergic to wheat, dairy products, eggs, and yeast. Several patients told "Inside Edition" that they had not been examined before being diagnosed and treated. To verify this behavior, an "Inside Edition" producer visited Berger as a patient while carrying a hidden camera. After a blood test, a five-minute consultation, and no examination, she was told she had chronic fatigue syndrome and candidiasis, charged $845, and advised to undergo six months of vitamin therapy that would cost thousands of dollars more. When Berger realized what had happened, he asked a federal court to forbid airing of the undercover tape, but he was not successful. The "Inside Edition" telecasts said that Berger was "under investigation" by the New York State Department of Health. As of this writing, however, he is still very much in business.

Television is not usually so on top of things. Quite the contrary. We can thank Phil Donahue, for example, for making Berger one of America's wealthiest physicians. Donahue has hosted Berger several times and always presents him favorably. In 1985 *People* magazine reported that during the three days following a broadcast boosting his *Dr. Berger's Immune Power Diet,* an additional 50,000 copies of the book were sold. During a recent show, Donahue held up Berger's latest vitamin-promoting tract, *Forever Young* [Morrow, 1989], and said, "There's a lot of good stuff in here about the reality of aging." Reputable nutritionists rarely are invited to present their views on "Donahue."

The Fruitcake Diet

The Beverly Hills Diet [Macmillan, 1979] is a classic of diet quackery—and illustrates the depths to which major publishers can sink to make a buck. Macmillan, primarily a publisher of academic and scientific books, decided that Judy Mazel was qualified to tell millions of people what foods were best for their health. The fact that she had studied drama in college and lacked training in medicine or nutrition apparently posed no problem for Macmillan.

Mazel says that her diet originally was a Beverly Hills beauty secret and offers a revolutionary approach to losing weight and feeling and looking better without going hungry. Mazel's great truth can be summarized as follows: Obesity is not caused by what or how much you eat but by adverse combinations that are poorly digested. She emphasizes that fat comes from undigested food; if food is fully digested, no weight gain will occur. If you avoid poor combinations, you will never get fat, because only undigested food accumulates and becomes fat. She also advises chewing foods thoroughly lest they stay in the stomach "festering, fermenting, rotting and ultimately turning into fat."

The combinations to avoid are starches and sugars, and carbohydrates and proteins. Carbohydrates should not even be eaten on the same day as proteins, she says, because once you have eaten the slightest morsel of a protein food, your carbohydrate metabolism will be shut down for the day and all sugar or starch you eat will turn to fat. In general, protein foods are the most fattening because they are the hardest to digest.

Mazel doesn't explain how food in the intestines is transformed and/ or delivered to the body's fat cells without being digested, but she assures us her diet plan "synthesizes the work of scores of scientists, nutritionists, and doctors." These are mostly unnamed, but she does "thank God" for Herbert Shelton, the "natural hygienist" of the early 1900s whose system of food-combining she adopted. Mazel's (actually Shelton's) system of "conscious combining" involves eating proteins with other proteins or fats, carbohydrates with other carbohydrates or fats, and fruits alone. If you violate these rules, food gets trapped and is not digested.

Artificial sweeteners are bad, Mazel says, because they too are indigestible and therefore fattening. Milk is also a problem, according to Mazel, because an enzyme from the thymus gland is required to digest it. In adults this gland is atrophied, so milk goes undigested and turns to (guess what?). Because it is not digested, we can't utilize its important nutrients—yet somehow its calories get transformed into body fat. Moreover, one drop of milk in your morning coffee will make subsequent carbohydrates indigestible and therefore fattening. And cheese is poorly digested, will trap other foods, causing a fermenting mass that will turn to fat! (By the way, did you know that the moon is made of green cheese? Mazel didn't state this in her book, but her grasp of biochemistry reminds me of this classic bit of childhood folklore.)

The Beverly Hills Diet is highly restrictive. For the first week it includes nothing but pineapples, bananas, mangos, papayas, prunes, strawberries, and watermelon—with a two-hour wait between different fruits. Nonfruit items are added gradually, but they must not be eaten within three hours of the fruit. Only after achieving your desired weight can you eat anything you want, but only in proper combinations.

Mazel says she favors fruits because they contain enzymes that aid digestion and burn off fat. But to get the full benefits of fruits you must eat their seeds, which are, she says, the storehouse of the enzymes and the focus of the nutrients. Yes, you are actually supposed to chew (or grind in a blender) and swallow seeds of watermelons, papayas, apples, grapes, and other fruits. Mazel apparently does not realize that this contradicts her advice not to eat proteins and carbohydrates together. It is also bad advice because seeds generally taste bitter and some contain toxins. Apple seeds, for example, contain cyanide.

The book's popularity waned sharply after the *Journal of the American Medical Association* published a devastating analysis by Gabe Mirkin, M.D., and Ronald N. Shore, M.D., two physicians practicing in Silver Spring, Maryland. After explaining in detail why Ms. Mazel's basic theory was nonsensical, they selected eighteen statements from the book and explained why each was wrong. Then they described how three of their patients had developed severe diarrhea, muscle weakness, and dizziness during their first week on the diet—which is not surprising, because eating large amounts of fruit usually will cause diarrhea. Finally, they indicated why more serious complications might well occur.[3]

The commercial success of Mazel's book is a sad commentary on the gullibility and scientific literacy of the American public—and the disgraceful greed and irresponsibility of the publishing industry.

More "Natural Hygiene" Cultism

The best-selling diet book of the 1980s, and perhaps of all time, was *Fit for Life* [Warner Books, 1985], by Harvey and Marilyn Diamond. This generated so much money that Warner advanced the authors a million dollars for their next book, *Living Health.*

According to the Diamonds, eating more calories than you burn off has nothing to do with obesity—people become overweight by eating foods at the wrong times and in the wrong combinations. This obstructs elimination (causes constipation) and causes toxins to seep into the body, which leads to obesity. As strange as they are, the Diamonds' ideas on food and nutrition are not original. Like Judy Mazel's *Beverly Hills Diet, Fit for Life* is mostly a rehash of Herbert Shelton's fancies about mucus-producing foods and food combinations that "clog up the system" and cause weight gain when poorly digested.

Cooked food, the Diamonds say, is altered from its original state. "We are not biologically adapted to deal with it, and the by-products of its incomplete digestion and assimilation form a residue in the body. The residue is toxic." As the toxic waste builds up, it "translates as overweight" by some unspecified process. Like Mazel, they do not explain how undigested food gets into the blood and the body's fat cells, or which "toxins" are converted to fat. Biochemists know no biological process by which an assortment of "toxins" (whatever they may be) are converted to fat.

According to the Diamonds, the key to avoiding poor digestion, toxin accumulation, and obesity is to eat foods with high water content and avoid concentrated foods. This means eating mostly fruits and vegetables rather than meat, dairy products, beans, or grains. If we don't eat mostly watery foods, the Diamonds tell us, our insides are not cleansed sufficiently. People develop cancer and heart disease because "the outside of the body is washed, but the inside, which is far more important, is not."

It's not good enough to just drink lots of water, because the water in fruits and vegetables is very special—it is "distilled water." (According to dictionaries and science texts, distilled water is pure H_2O without any minerals or other substances in it. How water in fruits with all those vitamins, minerals, flavors, colors, and sugars floating around could be considered distilled is beyond me.) In case you don't get enough water from your fruits and vegetables, you should drink only distilled water. Why? Because, the Diamonds say, just look at what regular water does to a steam iron. Yes, that's their scientific proof. Considering what a banana would do to my iron, I guess I better not eat any more bananas.

The Diamonds claim that any food subjected to temperatures above 130°F is "dead food, devoid of nutritional value." This is 82 degrees below the boiling point of water. Yet they provide dozens of recipes for stir-fried vegetables, broiled chicken, and the like, which are cooked at much higher temperatures and therefore, by their own logic, would be rendered nutritionally worthless. And did you know that "tofu is absolutely devoid of any nutrients whatsoever"? The Diamonds say that despite what government, industry, and university biochemists say, all of tofu's protein, calcium, iron, and other nutrients are destroyed by the heat used in making it. Yet they also provide recipes for breads, pastries, potatoes, rice, beans, and other foods that require prolonged cooking at high temperatures.

The Diamonds tell us that we should never eat carbohydrate and protein foods in the same meal. No fish with rice, bread with peanut butter, pasta with cheese, and so on. The digestive system cannot handle these combinations and the foods turn into a "putrefying, fermenting, rotting mass." Moreover, this stinking mass produces alcohol in your gut and has "the same consequences that come from drinking alcohol and with the same potential for liver damage." Hmm. Do you think that laws should be passed against driving under the influence of hamburgers or tortillas and beans?

The truth is that foods are utilized best if eaten together. Starch, for example, enhances the efficient utilization of dietary protein. Studies dating as far back as the 1830s prove that the human digestive system can handle combinations of food types without any trouble.

Human breast milk is, of course, a balanced combination of carbohydrates, proteins, and fats. The Diamonds don't explain how anyone survives infancy without becoming an obese drunkard. Nor do they explain why it's O.K. to drink unpasteurized (raw) milk, which has the same mixture of carbohydrates, fats, and proteins as the pasteurized kind—except to say that heat degrades calcium into "coarse" calcium, while the body can use only "fine" calcium. The chemists of the world know nothing of these two forms, the coarse and the fine, or that heat could degrade one into the other. Worse yet, raw milk, even if labeled "certified," is so dangerous that it has been banned from interstate commerce by the Food and Drug Administration. It often harbors salmonella bacteria that cause severe illness and even death. But the Diamonds advocate taking this very real risk in order to avoid nonexistent risks.

Other dangerous claims concern vitamin B_{12}. The book states that "most people who eat meat have vitamin B_{12} deficiency. It's not a problem for vegetarians. A million and a half Hindus don't have a problem." In reality, meat-eaters will not become deficient in vitamin B_{12} unless they can't absorb it—as happens in pernicious anemia. On the other hand, vegans (strict vegetarians who avoid all animal products) are at high risk for B_{12} deficiency unless their grains and vegetables contain sufficient insect fragments and dirt to supply the vitamin, which is the case for many vegans in developing countries.[4]

It would be hard to find books with a higher density of health misinformation than those by the Diamonds. I haven't space to cover it all, but here are a few more of their gems:

• Raw fruits are the ideal foods, the only ones that provide all the nutrients we need in the correct amounts. Our diets should be 90 percent sugar and 4 to 5 percent protein. (Actually, a diet of fruit alone would be seriously deficient in a number of vitamins, minerals, and amino acids. It could lead to stunted growth, miscarriage, permanent nerve damage, severe neurological defects, and death.)

• Digestion requires more energy than running, swimming, or any other function or activity of the human body. But combining foods properly can decrease the energy required to digest them. This frees energy to work on detoxification, which helps get rid of fat. (In other words, we can expend more energy by eating than by exercising!)

• Cooked fruit supplies no nutrients and is toxic and damaging to the body. This, of course, is false. Cooking leaves intact all the minerals and most of the fiber and vitamins, though it causes changes in the fibers and some decrease in vitamin content. And, of course, cooking does not decrease the calorie content of fruit.

• Pregnant women should not gain more than twenty to twenty-five pounds or the baby will be oversize and the delivery risky. Fifteen pounds is about right, they assert. This is an old-fashioned and dangerous idea. Most experts now believe a weight gain of thirty to forty pounds is more likely to produce a healthy baby.

• A cold is not a virus infection but the body's way of eliminating mucus and toxins produced by poor eating. (I know some researchers who induce colds in volunteers by using nasal swabs teeming with rhinoviruses. They would love to test the Diamonds' theory on the Diamonds themselves.)

• If you have appendicitis, even if diagnosed by a physician, you should not submit to surgery, but should fast instead. This is killer misinformation.

Phony Credentials

The Diamonds' credentials deserve scrutiny. Harvey obtained a "Ph.D." in "nutritional science," and Marilyn received a "masters degree" from the American College of Health Science, a correspondence school that was located in Texas. While most people must complete four to six years of training after college to earn their doctorate, Harvey whizzed through his in a few months— by mail. While most medical doctors require years of postgraduate training to become specialists, the amazing Diamonds acquired their basis for pontificating about AIDS, cancer, schizophrenia, and much more in mere days.

The dean of the American College of Health Science, now called Life Science Institute, is high-school dropout T. C. Fry, whom the Diamonds refer to as "Professor Fry." Harvey Diamond also calls him "today's most eminent, active proponent of Natural Hygiene . . . a most brilliant spokesperson for health." What does he teach that deserves such praise? Among other things, that viruses do not exist and that AIDS, polio, and cancer are inventions of a government–drug industry conspiracy designed to foist dangerous, worthless, and expensive drugs and vaccines on the public. According to Fry, the Rockefeller complex and the Centers for Disease Control (which he calls "the prostitute of the drug/medicine/hospital monster") have brainwashed the American people into believing the myth of viruses and the cynical lie of contagion.

What, then, causes AIDS? Cooked foods. The editorial in a 1985 edition of *Healthful Living,* the institute's official periodical, says, "AIDS is a medical/political fabrication . . . a nothing disease . . . a voodoo scare . . . a hoax," and adds that "Drug concerns and medical practitioners . . . orchestrate fear through the Centers for Disease Control . . . that works in behalf of medical/drug interests." It concludes that AIDS is really the "destruction of our white blood cell procreative faculties" caused by poisons, "including the deranged debris from foods subjected to heat."

T. C. Fry's school was not merely unaccredited; it also lacked permission to offer degree programs within Texas. Nonetheless, a flyer from the Diamonds' alma mater promised that even high-school dropouts can learn the Hygienic System of healing, which is 100 percent effective in curing and preventing cancer, schizophrenia, herpes, asthma, arthritis, heart disease, diabetes, and just about every other disease known to humanity. You can earn $50,000 per year working part-time keeping your friends and neighbors healthy with this miraculous method of natural healing. You won't even need a license or malpractice insurance because this is God's method and it's infallible. In 1986 Mr. Fry agreed to a permanent injunction barring him from representing his operation as a "college" or granting any more "degrees" or "academic credits" unless he acquired a certificate of authority from the Texas Department of Higher Education.

The Teflon Talk Show Stars

I often wonder about the cozy relations publishers have with talk-show producers and hosts. For several years the Diamonds were the darlings of the talk-show circuit and made dozens of radio and television appearances, usually to discuss weight control. Of course, any dingbat diet can lead to temporary weight loss, and since the Diamonds look almost anorectic, their theory may be given some credence. Hosts rarely investigate their dubious credentials or ask embarrassing questions about bizarre nutritional theories.

Throughout his career, Merv Griffin has plugged many quack diet books, some with theories the exact opposite of the Diamonds. Harvey has said, "We really owe a lot to Merv Griffin. He's constantly talking about our book on his show." Phil Donahue and Larry King also have enabled the Diamonds to reach vast audiences.

Skeptics and responsible diet critics rarely get on talk shows, perhaps because they ruin all the fun by exposing the scams for what they are. But in a rare example of an attempt at fairness, the "Larry King Show" let physician-nutritionist-attorney Victor Herbert say a few words about the Diamonds and *Living Health*. Herbert said, "It's a quack book, full of deceptions, misinformation, and fabrications, with a lot of advice harmful to your health if you follow it. Children can be killed by the advice in this book. . . . They are charismatic. They are charming. They are smiling. They are liars."

The Diamonds' books and their claims to expertise in nutrition and health sciences are hoaxes perpetrated for the purpose of making money. They are part of the "Natural Hygiene" cult, which profits from books, tapes, seminars, consulting services, classes, and the like. The participation of Warner Books and major TV and radio networks in profiteering with the cult is an egregious example of corporate irresponsibility.

The Name-dropper's Diet

Robert Haas, who has a "Ph.D." from an unaccredited correspondence school, has made a career of hyping himself and taking credit for the achievements of prominent athletes. His books, *Eat to Win: The Sports Nutrition Bible* [Rawson Associates, 1983] and *Eat to Succeed: The Haas Maximum Performance Program* [Rawson, 1986], advise eating lots of whole grains, potatoes, vegetables, fruits, low-fat dairy products, fish, and poultry. Although this is largely the same dietary advice advocated for years by scientific groups and government agencies, Haas calls this the Haas Peak Performance Program and claims it started a worldwide revolution in eating habits.

Where Haas differs from the experts, he is wrong. For example, he advocates avoiding peanuts, olives, and avocados. There is no evidence that inclusion of these nutritious and tasty foods in a balanced diet is detrimental to health or athletic performance. He also claims that his diet and supplements will protect people from radiation exposure during airline flights. There is not a shred of evidence to support this claim.

The back cover of Signet's paperback edition of *Eat to Win* calls Haas "a world-class nutritionist" and says he reveals the "secrets of the breakthrough diet that gives top athletes that unbeatable edge—and now can . . . even improve your sex life." Actually, Haas is little more than a world champion name-dropper who has brazenly hyped himself. He implies that drinking lots of water before, during, and after an athletic event is his invention. "I have told all those world-class tennis players," he brags, "about the single most important nutrient they need to enhance their athletic performance." Good coaches and good books on exercise, including those by Dr. Kenneth Cooper written long before Haas got his unaccredited degree, advocate great care to avoid dehydration. It is hard to believe that the careers of athletes like Martina Navratilova and Jimmy Connors depended on Haas telling them to drink up.

Haas also claims that his Peak Performance Program "teaches your muscles and liver how to clear lactate from your blood and convert it back to sugar through a biochemical process call gluconeogenesis." I hate to disappoint him, but the muscles and livers of prehistoric animals knew how to metabolize lactic acid long before they crawled out of the slime millions of years ago.

In *Eat to Win* Haas advises eating a diet that is balanced, low in fat and cholesterol, and high in starch. How is this stretched into a 350-page paperback? Lots of padding. He uses twenty-odd (very odd) pages to brag about his associations with Navratilova and other celebrities. Then come about 135 pages of mediocre meal plans and recipes for soups, salads, chicken, and the like. He takes twenty pages to say that women who eat well generally don't need iron supplements but might benefit from extra calcium. He also suggests that women shouldn't rely on just three meals a day but should snack between meals. He doesn't say why this would be more important for women than for men.

His chapter on "sports-specific diets" is forty pages of utter nonsense. He classifies fourteen popular sports into five categories and offers a plan to maximize performance for each. He gives detailed advice on how much beans, rice, milk, meat, and other foods are appropriate for each category. For example, jogging or swimming rates one more piece of fruit and a little more pasta per day than tennis or racquetball. But even this is contradicted by his advice to let appetite determine your portion sizes. Another Haas brilliancy is to eat when you are hungry and stop when you are satisfied. Haas also provides "revolutionary" precompetition and postcompetition meal plans. They are the same for all sports but omit fish and poultry from the precompetition meal. He provides no evidence that following his program leads to better performance.

Haas advises using a number of chemicals to enhance performance. Caffeine, he assures us, provides a definite edge. Long-distance runners, for example, should drink two cups of coffee just before a race. He cites no evidence that it really helps, and he ignores the potential problems such as dehydration or a full bladder (caffeine is a diuretic) or having to stop to urinate more or to drink more water. In some people, caffeine taken just before exercise can result in dangerous elevation of blood pressure during the workout. In others it can cause excessive adrenaline secretion and subsequent low blood sugar and weakness.

Haas also promotes the use of calcium lactate, octacosanol, ginseng, assorted B-vitamins, phenylalanine, calcium pantothenate, and other supplements to boost performance. He provides no evidence that they work, but he assures us his own (unspecified) research supports this. Haas calls PABA (para-aminobenzoic acid) a B-vitamin that prevents "certain types" of anemia. In fact, PABA is not a vitamin, and PABA supplements are a waste of money.

At the end of *Eat to Win* Haas provides more padding: a 25-page bibliography, listed alphabetically by author, with no indication of how they may be related to the book's contents. If you want to know, for example, what study supports Haas's notion that calcium lactate pills enhance endurance, you would have to wade through 300-odd titles with no assurance of finding one.

Eat to Succeed, the inevitable sequel, contains many contradictions. For example, Haas says that plant proteins are complete, while animal proteins have amino acid patterns "inconsistent with optimal health in humans." (The truth is quite the opposite.) But later in the book he says liquid meals should contain a "high-quality protein source—from nonfat dry milk or egg white."

The covers of *Eat to Win* and *Eat to Succeed* say that "Dr. Haas" is a "clinical nutritionist." Lately, however, he (or his publisher's marketing department) seems to have become a bit more modest. His most recent book, *Forever Fit* [Bantam, 1991], coauthored with Cher, the actress, uses neither of these labels.

Macrobiotic Malarkey

Macrobiotics is a quasireligious philosophical system that includes a semivegetarian, high-starch, low-fat diet. The early version, especially popular in counter-culture communities in the sixties, considered brown rice a perfect food and a panacea for all ills. Its guru, chain-smoking George Ohsawa, advocated going for weeks eating nothing but brown rice. This, he said, would cause the body to start making its own vitamin C, iron, and other essential nutrients lacking in rice. The earnest quest for this new and improved metabolism led many people, some with children in hand, down the garden path to malnutrition. In 1965, after a medical malpractice suit and an FDA raid, the Ohsawa Foundation in New York was closed.

The current version of macrobiotics, whose guru is Michio Kushi, includes a diet that is much more reasonable but still unnecessarily restrictive. Like its predecessor, it is based on the ancient Oriental concept of balancing the "yin" and "yang" (female and male) forces in one's life. Whole grains are emphasized because they are considered closest to neutral (neither too yin nor too yang). Generous amounts of certain vegetables and smaller amounts of fruits, nuts, and fish also are allowed. Ideally these are native to the area and are locally produced. Dairy products, eggs, land-animal meats, refined grains and sugars, and canned, frozen, "chemically treated" and irradiated foods are not allowed. Salty condiments, such as soy sauce, miso and pickled vegetables, are used generously, but fluid intake is limited.

Macrobiotic cookbooks contain excellent recipes for soups, breads, and vegetable dishes. Moreover, because it is very low in fat, calories, and cholesterol and high in fiber, the modern macrobiotic diet could be a big improvement for people who indulge in the worst of America's high-fat, low-fiber cuisine. Unfortunately, it is promoted to the general public *as a lifetime diet.* This is dangerous, because the diet has some major deficiencies. The very low fat content makes calorie deficiency a risk for children, pregnant and lactating women, athletes, and others who have a high energy requirement. The diet is low in protein, calcium, vitamins D and B_{12}, and perhaps some trace minerals. It may be too high in sodium for some. And those who take the taboo on imported foods seriously may end up with a monotonous and inadequate fare instead of the variety that ensures good nutrition and more enjoyment. The restriction of fluid intake is irrational and could be harmful to athletes, laborers, infants, the elderly, and those suffering from constipation, hemorrhoids, kidney stones, and other disorders.

Macrobiotics is more than just a diet; it offers a mystical system of medicine. Its dangers include more than malnutrition; they include misdiagnosis, inappropriate treatment, and unnecessary injury and death. Macrobiotics is also a thriving industry. The Kushi Institute and scores of affiliated and like-minded enterprises around the world do a brisk business in books as well as audiotapes and videotapes. And there are macrobiotic food stores, restaurants, classes, and health care. The latter is a hodgepodge of traditional Oriental medicine (such as pulse diagnosis and astrological diagnosis) and miscellaneous other mystical, psychic, and superstitious concepts such as diagnosis by aura, facial appearance, and movements of a pendulum held over "chakras" (alleged centers of spiritual energy located along the spine).[5]

In *Macrobiotic Home Remedies* [Japan Publications, 1985], Kushi states that "natural medicine is the medicine of energy and vibrations." He doesn't define energy or vibrations, but one consequence is that "two foods may be chemically identical but if, for example, their shape is different, then they are different and when consumed they will influence us differently." According to Kushi, the nutritional qualities and physiological effects of foods depend not on their nutrient content but on their shape, growth patterns (if plants), habitat and behavior (if seafood), flavor, and other characteristics that are mystical and incomprehensible to those not steeped in the dogma.

Foods are classified as having or being derived from energy that is either water, tree, fire, earth, or metal. They are further classified as having a character and effect that is "ascending" or "descending." Their medicinal uses are based on such attributes. For example, food poisoning from contaminated eggs (an earth-type food) can be cured by eating foods that are tree-type, such as onions and lemons, or fire-type, such as wine and green tea. Food poisoning from shellfish can be cured with horseradish and ginger. Roasted cockroach is great for colds, flu, bedwetting, and headaches. Snake skin cures all skin and eye diseases. Baked human hair is the remedy for blood in the stool, uterine bleeding, gonorrhea, and jaundice. The squeamish needn't worry: The last three and other distasteful remedies are usually powdered and available in capsules.

Probably the most significant vehicle for macrobiotic philosophy is *East West Natural Health* (formerly called *East West Journal)*, a monthly magazine founded by Kushi. Its articles promote acupuncture, homeopathy, past-life therapy, naturopathy, and other fringe healing systems. It also promotes distrust of scientific medicine. Ads in the magazine offer a wide range of supplemental nutrients, pseudonutrients, medicinal herbs, and such gimmicks and nostrums as aromatherapy, iridology, astrology, subliminal tapes, and psychic counseling. With about a quarter million readers, *East West Natural Health* is a significant source of health misinformation.

Of all the unproven claims made by macrobiotic proponents, perhaps the most dangerous is that the system can cure cancer. Those who believe this may be diverted from effective treatment. They may also become malnourished and lose weight at a time when they most need optimal nutritional support and preservation of lean body mass. In the 1980s the celebrated Anthony Sattilaro, M.D., wrote books and appeared on talk shows promoting macrobiotics as a cancer cure. In *Living Well Naturally* [Houghton Mifflin, 1985], Sattilaro claimed that his diet had put his own prostate cancer into permanent remission. The cover blurb for his book *Recalled by Life* [Avon, 1982] says, "Here is the inspirational true story of his complete recovery." Sattilaro died from prostate cancer in 1989. Bookstores and libraries still offer his books with no warning that his claims have been proven false.

The failure of macrobiotics to tame cancer and other diseases has not stopped Kushi from pontificating on AIDS. *The Way of Hope: Michio Kushi's Anti-AIDS Program* [Warner Books, 1988] claims that pressure-cooked rice has stronger "healing energy" than rice cooked by other methods. No such "energy" has ever been identified or measured by scientific means. The calorie deficiency of the macrobiotic diet can be especially harmful to AIDS patients. Other fallacies in the book include assertions that sugar, protein, and fat make the blood acidic; that the common cold is the body's way of eliminating (unnamed) toxins; and that sugar and fat weaken the immune response.

Rice Reports

Another rice-based diet deserves mention here. In the 1940s Dr. Walter Kempner of Duke University devised regimens, based on rice and fruit and low in calories, fat, protein, and sodium, for heart disease, kidney disease, severe obesity, and other life-threatening conditions. The clinic he founded is still treating patients with rice-based diets, apparently with some success.

A former patient, Judy Moscovitz, claims to have lost 140 pounds in nine months on a rice diet. A psychologist with no training in nutrition or medicine, she went on to write *The Rice Diet Report* [GP Putnam's Sons, 1986]. Unfortunately, it is just another irresponsible miracle diet book.

Moscovitz promises an average weight loss of 2 to $3^1/_2$ pounds per day and claims that some people have lost fifty pounds in the first two weeks. On this basis alone the book should be dismissed as not credible. In fact, the publisher should recall the book because weight loss that rapid would be dangerous. The loss is mostly due not to fat loss, but to dehydration and the breakdown of muscle tissue that is "cannibalized" for energy. The loss of muscle tissue can result in a lower level of fitness and fewer calories burned by exercise. Bone mass can decrease, which is most undesirable since recovery may be difficult. Moscovitz's diet can also cause gall bladder problems, liver dysfunction, heart attack, dizziness, weakness, lack of stamina, and other health problems. The rice diet is certainly not safe for children, as Moscovitz also claims.

Experts generally agree that long-term success against obesity comes from moderate exercise combined with moderate calorie restriction and a weight loss of one to two pounds per week. Ironically, rapid weight loss usually leads to rapid regaining of the weight—and often more is gained than was lost.

Vegetarian Extremism

John A. McDougall, M.D., has been America's most influential vegan zealot since the early 1980s. His most popular book is *The McDougall Plan for Super Health and Life-Long Weight Loss* [New Century Publishers, 1983]. He also has been a contributing editor of *Vegetarian Times* magazine and has appeared on many radio and television talk shows. In the late 1980s he went into the frozen food business with his own line of low-fat, low-protein, vegan meals.

"Vegan" means strictly vegetarian, without meat, fish, eggs, milk, or any other food from an animal source. Like the macrobiotic proponents, McDougall emphasizes whole grains, vegetables, and fruits. Unlike them, he excludes even small amounts of fish and low-fat dairy products. He takes the concept of low-fat vegetarianism to an extreme probably unmatched in human history, at least not voluntarily. Even Hindu vegans who avoid stepping on ants for fear of killing them have no problem with olives, nuts, peanuts, avocados, soybeans, and their oils. They even indulge in oily coconut milk when it's available. To McDougall these and most other oily foods are practically poisons. In his diet only 5 percent of the calories come from fat.

McDougall also claims that a moderate amount of protein in the diet is poisonous to the kidneys, so low-fat, high-protein foods like fish are excluded. Even plant proteins are severely restricted: beans and peas should be limited to a cooked cupful per day and should be avoided whenever we are sick, lest they slow our recovery, he says.

Dr. McDougall is a practicing internist, not a research clinician doing original studies. He supports his claims by citing studies reported in the medical journals. However, his interpretations and extreme recommendations are often at odds with those of the studies' authors. For example, he supports his protein paranoia by citing an article by kidney specialist Barry Brenner, M.D., that discussed possible hazards of protein foods for people with kidney disease.[6] Since the article said little about protein and normal kidneys, I asked Dr. Brenner whether he knew of any evidence that kidney disease can be caused by eating moderate amounts of fish, low-fat milk, beans, and tofu. He said he did not. Nor did he know of any evidence that eating beans while sick can slow recovery.

McDougall often refers to a study reported in February 1985 in the *American Journal of Clinical Nutrition* to support his contention that milk is actually bad for the bone health because its protein causes excretion of more calcium than the milk provides. But the authors of the study, which involved postmenopausal women, concluded that three cups of low-fat milk a day help improve calcium balance and maintain bone health.

McDougall's hatchet job on dairy products includes suggestions that they cause leukemia and multiple sclerosis (MS). While it is true that a leukemia virus sometimes infects cows, it is destroyed by pasteurization. There is no evidence that humans are being infected. His reasoning for the MS charge is that milk has little linoleic acid, which is needed for nerve development. He claims that if nerve development is poor, MS can result. Linoleic acid deficiency is very rare, however, and there is no evidence that it leads to MS.

To bolster his attack on dairy products he mentions that milk is made for calves, not humans, and that no other animal in nature drinks milk after it is weaned or drinks the milk of another animal species. He neglects to mention that no animal in nature eats cooked grains and vegetables, refrigerated foods, or fruits grown in orchards. And that grains and fruits are not made by nature for human consumption but for the nourishment of the seeds and the perpetuation of the plants. If we avoid all foods intended to nourish other species, all that is left is human milk.

In a public debate with me, Dr. McDougall summed up his argument against fat this way: The American Heart Association (AHA) tells us that smoking cigarettes and eating fat and cholesterol cause heart disease; we don't tell people to cut down to a couple cigarettes a day, we tell them to stop completely; similarly, we shouldn't tell them that a little fat and cholesterol are OK. The AHA, however, does not say fat and cholesterol cause heart disease; it says that *too much* of these can *help* cause heart disease.

If dietary fat and cholesterol were poisons, why would human breast milk supply forty percent of its calories via fat and have high levels of cholesterol? This is so because they are important nutrients for infants and young children. Fat is a normal constituent of our diet that should be consumed in moderation. Cholesterol is not an addicting poison like nicotine, but is an essential precursor of adrenal and sex hormones. It is a problem only if blood levels are too high for long periods.

McDougall's book says repeatedly that his plan causes weight loss without restricting food intake, that people can eat all they want and still get thinner. But the book is promoted to the general public, not just the obese. Where does this leave people who don't need to lose weight?

McDougall's followers risk deficiencies in protein, phosphorus, calcium, iron, zinc, vitamin B_{12}, and perhaps other nutrients. Children on the diet are especially at risk for calorie deficiency, which can have disastrous consequences. There have been reports of failure-to-thrive syndrome with very slow development and growth in infants and children of parents who put them on an overly restrictive diet in efforts to prevent obesity and atherosclerosis later in life.[7]

McDougall's enthusiasm for his diet extends far beyond the realm of obesity and heart disease. He is equally convinced that he has the answer to breast cancer and other malignancies. In *McDougall's Medicine* [New Century, 1985], he rails against conventional cancer treatment. Early detection and treatment, he says, is primarily for the benefit of the physician, who can reap the profits of treatment without improving the length or quality of the patient's life. He contends that we're being hoodwinked by our doctors, the American Cancer Society, National Cancer Institute, and cancer researchers around the world.

The notion that a "cancer establishment" wants Americans to keep dying of cancer is sheer poppycock. Doctors, researchers, administrators, and their families get cancer too, and they prefer the same early detection and treatment that they advocate for the public. One irate woman who called

McDougall on his Sunday radio program in Honolulu in 1985 summed it up succinctly. "Doctor," she said, "if I had followed your advice and not gotten a mammogram I would be dead now." Then she slammed down the phone.

References

1. AMA Council on Foods and Nutrition: A critique of low-carbohydrate ketogenic weight reduction regimens—a review of *Dr. Atkins' Diet Revolution. Journal of the American Medical Association* 224:1415–1419, 1973.
2. R.C. Atkins: Testimony at an administrative hearing on June 25, 1980 regarding a False Representation Complaint brought by the U.S. Postal Service against Great Life Laboratories, which had marketed an RNA product.
3. G. Mirkin and R.N. Shore: The Beverly Hills Diet—dangers of the newest weight-loss fad. *Journal of the American Medical Association* 246:2235–2237, 1981.
4. I. Chanarin et al.: Megaloblastic anemia in a vegetarian Hindu community. *The Lancet,* Nov 23, 1985, pp. 1168–1172.
5. J. Raso: A Kushi seminar for professionals. *Nutrition Forum* 7:17–21, 1990.
6. B.M. Brenner et al.: Dietary protein intake and the progressive nature of kidney disease. *New England Journal of Medicine* 30:652–659, 1982.
7. M.T. Pugliese et al.: Parental beliefs as a cause of nonorganic failure to thrive. *Pediatrics* 80:175–182, 1987.

2

"Experts" to Beware of

Freedom of speech and free enterprise are wonderful institutions. They make the pursuit of happiness possible. Without them the creative spirit is suppressed and social and material development are impeded. They come with a price, however—eternal vigilance, not just against tyrants who would take them away, but against misguided zealots and con artists who abuse these freedoms to mislead, confuse, and defraud the public.

The Bill of Rights guarantees all citizens the right to write and publish articles and books even if they even contain false, misleading, or dangerous advice. Almost anything can be published and presented as fact or opinion, even if the author knows it is false or absurd. Moreover, no education or credential is needed to distort facts or to express personal opinions on any subject.

This chapter describes the activities of eleven authors who have presented significant amounts of health-related misinformation to the public: Paavo Airola, Adelle Davis, Kurt Donsbach, Carlton Fredericks, Robert Mendelsohn, M.D., Earl Mindell, Gary Null, Kristen Olsen, Durk Pearson, Sandy Shaw, and Lendon Smith, M.D.

"Internationally Recognized Nutritionist" Paavo Airola

Paavo Airola, a self-proclaimed naturopath who was described on the jackets of his books as "an internationally recognized nutritionist," remains influential years after his death. His fourteen books and booklets, which have sold millions of copies, mostly in "health food" stores, promote many of the products sold in such stores. Airola claimed to offer miracle cures for arthritis, cancer, multiple sclerosis, and other serious diseases.

Airola's most comprehensive book is *How to Get Well* [Health Plus, 1974], which his followers consider a classic. The book's publisher has assured store managers that it will sell their megavitamins, herbs, juicers, and the like. One sales letter suggested that each copy sold could generate at least one customer who would spend about $300 several times each year.[1] Here is a brief analysis of some of the book's many fallacies:

• *Fasting and taking enemas are highly effective against acne, jaundice, parkinsonism, multiple sclerosis, alcoholism, and many other ailments.* All of these applications are irrational and potentially harmful, but Airola's advice about alcoholism is particularly ill-advised. Many alcoholics are already malnourished and suffer from liver disease. Fasting, especially for the two weeks Airola advocates, can seriously complicate their condition. The three enemas per day he recommends can adversely affect normal bowel function and cause mineral depletion.

• *Megadoses of vitamins are valuable treatments for a wide variety of ailments.* Many of Airola's recommendations are dangerous as well as irrational. For example, he suggests taking massive doses of vitamin A (up to 150,000 International Units) for psoriasis and acne, without warning that this can be very dangerous, especially during pregnancy. He also recommends potentially toxic doses of vitamin A for alcoholics, who may be sensitive to vitamin A and can suffer liver failure and death from it.

• *Adrenal cortical extract (ACE) is useful for hypoglycemia.* Quacks overdiagnose this rare condition by at least 10,000 percent. The treatment for genuine hypoglycemia depends on the cause but should never be ACE, which was abandoned by scientific medicine decades ago. Equally foolish are Airola's recommendations of laetrile, which he calls "vitamin B-17," as a preventive and cure for cancer, and of pangamic acid ("vitamin B-15"), another nonvitamin, as a remedy for angina, emphysema, and epilepsy.

• *Diabetics should eat a lactovegetarian diet with plenty of fruit.* This is nonsense. Diabetics can do very well eating some fish and lean meat. Airola also recommends that diabetics eat certain cactus leaves because of their "natural, organic" insulin content. This, too, is absurd. Cactus plants do not make insulin; and, even if they could, taking insulin by mouth would accomplish nothing because it would be inactivated by the digestive process rather than absorbed into the body. That's why it must be injected.

• *Raw skim milk and raw egg yolks are useful for treating jaundice. Raw eggs are useful against multiple sclerosis.* There is no conceivable justification for these recommendations. Both unpasteurized milk and raw eggs carry a substantial risk of food poisoning from *Salmonella* bacteria and other pathogens.

• *Brewer's yeast has the highest quality protein.* In fact, its protein is of rather poor quality, ranking far below that of milk, eggs, fish, meat, and even some legumes and grains.

• *Magnesium is good for diarrhea.* While it is a good idea to provide some mineral supplements during extended bouts of diarrhea, magnesium is a laxative whose use can *aggravate* the problem.

• *Garlic suppositories are good for hemorrhoids.* On the contrary, garlic suppositories have no proven benefit and can cause severe irritation and pain.

• *Gerovital can help impotence and slow aging.* Gerovital is a hoax, a classic among snake oils, which originated in Rumania decades ago. He also prescribes licorice, false unicorn, and elder to slow aging and says halvah (a sesame seed candy) and fertile eggs are special virility foods.

Although Airola said that people who know the principles of health can live to be 120, he died of a stroke at the age of 64. His books are likely to survive as long as they are marketable.

"Foremost Nutrition Authority" Adelle Davis

Adelle Davis was the founder, or at least an important cofounder, of megamania, the passionate belief that, in nutrition, more is always better. Her books, which have sold millions of copies and continue to sell, include *Let's Get Well* (1965), *Let's Eat Right to Keep Fit* (1954, 1970), *Let's Have Healthy Children* (1951, 1959, 1972), and *Let's Cook It Right*. Their covers promise nutritional help for arthritis, infections, kidney disease, sexual problems, and scores of other health problems. The books were published in hardcover editions by Harcourt Brace Jovanovich and in paperback by New American Library. Their covers tout Davis as America's "most celebrated," "most famous and acclaimed," and most "highly regarded nutritionist," as well as "America's foremost nutrition authority."

The truth is that although Adelle Davis had university-based training in nutrition, she was widely regarded by her colleagues and former professors as a disgrace to her profession. Her books consist of elaborate arguments for more, more, and still more of virtually every nutrient. She urged her readers to take handfuls of pills, drink buckets of milk-based concoctions, and gorge on high-protein, high-fat, high-cholesterol foods. Her recommended daily intakes for most nutrients ranged from about three to thirty times the RDAs.

Ms. Davis instilled in her followers a neurotic fear of going a few hours—or, God forbid, a whole day—without ingesting several times the RDA of every nutrient. Of course, if more is better, even more must be even better. Since anyone can advocate megamania, Davis has been eclipsed by imitators who recommend ever higher doses. Supplement manufacturers have profited enormously from the resultant mythology. There is now endless competition among the makers of stress, superstress, and supermegastress formulations to see who can pack the most vitamins and minerals into one pill. This nonsense has even spread to fortified foods, with some breakfast cereals supplying the RDA of ten vitamins in a few bites and tasting like vitamin pills.

Adelle Davis illustrates how a little knowledge combined with a lot of zeal can be a dangerous thing. She earned a bachelor's degree in nutrition and dietetics and a master's degree in biochemistry, but her learning must have been very superficial for she quickly abandoned science for pseudoscience. She adopted the notion that "more is better" and made a career of misinterpreting and misquoting scientific literature to support her dogma. Dr. Leo Lutwak, a nutrition expert who was professor of medicine at UCLA, said, "Her books are phony and her quotations are deliberate distortions of facts taken completely out of context."[2]

Dr. Edmund H. Rynearson of the Mayo Clinic came to the same conclusion.[3] He wrote to twenty of the scientists Davis referred to in *Let's Get Well*. Most said they were misquoted or misunderstood by Davis, and none recommended the book. Dr. Victor Herbert said that in each reference to a scientific paper by him she misrepresented what he wrote. Yet she had the gall to dedicate the book to "the hundreds of wonderful doctors whose research made this book possible." She would have been lucky to find a single nutrition scientist who could support even a small fraction of her claims.

Davis's books are so dense with factual errors and wild speculation presented as scientific fact that readers can safely assume that most of what she says is false. The following are but a small sample:

Eating too little fat is a major cause of overweight.
Most Americans eat far too little protein.
100,000 IU of vitamin A can be safely taken for many months and can cure warts.
Massive doses of vitamin E during pregnancy prevent miscarriage, mental retardation, and assorted birth defects.
Drinking lots of milk prevents cancer. (She died of cancer.)
Most Americans are deficient in the fifteen B-vitamins. (There are only

eight, and deficiencies are rare in the United States.)

Calcium is a tranquilizer.

Magnesium supplements can control epilepsy.

Fertile eggs are more nutritious than infertile eggs.

Inositol supplements can cure baldness.

Patients with failing kidneys should take potassium chloride. (This is a potentially lethal suggestion.)

PABA supplements can cure Rocky Mountain spotted fever, typhus, and other serious infections.

Abundant dietary cholesterol does not aggravate high blood cholesterol. People with high cholesterol levels and atherosclerosis should eat lots of cholesterol-rich foods such as eggs, livers, kidneys, brains, and cream. Atherosclerosis is not caused by excessive fat and cholesterol consumption, but by deficiencies of certain nutrients. (It is established beyond doubt that a high-fat, high-cholesterol diet can elevate blood cholesterol levels and increase the risk of death from heart disease.)

Supplements of lecithin and choline can prevent and reverse atherosclerosis.

Any bruise from a blow, no matter how severe, is a sign of vitamin C deficiency.

Vitamin E supplements can correct crossed eyes, cure muscular dystrophy, and increase sperm count.

Adelle Davis encouraged inappropriate self-diagnosis and self-treatment of symptoms with dietary changes and supplements, which is inherently dangerous. Despite all this, her books still refer to her as "America's foremost nutritionist" and are marketed without warning that her theories are not supported by scientific evidence.

Her advice regarding children was especially irresponsible. At least one infant died due to an overdose of potassium recommended by her book *Let's Have Healthy Children.* Another child's growth was permanently stunted after she was given excessive vitamin A in her first year. Following lawsuits, settled out of court, the book was revised by a physician aligned with the health food industry and was returned to the marketplace.[4] Although most of the directly dangerous misinformation was removed, much of the nonsense remains. Her other three books have not been revised to remove even the most preposterous claims. I can see their publisher's dilemma, though. Any serious revision might result in the books being taken out of print. That would be the moral thing to do, but is unlikely as long as they remain profitable.

"Vitamin King" Kurt Donsbach

Kurt W. Donsbach has been one of the most energetic and prolific promoters of quackery during the late twentieth century. He calls himself Dr. Donsbach and frequently appends "D.C., N.D., D.Sc., Ph.D." to his name. Only the D.C. appears to be valid, though he does not appear to have practiced chiropractic for many years. While Donsbach has been convicted of practicing medicine without a license, his activities extend far beyond such individual counseling and include leadership roles in the quackery industry.[5] He has marketed the ideas of others with such vigor and financial success that the *Los Angeles Times* once dubbed him the "Vitamin King."

Donsbach's career has consisted of marketing miscellaneous crackpottery to the public and to fellow unscientific practitioners in just about every conceivable way. His books, pamphlets, and articles are widely distributed. After graduating from Western States Chiropractic College in Portland, Oregon, and practicing for a few years in Montana, Donsbach went to work for Royal Lee, a supplement manufacturer who soon afterward was convicted of misbranding 115 products with false claims that they were effective against more than 500 diseases and conditions. Lee, a nonpracticing dentist, was a pioneer in the sleazy business of writing pseudoscientific books and pamphlets to promote supplements in which the author has a financial interest. In 1963, an FDA official said that Lee was "probably the largest publisher of unreliable and false nutritional information in the world." So much more nonsense has been published since that time that it would be difficult to identify a single market leader. But Donsbach certainly has followed in Lee's footsteps. The following is a partial account of his activities.

In the late 1960s, Donsbach started a "health food" store and a supplement packaging business in California. In 1970 he was prosecuted by California state authorities for telling customers in his store that heart disease, cancer, arthritis, and other serious diseases could be remedied by his line of supplements and herbal medicines. He was assessed $2,750 and served two years' probation. In 1973 he was charged with nine counts relating to making, misbranding, or selling new drugs illegally. He again paid a small fine and was placed on two years' probation. A year later he was caught violating his probation and was fined yet again.

Donsbach then sold his company and the rights to the "Dr. Donsbach" line of supplements to RichLife, Inc., for $250,000. He stayed on the payroll as a part-time consultant and speaker while he started (and soon sold) another supplement business, Metabolic Products. In 1975 he started producing booklets on a wide variety of ailments, from the irksome to the lethal. Not surprisingly, these are full of misinformation promoting supplements and other unproven remedies. Millions of copies have been sold, and they can still be found in "health food" stores and even in some pharmacies throughout the United States. The proprietors love them because they not only turn a tidy profit in themselves, but they help boost sales of vitamins, minerals, herbs, and the like.

In 1977 Donsbach became Dean of the new Department of Nutrition at Union University in Los Angeles, an unaccredited school that is now defunct. Never one to stagnate, Donsbach then opened Donsbach University, which offered correspondence courses in pseudonutrition. Students paid nearly $4,000 for Ph.D. degrees they earned by reading mostly classics in paperback nutrition quackery, such as the works of Donsbach, Lendon Smith, and Robert Atkins. Some graduates went on to practice "nutritional medicine" on the unwary public. For about $500 Donsbach also offered a "Dietary Consultant" certificate primarily for "health food" store clerks. Although Donsbach University no longer exists, some of its "graduates" continue to misrepresent themselves to the public as qualified nutritionists.

At various times and in various capacities, Donsbach has: published the chiropractor-oriented *Journal of the International Academy of Nutritional Consultants,* which later became *Health Express;* produced and marketed Dr. Donsbach's Tapes, a line of cassette tapes promoting pseudonutrition; served as chairman of the American Association of Nutritional Consultants; published the *Journal of Ultramolecular Medicine,* which specialized in homeopathy and phony electrodiagnosis; published a newsletter called *HerbLetter;* run Health Resources Group, a supplement wholesaler; hosted a syndicated radio show called "Let's Talk Health"; repurchased the right to his name from RichLife; conceived and marketed Orachel (for heart disease), Prosta-Pak (for prostate problems), C-Thru (for cataracts), and other unproven remedies for serious diseases; and served as "therapy coordinator" for the Bio-Genesis Institute, a clinic in Mexico that specialized in an assortment of expensive quack treatments (such as laetrile, chelation therapy, live cell therapy, and homeopathy) for a wide variety of serious diseases. Currently, he administers the Hospital Santa Monica in Baja, Mexico, which is apparently a bigger, fancier version of the Bio-Genesis Institute.

In 1985 the New York Attorney General Robert Abrams ordered *Orachel* seized from retail outlets and brought actions against Donsbach and his school for illegally advertising unaccredited degrees and for scheming to defraud consumers with a phony questionnaire that allegedly determines nutritional deficiencies. The test has no validity and it prescribes supplements no matter how the questions are answered. Donsbach agreed to cease and desist and pay a small fine.

Donsbach's latest brush with the law involved hydrogen peroxide products sold through the mail. He would buy 35 percent hydrogen peroxide in bulk and bottle it for consumers for drinking, douching, taking enemas, brushing teeth, and so on, as well as for use in cancer, AIDS, and many other diseases. In his hospital he injected it intravenously in some patients. In 1988 the U.S. Postal Service charged that certain products were being falsely advertised. Donsbach said that the company marketing the products was owned by his nephew, but both of them agreed to stop making the challenged advertising claims. Of course, this puny measure didn't exactly bring Donsbach to his knees. With the bulk of his operation now in Mexico, he is out of the reach of U.S. authorities.

"Foremost Nutritionist" Carlton Fredericks

Carlton Fredericks, on the basis of a Ph.D. in communications, called himself "Dr. Fredericks" and gave nutrition and medical advice to millions through his books, lectures, and radio and television broadcasts. He also practiced medicine one-on-one, and claimed "no other author has had more years of experience in the diagnosis and treatment of hypoglycemia." He not only admits to practicing medicine, he brags about it. Although he had absolutely no training in medicine or nutrition, some of his book jackets have proclaimed him the "world's foremost nutritionist" and described him as the "world's foremost expert" in the treatment of several serious medical problems.

Fredericks was obsessed with the idea that chronic reactive hypoglycemia, or low blood sugar, is the cause of dozens of diseases and symptoms. He helped popularize this notion almost to the point of national hysteria. He and other proselytizers had thousands of people diagnosing themselves as hypoglycemic, demanding that their doctors do expensive testing to prove it, and eating according to Fredericks's dictates whether tested or not and regardless of what any tests showed.

Fredericks saw his dietary recommendations as a preventive and treatment for epilepsy, schizophrenia, obesity, allergies, depression, anxiety disorders, sexual dysfunctions, headaches, insomnia, forgetfulness, chronic fatigue, and many other ailments. The fare is low in starch and sugar, with refined sugar forbidden altogether. It is somewhat high in fat and especially cholesterol, and it calls for much more protein than we need. The excessive protein may or may not be harmful, but it definitely costs more than the starchy foods, such as whole grains and potatoes, generally recommended by scientific nutritionists. Fredericks also recommended injections of adrenal cortical extract on the theory that the gland is weakened in hypoglycemia and needs a boost. Fredericks thus compounded nonsense with dangerous nonsense.

In reactive hypoglycemia, excessive insulin is produced in response to eating sugar and starch. Blood sugar then drops too low, and a variety of symptoms, especially weakness, fatigue, and drowsiness, can occur. However, reactive hypoglycemia is not nearly as common as Fredericks said. He claimed many millions suffer from it, but, according to the American Diabetes Association, the Endocrine Society, and other experts, very few people have the problem. Moreover, it does not cause the ailments he attributed to it. While in rare cases it may aggravate some of the symptoms he mentioned, it is certainly not a cause of schizophrenia, allergies, epilepsy, or any other disease.

As the hypoglycemia fad faded, Fredericks put more emphasis on other fringe ideas such as so-called yeast allergies and megavitamins. He once examined the palms of a friend of mine and, based on this alone, recommended extremely high doses of B vitamins and other supplements. He also promoted quack diagnostic methods such as applied kinesiology and cytotoxic testing. As a nutrition consultant for the Atkins Centers for Complementary Medicine, he charged $200 and very likely recommended supplements for everyone. While Fredericks devoted himself to promoting his version of healthful living, he was a chain smoker throughout most of his life.

Fredericks began his career in quackery in 1937 writing ad copy and giving sales talks for the U.S. Vitamin Corporation. At that time he adopted the title of "nutrition educator." He soon began seeing patients, diagnosing diseases, and prescribing vitamins as cures. In 1945 he pleaded guilty to the unlawful practice of medicine and paid a $500 fine. He later became "Chief Consultant" to Foods Plus, a vitamin company repeatedly charged by the FDA with misbranding its products as effective against dozens of diseases. In one of these cases, the judge concluded that Fredericks had been telling his radio audience that supplements can cure many diseases, including epilepsy, multiple sclerosis, and arthritis. The judge also permitted expert testimony that he was a charlatan rather than a nutritionist.

For many years Fredericks wrote a column for *Prevention* magazine, which identified him as Carlton Fredericks, Ph.D., without informing its readers that the Ph.D. had nothing to do with expertise in nutrition or medicine. One of his publishers, Putnam Publishing Group, touted Fredericks as "America's foremost nutritionist." Grosset and Dunlap hyped his "revolutionary" approach to breast cancer and psychological disorders. Merv Griffin introduced him as a leading nutritional consultant, and the Mutual Broadcasting System aired his show to millions of listeners all over the country. Radio station WOR in New

York broadcasted his one-hour show six nights a week for nearly thirty years.

On the radio "Dr." Fredericks didn't tell people he wasn't a medical doctor or a real nutritionist, which many listeners assumed he was. When one of my associates called his show, an assistant wanted to know the question before letting her on the air. When she said she wanted to know whether Fredericks had a degree in nutrition, she was disconnected.

Why would a major radio network be so irresponsible when it could just as easily have a real nutritionist do a show? Probably because its directors believe that nutrition "magic" can outdraw nutrition science. Years ago, Mutual Broadcasting was owned by Amway Corporation, which makes hundreds of millions of dollars peddling unnecessary supplements. Fredericks's radio show was great advertising for the supplement industry because it could spread claims that were illegal for manufacturers to make about their products. Amway no longer owns the network, but talk shows that promote the use of supplements have no difficulty attracting sponsors who market them.

"Medical Heretic" Robert Mendelsohn

The late Robert S. Mendelsohn, M.D., was one of the most vicious medical paranoia peddlers ever to make a buck on a bestselling book. His *Confessions of a Medical Heretic* [Contemporary Books, 1979] describes the physicians of America as the "Devil's Priests" carrying out "Holy War on the Family." They and their "Temples of Doom" (hospitals) could disappear from the face of the earth and our health would not suffer, he says. In fact, we would all be better off, because "the God that resides in the Temple of Modern Medicine is Death." Practically all doctors, he says, will addict you to worthless and dangerous drugs, slice you up for no good reason, dose you with unnecessary x-rays, infect you with deadly germs, and rob you blind while doing you in. All the while they unfairly suppress unorthodox but effective methods such as chiropractic, homeopathy, laetrile, and applied kinesiology.

Mendelsohn's solution was nothing less than completely eliminating modern medicine and replacing it with the New Medicine and New Doctors who would be trained at a New Medical School, which he talked about founding. The New Doctor would be truly prevention-oriented, so hospitals would not be needed. Babies would be born at home, and the fields of obstetrics, gynecology, and pediatrics would disappear. Modern cancer therapy with its drugs, surgery, and radiation would vanish, as would psychiatry and internal medicine. The New Doctor would be a generalist, not a specialist, and would help educate and motivate people about good health habits. Mendelsohn provided no references to support his contentions, but said they were based on common sense. He added that he had not ignored unorthodox sources of medical information such as the *National Enquirer*.

Mendelsohn did much of his hatchet work on straw men he had set up. For example, he praised breast-feeding as the greatest of preventive medicines and railed against modern medicine for forcing bottles on mothers and their kids. He said pediatricians were especially guilty, because they know the bottle-fed children will get sick more often and this generates more business. He didn't mention that the American Academy of Pediatrics has long encouraged breast-feeding, which has increased steadily now for some three decades. Mendelsohn accused modern medicine of labeling persons interested in nutrition as faddists, freaks, and quacks. In reality, the American Medical Association, the American Heart Association, and scores of other prominent professional groups have advocated scientific nutrition for many years. Their criticisms of the advice of faddists and quacks have been fully justified.

Mendelsohn served a year as president of the National Health Federation and participated actively in the American Quack Association, two groups that have shamelessly promoted unproven methods and opposed important public health measures. He also spent a great deal of time on the talk-show circuit and was a favorite guest of Phil Donahue and radio talk-show host Michael Jackson. To responsible health professionals, he sounded like a whiney-voiced crank preaching hatred against his chosen profession, because of some unspecified personal grudge. To tabloid talk-show producers, his sensationalizing sounded like ratings sweeps. He never got around to founding his New Medical School.

Contemporary Books once advanced me several thousand dollars to complete a handbook of preventive medicine, but when they saw the first draft they dropped the idea and wrote off the advance. I had included chapters critical of the quackery Mendelsohn promoted, as well as comments critical of the doctor and his paranoia-peddling.

It would be interesting to know whether the editors and executives of Contemporary Books and Warner Books, which markets the paperback edition of *Heretic*, follow the advice they so readily foist on the public. Do they keep their kids from getting vaccinated, as Mendolsohn recommended? Do they avoid screening tests for high blood pressure, high cholesterol level, colon cancer, and the like? And if they get cancer, will they go to a cancer specialist, or will they seek out laetrile peddlers and homeopaths, as Mendelsohn suggests? Ironically, Mendelsohn died of a heart attack at the age of sixty-one, about ten years sooner than would be expected for an average male in the U.S. It would be interesting to know whether his life could have been prolonged by modern medical care.

"Vitamin Expert" Earl Mindell

Would you like to get rich in a relatively low-risk business? Here's how. First, get yourself a Ph.D. from an unaccredited school; there are a dozen or so in the country. With the degree you can call yourself "Doctor." Few publishers, reporters, or talk-show hosts will question the validity of your credentials if their source has an official-sounding name. Most don't care whether it's accredited or just an office running a mail-order business.

Next, open a "health food" store. It can be small at first. You can stock your store with a few food items like nuts, seeds, fruits, and juices, but your big profits will come from your pills and powders—vitamins, minerals, amino acids, and pseudonutrients. These don't spoil quickly, they take very little shelf space for their value, and they have high profit margins.

Now start writing articles, pamphlets, and books—by "Dr." You, of course—on the importance of taking huge doses of every kind of supplement you sell. Claim that taking these pills and powders can help prevent and cure arthritis, asthma, allergies, colds, diabetes, female disorders, skin diseases, sports injuries, and dozens of the most common health problems people face. Also say that supplements will make you sexier, more beautiful, more energetic, and happier.

Finally, hire an agent to get you on radio and TV talk shows as often as possible. Always dress nicely and cultivate a sober, professional demeanor. Have your agent make sure the hosts always address you as "Dr." While on the shows take every opportunity to promote the types of products your store sells, but don't be so obvious that the show seems like a commercial.

Master of the Media Nutrition Game

In recent years several "nutrition experts" have played this game very well, but none better than "Dr." Earl Mindell, cofounder of the Great Earth "health food" stores, the second largest such chain in the country. He passes himself off as a Ph.D. nutritionist on the basis of a certificate from the University of Beverly Hills, which was never accredited and no longer exists. *Earl Mindell's Vitamin Bible* [Rawson Wade, 1979] and other books by Mindell are little more than commercials for the products sold in "health food" stores. Mindell has appeared frequently on talk shows where the host and members of the audience call him Dr. Mindell and ask disease-related questions.

There is no limit to the nostrums Mindell has huckstered. His writings promote cytochrome C, octacosanol, and bee pollen as energy boosters;

spirulina for hunger control; and assorted nutrients and herbs to enhance one's sex life. His *Vitamin Bible lists* twenty-three vitamins; there are actually only thirteen. He also claims that large doses of a wide array of dietary supplements are effective against hypertension, depression, hemorrhoids, psoriasis, back pain, athlete's foot, premenstrual syndrome, vision problems, AIDS, eating disorders, arthritis, heart disease, diabetes, obesity, sprains, hair loss, hair graying, dandruff, tonsillitis, warts, acne, poor memory, and sexual dysfunctions, all without a shred of evidence. He has even recommended large doses of B vitamins as an antidote to habitual lying by children.

During the mid-1980s Mindell formulated a product called "Metabolean," which Great Earth advertised as a "clinically proven" appetite suppressant and weight-loss aid. The product is primarily ground up cow intestine and has never been proven effective against any health problem. It may contain small amounts of cholecystokinin (CCK), a small protein molecule produced by the intestine of all mammals. CCK made within the body is involved in appetite control. When taken orally, however, it is digested and exerts no pharmacological effect. The animal experiments showing that CCK suppresses appetite involved injecting highly purified CCK intravenously before each meal.[6]

Self-Serving Propaganda

Mindell has edited a large series of pamphlets called "Good Health Guides" with "Dr." Richard Passwater, who represents himself as a Ph.D. biochemist and nutritionist on the basis of a bogus "degree" from Bernadean University, a correspondence school that not only was unaccredited but never had state authorization to operate. Passwater is research director for Solgar Corporation (a vitamin supplement manufacturer) and writes a regular column, boosting supplements, for a "health food" industry trade magazine. In *Supernutrition* [Pocket Books, 1975] he recommends megadoses of vitamins for everyone.

The "Good Health Guides" are cesspools of nutrition misinformation and deceptive promotion. One promotes dehydroepiandrosterone (DHEA) as a weight-loss miracle, which it isn't. (In the mid-1980s, the FDA ordered manufacturers to stop marketing it as such.) Another promotes glucomannan (a plant fiber) as an effective appetite suppressant, which it isn't. Another suggests (falsely) that lecithin can prevent and treat heart disease, muscle weakness, psoriasis, poor memory, and multiple sclerosis. Yet another promotes superoxide dismutase (SOD) pills for arthritis, atherosclerosis, cancer, and senility. In fact, SOD is digested in the stomach and doesn't do anything for any disease. Some of Mindell's recommendations are potentially dangerous, especially those for vitamin A, vitamin D, niacin, vitamin B_6, and zinc.

The manuscript for *Earl Mindell's Vitamin Bible,* originally written as Mindell's "Ph.D." thesis, was reviewed by James Kenney, Ph.D., R.D., a real nutritionist. Although Dr. Kenney told Mindell his work contained over a hundred important errors, most of them remain in the published book.[7] Nevertheless, the book's acknowledgments thank Kenney, as well as the American Medical Association, the National Academy of Sciences, the National Dairy Council, and the American Academy of Pediatrics, none of whom would agree with most of the book's contents. Another of Mindell's books, *Earl Mindell's Shaping up with Vitamins* [Warner Books, 1985] thanks these groups plus the American Dietetic Association, even though he must know that the ADA strongly opposes the megadoses and pseudonutrients he promotes. The book's jacket calls Mindell "America's #1 Vitamin Expert" and assures the reader that Mindell's hundreds of suggestions on supplements for health and athletic performance are "proven." This is gross and deliberate deception.

In 1987 the FTC finally stopped Great Earth from falsely claiming that its products can cure or prevent diseases, assist in weight control, strengthen organs or their functions, or eliminate harmful substances from the body. The company is also prohibited from claiming its amino acid formulas can stimulate the production of human growth hormone or promote muscle development, muscle tone, fat burning, or weight loss during sleep.[8]

"Health Crusader" Gary Null

Gary Null, who bills himself as "America's #1 Health Crusader," is in reality one of America's foremost promoters of dangerous health misinformation and a peddler of supplements as well. Long before Null had so much as a bachelor's degree, he was promoting himself as a "Health and Nutrition Expert." Inquiries and skepticism about his credentials generally have been met with silence or threats of lawsuits. One would think that a person who holds himself up to the nation as a learned nutritionist and health expert on radio and television and in books published by major publishers would be willing to inform his audience about his claims to expertise. I have repeatedly inquired about his educational background, but my certified mail has gone unanswered.

On the Morton Downy, Jr., show in January 1989, Null claimed he would have a Ph.D. in a few months. When physician-attorney Harvey Wachsman asked from what college he had a bachelor's degree, Null replied, "None of your damned business!" He then walked over to Wachsman, mocking and gesturing at his ample belly, and said, "I would like to see Dr. Wachsman hold himself up as an authority on good health!" Null finally said he had a bachelor's degree from Edison State College in New Jersey. Recently, he acquired a Ph.D. in human nutrition and public health sciences from Union Graduate School. Both of these schools are accredited but "nontraditional." At Union Graduate School, the student decides the title of the degree and the content of the program, which is largely self-administered. The course of study is not as stringent or comprehensive as a university-based science program.

But enough about Null's credentials—let's look at what he says. Probably the best indication of his philosophy is a large series of articles on "Medical Genocide," which he wrote for *Penthouse* magazine.

Cancer and AIDS Quackery

Null preaches that practically all cancer therapies approved by the American Cancer Society, the National Cancer Institute, and practicing oncologists are worthless and dangerous and that practically all the unapproved therapies are beneficial. Moreover, he promotes the extremely dangerous idea that the latter should be used not as a last resort after conventional therapies have failed, but *before and instead of* such therapies. He has endorsed laetrile (which can cause cyanide poisoning and has been proven worthless in several studies); krebiozen (extracted from horse urine); zoologist Lawrence Burton's "immuno-augmentive" therapy (extracted from tumor tissue and blood and reported to have transmitted serious infections); fasting (even though many cancer deaths are ultimately caused by cachexia, or starvation); Max Gerson's diet of raw juice and raw calf liver; coffee enemas (which can cause lethal potassium depletion); and massive doses of vitamin C (proven worthless in controlled trials at the Mayo Clinic). Null falsely claims spectacular success rates for these therapies, all of which the American Cancer Society considers questionable.

His rave review of the Gerson method in *Penthouse* quotes Dr. Curtis Hesse, former director of a Gerson clinic. "Ironically," Hesse says, "the main problem we usually have is not always cancer, but the other medications and treatments that the patients have already undergone. . . . In cancer, we do not, as a general rule, accept any patient who has undergone chemotherapy. . . . Malignant melanoma, considered to be incurable by conventional methods, is one of the most deadly cancers known, yet we see within two to three weeks a good response."

This is potentially killer misinformation because it encourages people with melanoma (and other cancers) to avoid medically recognized therapy and use an unproven dietary regimen instead. Melanoma is curable about 75 percent of the time by simple surgery alone, and the cure rate approaches 100 percent if surgery is done early enough. There is no evidence whatsoever that diet has any effect on melanoma. If you believe Hesse, you could waste precious time drinking vegetable juice instead of getting the cancer removed surgically.

Null has much the same attitude about AIDS. He claims there is a massive government cover-up of effective treatment. "The most successful treatment," he says, "would begin with detoxification. . . . fasting would accomplish this." Then he would give them raw foods, juices, garlic, and vitamins. He is especially fond of massive doses of vitamin C. Does he believe that AIDS patients who already are emaciated will benefit by a regimen that begins with starving themselves?

Null claims that the "medical establishment" is suppressing effective AIDS and cancer treatments so doctors, hospitals, and the pharmaceutical industry can make more money. Null apparently believes there is a conspiracy involving thousands of people who study for years to master complex sciences, not so they can save lives, make their families proud, and gain the admiration of their colleagues, but so they can secretly suppress cures for diseases that might kill them and their loved ones. On one of his radio shows Null expressed exasperation that the media ignored a press conference he called to tell the world how to cure AIDS and end the epidemic in three months. "*The New York Times*," he said, "won't move unless the American Medical Association gives it permission."

I guess in some people's minds, almost anything is possible.

Public Health Enemy #1

Lest you think that Null specializes in just AIDS and cancer, let me assure you he promotes unfounded ideas in many other areas. Among the most dangerous is that vaccinations are bad. "I am passionately opposed," he said during a show in August 1987, "to thousands of people getting DPT shots every day. . . . The vaccine causes death, paralysis, and sudden infant death." He erroneously said the "T" stands for typhoid. Actually, it stands for tetanus, a preventable disease that is almost always fatal.

On his radio show in October 1987, Null said, "I would never get vaccinated for anything—polio, smallpox, measles." Of course, no one has to get smallpox vaccinations anymore, because it was eradicated from the face of the earth by a worldwide vaccination campaign—one of the great triumphs of modern scientific medicine. Paralytic polio is also nearly a thing of the past, thanks to vaccination. Measles might also be wiped out if people took the disease more seriously and everyone got vaccinated. However, thanks in part to antivaccination propagandists like Null and Dr. Robert Mendelsohn, measles and pertussis (whooping cough) outbreaks are on the upswing. While the pertussis vaccine is not perfect and sometimes causes side effects, all experts agree that its benefits far outweigh its risks. But Null is certain his wisdom is greater.

Null also says that the interlocking bony plates of the skull can become misaligned and cause all kinds of serious health problems. This notion is preposterous because the bones of the skull become firmly fused to each other during infancy. (See cranial osteopathy in Chapter 5 for further information on this subject.)

Nutritional Nonsense

For someone who claims to be an expert in nutrition, it is astonishing how many absurd notions about food, nutrition, and physiology Gary Null has. For example, he says fat from meat is difficult to digest. If that were true, fatty meat would not be a major contributor to obesity and high cholesterol levels. Null's claim resembles Judy Mazel's notion (see Chapter 1) that people store fat only from the foods they don't digest. But what can we expect from an "expert" who would starve AIDS patients?

Null often says he has discovered this or that in his laboratory. In December 1987, for example, he said that his laboratory studies prove that meats have no energy. This would mean that meats would not provide calories to the human body. Is Null's laboratory in the Land of Oz?

Null says there is a vitamin B_{15}, and he has even peddled dimethylglycine (DMG), one of several substances promoted as B_{15}. But there is no vitamin B_{15}. The concept is a fraud perpetrated by members of the Krebs family who also developed the laetrile fraud. Null says that vitamins are absorbed best if you take them sublingually. That is, it's best to open the capsules or crush the tablets and put them under your tongue. There is no evidence to support this claim. He also says potatoes provide as much vitamin C as oranges. Actually, oranges contain more than twice as much vitamin C per pound.

According to Null, vitamin C supplements increase the body's requirement for iron, so if you take the vitamin you should take more iron. The truth is just the opposite. Vitamin C is well known to increase the absorption of iron from the diet. Taking large doses of both, which Null advocates, can cause some people to accumulate excess iron in body tissues, especially in the heart, and can cause serious health problems.

Null said on one of his shows that he normally takes ten grams of vitamin C each day and takes up to fifty-five grams for such stresses as running a marathon and excessive exposure to the sun. He says large doses of vitamin C can cure a bad sunburn in an hour, as well as cure cancer, AIDS, kidney stones, pneumonia, chronic mononucleosis, drug addiction, and many other ailments. This information is being suppressed, he claims, because it would deprive drug companies, doctors, and hospitals of profits. Null also happens to market his own brand of vitamin C. His Suprema-C, "the supreme vitamin C formula," is superior, because it supposedly is more efficiently absorbed and better utilized by cells. Of course, he provides no data to support these claims.

Null claims that some nutrients, including thiamine, folic acid, vitamin E, zinc, and iodine, are catabolic and should therefore be taken in the morning, while others, such as vitamin A, calcium, and magnesium, are anabolic and should be taken in the evening. His supplement line includes formulas for both morning and evening use. He also claims that swimming in chlorinated pools increases vitamin requirements. So all you morning dippers better stock up on Null's AM Vitamin, and you evening swimmers better use his PM Vitamin. His literature doesn't indicate what middle-of-the-day swimmers should do. Perhaps they should play it safe and take both.

Null blames many ailments on "toxins," but he never names them or explains how they cause the problems he attributes to them. He promotes and/or peddles various substances that he claims "detoxify the body" and "cleanse" and "purify the blood." While he claims his recommendations are based in science, he uses the language of medieval bloodletters and herbalists. His Rebalancer formula, which he calls a "cleansing formulation," contains vitamin C from sago palm, which he says is a "superior ingredient because some individuals have a sensitivity or hidden allergy to corn, the usual source of vitamin C formulations." He doesn't mention that sago palm contains toxins that are believed to cause brain damage and neurological disease and that such disease is common in the South Pacific where the palms are eaten. I don't know whether the specific plant used for his formulation contains the toxins or whether they are removed in the processing, but this should be of far greater concern than sensitivity to corn.

During a program in February 1988, Null said that the calcium from milk is not absorbed and therefore does nothing for your bones. He also said that grains are an excellent source of calcium. Of course, milk is an excellent source of bone-building calcium, and most grains are only a poor to fair source of calcium compared to dairy products, almonds, broccoli, tofu, and spinach. How can one "Health and Nutrition Expert" be so wrong about so many nutrition issues? *Gary Null is wrong so often that the average person who listens to him might be better off believing the opposite of what he says.*

Media Malpractice?

On another of Null's radio shows to which I listened, a caller said she had a kidney disease. Without asking what kind of problem she had, Null immediately told her she had to eliminate all protein from her diet. Although decreasing protein intake is appropriate for some people with kidney disorders, it is not appropriate for others. Regardless, since components of protein (amino acids) are essential nutrients, complete elimination could be disastrous.The caller should have been told to follow her doctor's advice.

In another case, a woman caller said she suspected she had Epstein-Barr virus, sometimes called "chronic mono." Null told her she should be on an "anti-Candida diet" and needed daily intravenous treatments of 200 grams of vitamin C. *Candida albicans* is a yeast that can cause vaginal infections. There is no evidence any diet works for *Candida* infection, which most supposed victims don't have anyway. If there were such a diet, why should it also work against a virus, which is a completely different type of organism? The daily 200-gram dose of vitamin C Null recommends is 3,333 times the RDA—more than a nine-year supply for an average individual! Smaller doses given intravenously have killed people.

Instead of detailing more here, I refer you to other parts of this book for a look at the following, all of which Null has promoted: catalyst-activated water, colonic lavage (including coffee enemas), clinical ecology, homeopathy, applied kinesiology, barley greens, wheat grass juice, hyperbaric oxygen for virus infections, germanium for athletic performance and a variety of serious disease. He has also expressed admiration for Adelle Davis, Carlton Fredericks, and Herbert Shelton. Null is even fond of electronic quackery. He owns an electromagnetic pulsation device, which, he claims, redirects and realigns the electrical poles of the body (whatever that means) and thereby improves health and stamina.[9]

Supplement Peddling

Null likes to portray himself as "America's #1 health crusader fighting for consumer rights."[10] He has dedicated at least two of his books to Ralph Nader to further the illusion that he is a consumer advocate. But I don't see Nader peddling pills and powders, or promoting pseudoscientific rubbish to the public. Nader could make millions endorsing automobiles, but he doesn't.

Null, on the other hand, owns a supplement business and promotes the ingredients in his products in an unfair and misleading manner. He sells several dozen formulations of nutrients, pseudonutrients, bee products, and herbs, as well as a dozen snacks, protein powders, and cereals. His promotional literature describes them as "scientifically formulated," "synergistically combined," "better absorbed," "better utilized," and "actually tested." His products can, he promises or implies, improve health, increase energy and stamina, boost immunity, cleanse the system, help the heart and skin, and "strengthen the cellular membranes of vital organs."

For athletes he offers "Gary Null's Competitive Edge Supplement System," which includes Sublingual Ge Oxy-132, Coenzyme Q_{10}, Sport DMG, and several other supplements. His various products will do just about everything advertisers can dream up to appeal to people looking for fitness in a bottle: improve performance, reduce fatigue, improve heart function, and enhance oxygen utilization, muscle metabolism, muscle growth, and muscle repair.

How much will Null's recommended supplement program cost? (Not that it really matters, of course, since your health is worth whatever it costs.) It's hard to be precise because Null's brochures and order forms don't provide enough information on daily doses to figure out cost per day. However, giving him the benefit of the doubt and taking a low estimate, even counting just one of his "irresistible" snacks per day, the cost per person would be about $325 per month. Some Nullites might have to spend about $450 per month for Null's nutritional products plus additional funds for Null's books, newsletter, seminars, marathon runs, audio cassettes, and "healthy singles parties."

Null is fond of fasting, or at least of advocating fasting. He claims that the Hunzas (mountain people of Pakistan) benefit greatly by fasting for up to six weeks at a time each year. This amount of fasting can cause serious health consequences.

I hereby challenge Gary Null to fast for six weeks and submit to periodic medical examinations to determine the consequences.

"Health Educator" Kristin Olsen

Kristin Gottschalk Olsen is one of the latest "health experts" to embrace and help popularize the whole gamut of alternative medicine. She is billed as a "journalist, health educator, and private consultant" with a master's degree in "holistic health education" from an accredited college. Her book, *The Encyclopedia of Alternative Health Care* [Simon and Schuster, 1989], is a love feast of past-life therapy, iridology, homeopathy, polarity therapy, pseudonutrition, and dozens of other irrational and silly practices. The front cover promises the book will tell how each of these methods works. Ms. Olsen does not seriously question *whether* they work; most of her discussions simply parrot the claims of the promoters. I have included her in this chapter, not because she is particularly influential, but because she is typical of the authors who write books promoting "alternative" methods.

While Olsen's book is a poor source of evidence or advice on the subjects it covers, it is fascinating for what it illustrates about the behavior of a "true believer." The book describes how she samples scores of quack nostrums now in vogue, much like a food critic goes from restaurant to restaurant. But while the connoisseur of food and wine is a hedonist and a skeptic, Olsen's quest is submissive and credulous. She submits to poking, prodding, needling, joint cracking, enemas, and brainwashing, and she proclaims them all wonderful. She even uses the term "guinea pig" to describe herself. Everything she tries makes her better, yet she apparently remains unwell enough to continue seeking treatment. The incongruity of this situation completely escapes her.

Olsen says past-life therapy "has been a profoundly healing influence" in her life. She says polarity therapy, a kind of astral body massage, is an energy tuner and balancer, a liver balancer, and a chakra balancer (whatever all this means). Similarly, her chapter on iridology reads like a promotional pamphlet from an iridologist's office. Analysis of photographs of the iris can, she assures us, give a complete profile of a person's nutritional and other health-care needs and act as an early warning system by detecting constitutional weaknesses and problems in specific organs. Incredibly, she mentions the controlled studies in which iridologists have failed miserably, but she parrots their excuse that some of the photographs were of poor quality. Actually, before the test the iridologists were permitted to reject all photographs they deemed unacceptable for any reason whatsoever.[11] Olsen fell under the spell of a California Christian faith healer who sees all illness as spiritual problems and claims to help even in cases of cancer and AIDS. While interviewing him, she claims, he sent "waves of energy" through her. She felt "palpably charged with a new perspective...in my heart." She knew that from then on she would turn to him for help with any illness, "physical or otherwise." It appears that Olsen is at least vaguely aware of her susceptibility to illnesses that are other than physical.

Olsen attributes the usual magical properties to medicinal herbs. They cleanse, purify, tone, invigorate, etc. She displays an abysmal ignorance of certain basic facts. For example, she says morphine and quinine are modern drugs synthesized in a laboratory. In fact, they are natural constituents of the opium poppy and cinchona tree bark, respectively, from which they are extracted. She says salicylic acid is "the active ingredient of aspirin." In fact, the two are different molecules. Aspirin is the acetyl salt of salicylic acid and does not occur naturally.

Taking an enema, especially a high-volume colonic lavage, Olsen says, "is one of the healing arts I use often when facing a health challenge." She claims her early ones "cleared out years of encrusted feces and some pockets of very warm, infected or decomposed material," more than a pound each time. She doesn't explain how she reached these conclusions or mention a pathology report or fecal analysis. Did she actually weigh the fecal material, take its temperature, or measure its water content? How did she determine its age? Why was she surprised the material was "decomposed"? Did she expect big chunks of undigested foods?

Olsen describes one colonic session as though it was a form of psychotherapy. She said that as she talked about incidents that bothered her, she experienced "a tremendous release of impacted material" and "a sudden release of energy that had literally been captured in my intestines all that time. I shook as the energy was released and cried the tears I had not allowed myself to show."

Yes, Olsen suggests that enemas cleanse the body and mind, enhance immunity, balance the glands, and provide "sudden energy release" followed by "internal calm or quietness." She recommends the procedure for a wide variety of gastrointestinal symptoms and disorders, chronic diseases, improvement of the circulation, and problems with the eyes, skin, muscles, joints, and urinary tract. She presents no evidence to support her recommendations, but since she, the "health educator," often uses enemas when facing a health challenge, that should be good enough for readers to sign up for a series of treatments.

Olsen seems to have health crises so often and to have so many favorite alternative methods that it occurs to me she could save time by undergoing several treatments simultaneously. For example, she could get polarized while a faith healer sends his healing vibes, and a past-life therapist carries her a few centuries into the past, all while an enema helps her explosively release impacted feces and impacted emotions. Now, if that doesn't finally get her well, I don't suppose anything ever will. Olsen is no more a health educator or responsible health journalist than a junkie shooting up street drugs is a pharmacologist. Doesn't her publisher (Simon and Schuster) know this?

Ms. Olsen says she focused primarily on thirty-three major wholistic practices because they are "the classics, the ones that have set the direction of the new health care." But, she also assures us, "these are by no means all there are. . . . There are many more types of health care practices to investigate." She says that the practitioners she describes are "at the leading edges of the holistic industry . . . using conferences, summit meetings, the media, courts, and legislatures to promote, define, standardize, and license their particular practices." They are networking, registering trademarks, organizing into guilds, and "providing a wide range of services and products. Wholistic health seems to have come of age."

Ms. Olsen appears to be correct on this particular point. "Alternative" health practices do seem to have come of age. But I certainly don't share her enthusiasm. America is riding a tidal wave of hogwash and health fraud that poses a real threat to our society.

"Research Scientists" Durk Pearson and Sandy Shaw

Durk Pearson and Sandy Shaw, neither of whom has credentials in the health field, have presented their notions of aging and longevity in the book, *Life Extension: A Practical Scientific Approach* [Warner Books, 1982], and on scores of talk shows starting with Merv Griffin in 1978. They suggest that people can greatly improve the length and quality of their life by taking supplements. Brain power can be increased; cardiovascular disease, cancer, arthritis, and other diseases can be prevented; and smoking, drinking, and breathing polluted air can be made safer. Skin aging can be slowed and even reversed, and sexual capacity and athletic prowess increased. We can combat baldness, prevent hangovers, and even develop our muscles without exercise.

Pearson and Shaw attribute these miraculous properties to certain vitamins, amino acids, minerals, food preservatives, and prescription drugs. Most of them are antioxidants, substances that tend to retard oxidation reactions in plant and animal tissues. The recommended doses are large—in the megavitamin range for the nutrients and far in excess of the usual doses for the drugs.

Pearson and Shaw speculate that antioxidants protect cells from the ravaging effects of highly reactive chemicals, known as free radicals and peroxides, which create abnormal chemical bonds in various tissues. These abnormal bonds cause brittleness in arteries and lung tissue, wrinkling and spotting of the skin, nerve and brain damage, and other symptoms of aging. Flooding the body with antioxidants, we are told, can greatly reduce damage and retard or even reverse aging. Pearson and Shaw have parlayed this idea into a multimillion-dollar writing and pill-peddling enterprise.

The authors say their book is a "practical how-to-do-it-yourself book on life extension." They make the obligatory disclaimers and say that we are all biochemically distinct, so each person must experiment and explore to find the formula best for him- or herself. But there is no rational way for the individual to choose between, say, 100 and 1,000 units of vitamin E or 5 and 50 milligrams of Hydergine, to get the alleged benefits. If one is taking several dozen pills each day, how can one know which pill is doing what? Naturally, most people who decide to follow Pearson and Shaw's lead will try to mimic the formula they themselves use, even though they say it is strictly experimental and recommended only for themselves. If the authors didn't intend for other people to load up on chemicals, why did they write a book about them for the general public and list doses.

Nearly one hundred of the book's eight hundred pages are devoted to a tirade against the Food and Drug Administration for its restrictive policies on nutritional supplements and new drugs. They even blast the FDA for banning thalidomide, the sedative that caused thousands of children to be born with horrendous birth defects in West Germany, which permitted its use during the 1950s. They reason that, except for unborn children, thalidomide is safer than barbiturates, which cause about one thousand deaths each year in the United States. However, most barbiturate overdoses are either intentional or subsequent to illicit use of the "downers" obtained from drug pushers. Legalizing thalidomide would not affect these cases. Pearson and Shaw say nonpregnant women should have access to this "safe" tranquilizer. But women often don't know they are pregnant in the first month, the very period during which the fetus is most vulnerable to thalidomide.

Unscientific and Unsafe

Pearson and Shaw do a very peculiar job of providing references to back up their fantastic claims. Although they list lots of studies from the scientific literature, the references are not presented in the standard manner in which specific statements are backed up with specific studies. Instead, they just list a lot of references for each chapter and leave it to the reader to figure out which studies support which assertions. Those who puzzle this out will find that the articles listed generally do *not* support the claims made in the book's text. For example, they claim that the famous Framingham study on heart disease showed "no clear relation between serum cholesterol and deaths due to heart disease." Scores of articles in the scientific literature from the Framingham group come to the exact opposite conclusion.

The authors' other leg of support consists of anecdotes, which have about as much validity as hearsay has in a court of law. While the authors concede that anecdotal case histories are scientifically worthless, they devote more than fifty pages to them.

Scientific or not, Pearson and Shaw have increased the use of nutritional supplements and created a demand for routine use of certain prescription drugs. So let's look at some components of their "life extension formula" and the evidence regarding their use.

Vitamins A, most of the Bs, C, and E are recommended in daily doses up to six hundred times the RDA. The evidence they rely on to support the megadoses is very poor and even includes an account of how large doses of riboflavin—taken on the advice of Kurt Donsbach—relieved symptoms of Pearson's allergy to cats. (During the early 1980s, Pearson and Shaw wrote columns for Donsbach's magazine *Health Express*.) They scarcely mention or seriously underestimate the risks of taking such huge doses of supplements.

The amino acids in their formula include arginine, ornithine, cysteine, tryptophan, and sometimes phenylalanine and tyrosine. These supposedly promote normal sleep, prevent depression, and provide stamina. Several of them are also erroneously alleged to release growth hormone, increase muscle mass, and stimulate the immune system to help combat infections, cancer, and even atherosclerosis.

Their formula includes a fantastic seventeen grams of the amino acid arginine. The long-term effects of taking such large doses of isolated nutrients are not known.[12] Even if the amino acids did increase growth hormone levels, the dangers would outweigh the benefits since an excess of the hormone can have a host of deleterious effects. Moreover, it is well established that the amino acids compete with each other for absorption and utilization, so excessive intake of one or more may induce relative deficiencies of others. The authors make no mention of this or other potential hazards.

Dangerous Games with Drugs

Pearson and Shaw recommend BHT and other antioxidant food preservatives in much larger amounts than those available in foods. Besides slowing aging, the authors say, BHT reduces sleeping time and prevents alcoholic hangovers. But excessive BHT may be dangerous; doses smaller than those recommended by the authors have been shown to be toxic to the liver of animals, and some countries have banned even the very small amounts used in foods to prevent fat from becoming rancid. An overdose of BHT can be lethal; about one gram will kill a rabbit. Pearson and Shaw suggest two grams a day.

They also recommend the antioxidant prescription drugs Hydergine, Deaner, bromocriptine, and L-dopa and the prescription hormones vasopressin and thyroid extract to improve memory and learning, stimulate the immune system, and scavenge free radicals to slow aging. Their claims about these drugs are preposterous. For example, they say that Hydergine is "very effective in preventing brain damage from hypoxia (insufficient oxygen) in emergencies such as drowning, and smoke or carbon monoxide poisoning" and that it "can be injected intravenusly or, better yet, directly into the carotid artery in the neck." But officials at Sandoz Pharmaceuticals, the company that makes Hydergine, know of no evidence that any of this is true. In letters to Jack Yetiv, M.D., Ph.D., author of *Popular Nutritional Practices,* a Sandoz official also contradicted Pearson and Shaw's claims that (a) Diapid (another Sandoz product) improves memory and learning and aids in recovery from accident-induced amnesia; (b) in Europe Hydergine is commonly administered before surgery to reduce the chance of brain damage; (c) Hydergine helps 60 percent of asthma patients; (d) Sandoz spends about 40 percent of its research budget on Hydergine (it spends 2 to 3 percent, mostly for new dosage and delivery systems); and (e) Parlodel (another Sandoz product) normalizes growth hormone levels.[13]

Pearson and Shaw present antioxidants as the cure-all and prevent-all for humanity. No discussion is given to possible consequences of all this antioxidant power flooding our bodies, but it is oxidation within the cells that provides the energy to drive bodily functions. Why must we assume that the body's own mechanisms for balancing oxidative and antioxidative forces are incompetent? Might not an overdose of antioxidants interfere with vital cell oxidation or cause the body to slow down its own antioxidant production? Is the thyroid extract (which promotes oxidation) in the formula necessary to combat the excess of antioxidants? Incidentally, even slight overdoses of thyroid hormone may greatly increase the risk of osteoporosis by leaching minerals from the bones.[14] The authors don't mention that free radicals have some beneficial functions in the body. For example, infection-fighting white blood cells kill bacteria by generating free radicals. Thus, it is reasonable to suspect that megadoses of antioxidants (such as vitamin C) might hinder the body's ability to fight infection.

More Unsupported Claims

Pearson and Shaw claim that men and women who cannot reach orgasm often respond to large doses of niacin, which can cause a flush resembling the flush of orgasm. They cite no studies and provide no evidence. They do mention, though, that they often ingest niacin before sex in order to enhance the flushing. Most people find the niacin flush uncomfortable, however, because it is often accompanied by itching and burning of the skin. These side effects are certainly not erotic.

Pearson and Shaw also claim, on the flimsiest anecdotal evidence, that BHT is an effective antiherpes medicine. They say they recommended it to several people, and, lo and behold, their herpes subsided in a week. But, since herpes sores come and go frequently, no remedy should be proclaimed effective without carefully controlled studies.

These authors also claim that large doses of vitamins E and C and other antioxidant nutrients can maintain sexual capacity into older age and increase a depressed sex drive. They cite no evidence to support this claim. Nor do they support their claims that the amino acid phenylalanine is twice as effective as the antidepressant drug imipramine, that vitamin-containing creams can increase hair growth in balding men, that old rats can be made to swim like young rats if given the right antioxidants, that smoker's cough can be alleviated in twenty-four hours by large doses of vitamins A and C, or that raw pineapple and papaya applied to the skin can make it look younger.

Pearson and Shaw say that children with cystic fibrosis have low blood levels of vitamins A and E because of an excess of free radicals. It is well known that the low levels are due to poor absorption caused by pancreatic disease. They say human white blood cells often live a couple of years in the body. In fact, the life-span of these cells is about two weeks. They say PABA (para-aminobenzoic acid) is a vitamin, but it is not. They say ingested PABA is a good sunscreen, but it isn't.

Body Image Distortion?

Pearson (thirty-seven years old when *Life Extension* was published) says he remains in a chair or water bed 85 percent of the time and exercises only thirty seconds a day with a pair of dumbbells. Yet he claims to be more muscular than he was as a teenager. This he attributes to his use of the nutrients and drugs that purportedly release growth hormone. The book contains a photograph of him scantily clad and posing with his arm mucles flexed, with the caption, "It took me a total of about thirty minutes of exercise (over two months) to build these muscles." But most people who look at the picture wonder "what muscles?" Pearson certainly doesn't look like a trained athlete with only 13 percent body fat (as he claims). Nor does the book include a "before" picture to compare.

Both Pearson and Shaw (who was thirty-seven also) claimed that their skin had the appearance of people in their early twenties, a quality they attributed to the antioxidants in their formula. As evidence of this claim, they said that, when pinched, their skin snaps back in place about as quickly as that of a teenager's. They make no mention of the many variables than can affect such a test, such as muscle tension, sun damage, and hereditary factors. Nor do they provide any measurements or even anecdotal information to support their "younger skin" contention. They claim to have witnessed age spots gradually disappear from an elderly man's skin after he started taking one of their recommended drugs. But in just the case where photos might provide documentation, there were none.

"Research Scientists"?

Pearson and Shaw like to suggest they have special knowledge and status as "research scientists" in the field of aging. However, they have not had training or done scientific studies in gerontology, do not have any degree in the field, and have not been published in scientific journals. Their sole claim to being researchers is that they read and interpret scientific literature. (Their interpretations, of course, differ from those of the scientific mainstream.)

Their arrogance is illustrated by their claim that "as scientists, we have access to many drugs that are unavailable to pharmacists, physicians, and their patients due to FDA regulations."[15] Even if they were legitimate research scientists, they would have no special status with the FDA or access to drugs unavailable to pharmacists and physicians.

While physicians train for six to ten years after college, Pearson and Shaw don't even have graduate degrees. Pearson has an undergraduate degree in physics, a field unrelated to the one he now claims expertise in. Shaw has an undergraduate degree in chemistry. Although neither has the minimal credentials to teach health education at a legitimate university, they have made millions from book royalties plus additional money giving lectures and licensing their formulas.[16]

Impractical and Expensive

It should be clear that *Life Extension—A Practical Scientific Approach* is not scientific as its title claims. Is it practical? In 1984, William Bennett, M.D., editor of the *Harvard Medical School Health Letter,* calculated that with careful shopping and bulk purchases, the cost of its recommended pills and powders would be $64 a day.[17] In addition, there would be the cost of regular visits to a physician to get the necessary prescriptions plus the cost of the extensive laboratory tests, which, the authors emphasize, are absolutely essential. Thus the total expense would be quite high.

Could physicians be talked into prescribing large doses of powerful drugs with potentially serious side effects for people who do not exhibit the usual indications for using the drugs? Pearson and Shaw's recommended Hydergine dose, for example, is 40 milligrams a day, seven to ten times the usual dose for therapy in age-related forgetfulness—for which, incidentally, the drug is ineffective. Doctors with whom I have spoken say they would consider it extremely irresponsible—even malpractice—to administer what Pearson and Shaw recommend.

Weight-Loss Miracle

The fact that the authors' first book doesn't live up to its claim of being practical and scientific did not stop it from selling over a million copies. Having made millions of dollars for themselves and Warner Books huckstering a miracle antiaging regimen, it was only natural that Pearson and Shaw would follow up with a miracle weight-loss program. *The Life Extension Weight Loss Program* [Doubleday and Co., 1986] promises you can lose fat without dieting, hunger, or exercise. You can eat lots of meat, eggs, dairy products, fatty sauces, and desserts and still lose weight. The back cover shows the authors holding huge ice cream cones dripping with hot fudge. They emphasize over and over that they hate exercise and are totally sedentary, yet they stay fit. You can do the same by using their methods, primarily taking a bunch of pills, many the same ones they tout for alleged antiaging effects. The evidence they muster for their regimen is as flimsy as that for their life-extension program.

Pearson and Shaw's denigration of exercise is as irresponsible as their recommendation to take buckets of pills. They repeatedly say they hate exercise and love to sit or lie around all day. They assure their readers that exercise isn't necessary for weight control or good health.

Ironically, the scientific evidence for exercise as a means to control weight and slow aging is far stronger than the evidence for their pill-popping regimens, which they don't even pretend can strengthen the heart or increase vital capacity, perhaps the two most important indices of age. Effects of aging that can be modified by exercise include increased blood pressure, decreased cardiac output, increased blood fat and cholesterol, fatty degeneration of the arteries, reduced vital capacity, loss of muscle and bone tissue, poor glucose tolerance, sleep disturbances, tendency to depression, decreased immune function, and lower testosterone levels. Moreover, by burning calories and increasing lean body tissue and fat burning capacity, exercise helps control body fat.

Instead of utilizing and promoting exercise, which is free and of proven benefit, Pearson and Shaw encourage their readers to embark on an expensive, hazardous, impractical and unproven pill-popping program. Forty dollars for their books is just a start for the believers.

An additional irony here is that their program is far more troublesome and time-consuming than a moderate exercise program. A brisk twenty-minute or half-hour walk is simplicity itself compared to looking up references at a medical library, talking doctors into writing prescriptions, shopping for the pills, figuring out a dose schedule that doesn't make you nauseous or burn a hole in your stomach, and earning the money to pay for the pills. The one disadvantage of walking, from Pearson and Shaw's perspective, may be that it's free.

Their Regimens May Actually Accelerate Aging

Pearson and Shaw's disdain for exercise is so profound that I can't help but wonder whether all their drug-taking has deprived them of a normal *joie de vivre*. They see only misery in physical activity. Such an aversion may be common in people over seventy, but most younger people enjoy getting physical and working up a little sweat. Could Pearson and Shaw's overdosing on antioxidant chemicals and drugs be interfering with their normal muscle metabolism and brain chemistry to such an extent that any exercise is a chore? Are they aging faster than normal? Their appearance suggests that this is possible. Durk, especially, often is asked why he looks so old.

"Foremost Pediatrician" Lendon Smith

The famous Dr. Lendon Smith, the author of several bestsellers (mostly from McGraw-Hill), is a traveling salesman who pretends to be a practicing physician with a bag full of miraculous treatments most physicians don't know about. In 1973 the Oregon Board of Medical Examiners revoked his narcotics license and put him on probation for ten years for improper drug prescribing practices.[18] He was unable to prescribe drugs with a high abuse potential and was limited to pediatric practice. Restrictions were eased in 1974, but he again got into trouble for prescribing Ritalin for too many children. He then allied himself with chiropractors, homeopaths, naturopaths, and the "health food" industry.

In 1987 Smith voluntarily surrendered his medical license to the Oregon Board of Medical Examiners rather than face charges of "obtaining any fee by fraud or misrepresentation" and "making a fraudulent claim." The board has not released details of the case, but it apparently involved allegations of inappropriate and dangerous practices such as signing authorizations for insurance payments for patients he had not seen.

In spite of the lack of scientific support for his ideas, the media helped him unload tons of baloney on the public. He spoke to PTAs and clubs and was a regular guest of Phil Donahue, Johnny Carson, and other television and radio talk shows. Smith's miracle-mongering books have misled and endangered millions of people and made McGraw-Hill and himself a great deal of money.

His books include *Feed Yourself Right, Dr. Lendon Smith's Low-Stress Diet, Feed Your Kids Right, Dr. Lendon Smith's Diet Plan for Teenagers,* and at least six others. The Dell edition of *Feed Your Kids Right* calls him "America's leading pediatrician." His books are crammed so full of hogwash that a thorough refutation would take a book in itself. For our purposes a brief look at some of the quack nostrums he promotes should suffice. Many of these are discussed further in Chapter 5.

The core absurdity of Smith's medicine is the assertion that for virtually every symptom, disease, disorder, or simply unpleasant event, physical or mental, a specific megavitamin-mineral approach may help. His books are compendiums of his prescriptions for hundreds of conditions, from life-threatening and crippling diseases to minor tics and unhealthy nails. He even has specific formulas for dozens of occupations such as cab drivers, firemen, actors, musicians, surgeons, and housewives, and also for stressful events, such as living with the in-laws, taking exams, the first day of nursery school or kindergarten, going to a dentist, and going to a party. Unlike Adelle Davis, he barely pretends there is scientific support for his claims. Whereas Davis cited hundreds of research papers, most of which she misinterpreted, Smith rarely refers to studies other than his own personal observations.

Smith's prescriptions for scores of health problems are remarkably similar to each other, with just slight variations in doses. For practically everything that ever happens or might happen, the remedy is lots of vitamins and minerals. For some conditions, the recommended doses are enormous. For canker sores, he suggests 20 to 50 grams of vitamin C per day, while for genital herpes he suggests 10 to 20 grams per day. He also recommends dangerously high doses of vitamin A for a variety of conditions.

He seems fond of injecting the supplements, especially for misbehaving kids. He admits this is painful, but believes the alleged improvement in behavior is due to a therapeutic effect on the child's metabolism. It doesn't occur to him that perhaps the child does whatever his parents and Dr. Smith want to avoid getting another painful shot. Aversion therapy may appear to be effective, but it can also be cruel. Smith also recommends shots for the treatment of obesity, depression, infertility, and other problems, but cites no evidence to support his faith.

While megavitamins are Smith's main snake oils, they aren't his only ones. He claims that many people get muscle cramps and have insomnia if they drink homogenized, pasteurized milk. "The assumption is," he claims, "that they cannot absorb the calcium from the milk thus treated." Drinking raw milk may solve these problems, Smith suggests, provided you "know the cow" and are assured it is disease-free. This advice is both silly and impractical because it is virtually impossible to maintain uncontaminated herds. Although the sale of raw milk is still legal in some states, the FDA has banned interstate sale of raw-milk products, and a California judge has ordered the country's largest raw-milk producer to place warnings on its product labels.

Smith falsely claims that food allergies are extremely common and a major cause of obesity. He says we become addicted to foods we are allergic to and overeat them—and that we must stop eating these foods gradually or suffer severe withdrawal symptoms. He has advocated cytotoxic testing to determine allergies and hair analysis to determine nutrient levels and health status. On the basis of hair analysis he has claimed to diagnose, for example, hyperactivity from low calcium and magnesium levels. The remedy, of course, is calcium and magnesium supplementation. Neither cytotoxic testing nor hair analysis has any clinical value for determining people's nutritional status.[19,20]

Smith has claimed that many people have a stubborn weight problem because their thyroid gland does not produce enough thyroid hormone. He suggests that they diagnose themselves, beg their doctors for pills of the hormone, and take tyrosine and iodine supplements, as well as several toxic herbs. Others need to take pills of raw adrenal and thymus tissue, so-called glandulars that allegedly strengthen our corresponding glands. He also believes many people suffer from so-called yeast allergy, or chronic candidiasis, and need to take the drug nystatin and go on a very restrictive diet. By his reckoning, most of us are allergic to dozens of foods and must avoid dozens more because of "yeast allergy."

Smith accepts naturopathic dogma about fasting to rest and cleanse the liver and break supposed allergic addiction. In *Dr. Lendon Smith's Low-Stress Diet* [McGraw-Hill, 1985], he advocates taking nothing but distilled water and supplements for several days. Or, he claims, the liver can be "cleaned" with a beet-juice fast—and if your urine turns red you are anemic. He offers no evidence for this nonsense. Smith perpetrates the potentially dangerous naturopathic myth that the sicker a person feels during days of fasting, the more good the fasting is doing because this means toxins are being eliminated. Actually, fasting (also known as starvation) makes people feel sick because their brain lacks sugar, their metabolic machinery is forced to cannibalize muscle and liver tissue, and their bloodstream is flooded with toxic protein and fat breakdown products. Fasting doesn't cleanse and rest the liver, but overworks it by saturating it with toxins, which are produced not by poor diet but by starvation itself. Fasting also can be harmful to all organs and to overall health, especially for people who are already malnourished from adherence to fad diets or debilitated by chronic illness.

Encouraging fasting to the point of sickness is clearly irresponsible.

Yet Smith says, "If withdrawal symptoms are devastating, it is surely an encouraging sign to the faster that he or she is on the right track." It helps, he says, to use enemas to gain some relief from the sickness associated with fasting; the enema eliminates yeast, allergens, and toxins. Obese people and those with eating disorders are thus inspired by Smith to indulge in repeated rounds of fasting and enema taking in desperate and dangerous attempts to lose weight. He also accepts naturopathic dogma about food-combining, which is discussed in Chapter 1 of this book.

Smith's *Low-Stress Diet* contains thirteen affirmations to stay healthy. Item #9 says, "I will observe the food and even assign it to parts of my body that might need it. . . . If you eat carrots tell them to go to your eyes and your skin where they belong. If you are swallowing some bran or roughage, assign it to your colon, tell it to hold onto some moisture and make your next bowel movement soft and easy." But, he warns, say the affirmations to yourself rather than aloud, lest you swallow air and thus pass wind. (Not to mention that others might think you've gone bonkers.)

Doesn't Dr. Smith know that the blood carries nutrients to organs and tissues without conscious traffic directions from the person? Doesn't he know that bran that is eaten has nowhere to go but the colon and will absorb water whether we tell it to or not? Regardless, can't publishers like McGraw-Hill (a leading medical textbook publisher that surely has the resources to separate scientific facts from utter nonsense) find the moral strength to stop publishing unfounded health advice?

References

1. D. Forrester and S.L.T. Thompson: The legacies of Paavo Airola. *Nutrition Forum* 4:9–11, 1987.
2. J. Fried: *Vitamin Politics*. Buffalo, Prometheus Books, 1984
3. E. Rynearson: Americans love hogwash. *Nutrition Reviews*, Supplement, July 1974.
4. C.W. Marshall: *Vitamins and Minerals: Help or Harm?* Philadelphia, George F. Stickley Co., 1985.
5. S. Barrett: The mercurial Kurt Donsbach. *Nutrition Forum*, Oct. 1987.
6. CCK: Weight-loss breakthrough or hoax? *NCAHF Newsletter*, Jan./Feb. 1985.
7. J.A. Lowell: An irreverent look at the *Vitamin Bible* and its author. *Nutrition Forum* 3:46–47, 1986.
8. Franchisor of food supplement stores prohibited from making false claims,

under consent agreement with FTC. FTC news release, Jan. 4, 1988.

9. T. Monte: The Gary Null Show. *East West* 19(9):53–57, 109, Sept. 1989.

10. Promotional flyer, undated.

11. A. Simon et al.: An evaluation of iridology. *Journal of the American Medical Association* 242:1385–1389, 1979.

12. B.H. Jacobson: Effects of amino acids on growth hormone release. *Physician and Sportsmedicine* 18:63–70, 1990.

13. J. Yetiv: *Popular Nutritional Practices: A Scientific Appraisal*. New York, Dell Publishing, 1987.

14. *Harvard Health Letter*, March 1991.

15. D. Pearson and S. Shaw: *Life Extension: A Practical Approach*, New York, Warner Books, 1982, p. 594.

16. R. Rapoport:: Life extension's #1 couple. *Longevity* 3(1):54–60, Nov. 1990.

17. W. Bennett: Gurus of longevity. *American Health* 3(3):85–89, May 1984.

18. D. Lund: Lendon Smith loses license! *Nutrition Forum* 4:56, 1987.

19. S. Barrett and G. Monaco: Cytotoxic testing. *Nutrition Forum* 1:17–9, 1984.

20. S. Barrett: Commercial hair analysis: science or scam? *Journal of the American Medical Association* 254:1041–1045, 1985.

3

Chiropractic:
A Cancer of the
Health-Care System

For nearly a hundred years chiropractors have insisted that spinal misalignments can cause and/or aggravate a wide assortment of diseases by impinging on nerves as they exit the spine. According to chiropractic theory, this impedes the flow of "vital energy" (often called "Innate Intelligence") to organs and tissues throughout the body. Moreover, claim many chiropractors, "adjusting" the spine can help hasten recovery from practically any disease by improving nerve function. A large proportion of chiropractors say that everyone needs regular spinal adjustments to optimize nerve function and thereby prevent disease. They would like you to believe that whatever ails you—or even if you feel perfectly healthy—you can benefit from regular chiropractic care.

However, instead of doing scientific studies to test beliefs like these, chiropractors have relentlessly waged what *Consumer Reports* has called a "war with science."[1] Thanks to victories in legislatures and courts, their number, privileges, and income continue to grow, even though their underlying theory has been thoroughly discredited.[2-4]

The medical profession, concerned about chiropractic's dangers, shunned chiropractors and did its best to educate legislators and the public about chiropractic's absurdities and dangers. But intense lobbying enabled chiropractors to become licensed as independent practitioners in every state, gain inclusion under Medicare and many other insurance programs, and achieve the freedom to shower the public inappropriately with x-rays.

Chiropractic's political success has set the stage for similar actions by naturopaths, homeopaths, acupuncturists, and the like. Unless Americans wake up, we may be headed for a new Dark Age in which the legal status of cultists is equal to that of scientific practitioners.

Dark-Age Philosophy

Most chiropractors cling tenaciously to century-old philosophy for which there has never been any evidence or theoretical support and which has been disproved beyond reasonable doubt. From time to time they have modified their pronouncements in an attempt to appear less archaic. But they refuse to abandon their dogma and discard unscientific methods of diagnosis and treatment or to do significant research. Instead, they continue to pretend that chiropractic is based on science.

As with astrology, chiropractic has established no scientific standards. There is a very wide range of philosophy, theory, and practice. Some chiropractors believe that their professional role is to detect what they call "subluxations" and to adjust the spine to correct them. "True believers" in this philosophy may even say that the patient's history is irrelevant because they neither diagnose nor treat diseases. Some chiropractors limit their practice to the treatment of musculoskeletal disorders and make appropriate referrals to medical doctors when they encounter other conditions. Some do acupuncture, physical therapy, applied kinesiology, high colonics (enemas), iridology, and nutrition counseling (mostly supplement peddling), and/or anything else they can make a buck on. Some believe all spinal misalignments can be detected by hand, but most believe x-rays are essential. Even spinal-adjustment techniques vary widely. There are dozens of different methods, none of which has been scientifically validated or proven better or worse than the rest.

Despite the wide variations, most chiropractors adhere to the following false tenets:

• The human spine is subject to frequent and significant misalignments ("subluxations") from a wide variety of causes, including practically all simple daily activities, as well as strenuous work, sports, and minor and major accidents of all kinds. Even malnutrition, air pollution, cigarette smoking, and pesticides in food can cause or aggravate subluxations. Subluxations occur throughout life, no matter how strong and healthy a person may appear to be.

• Subluxations interfere with the normal flow of "nerve energy" through the nearby nerves. This causes or aggravates malfunction of the organs and tissues that they supply and can lead to disease and death.

• Spinal manipulations ("adjustments") can fix misalignments, thereby normalizing the flow of nerve energy and restoring normal nerve function and normal organ and tissue function.

• Chiropractors have a unique ability to diagnose and correct spinal subluxations. These lesions can cause or aggravate not only pain, but practically every health problem known to humans. Among those specified in widely distributed pamphlets and books are heart disease, cancer, asthma, hypertension, rheumatoid arthritis, hyperactivity, sinusitis, colds, and emotional, neurological, gastrointestinal, and skin disorders.

• Medical doctors treat only symptoms, but chiropractors get to the root of health problems by finding and treating subluxations.

• Chiropractors are uniquely qualified to prevent disease by regular spinal manipulation, which keeps nerve flow and organ function normal. Therefore, chiropractic is the supreme form of preventive medicine.

• Chiropractors should be considered primary-care family physicians, as capable as medical doctors of dealing with common health problems. They should, therefore, be included in all health insurance plans, both private and government-sponsored, and should be permitted to have full hospital privileges.

Typical Books

Everybody's Guide to Chiropractic Health Care [J.P. Tarcher, 1990], by Nathaniel Altman, is a typical presentation of chiropractic thought. This book is heavily promoted by chiropractors. Altman considers chiropractic superior to medical care in scores of crippling, incapacitating, and lethal diseases (even cancer and AIDS) on the strength of the chiropractic subluxation theory. He assures us that chiropractic treats the cause of disease, not just the symptoms, so it is preventive and wholistic.

The book's lengthy foreword was written by Fred H. Barge, D.C., then president of the International Chiropractors Association. He says, "No other book today explains so well the many complexities and forms of practice of this emerging profession." He adds that the true cause of disease is misalignment of the spine, not "germs, viruses, allergens, insects, and carcinogenic chemicals." These things are harmful only when misalignments weaken the body's resistance.

Barge strongly recommends Altman's book as an antidote to ignorance of the real cause of disease. "This awareness," he says, "will stop the foolish and costly war against germs and agents of disease." Does Barge really believe that research on AIDS, cancer, pneumonia, tuberculosis, herpes, and scores of infectious diseases and cancers should stop and the resources be diverted to chasing phantoms in the spine? Much of his foreword consists of long quotes of Daniel David Palmer, founder of the chiropractic cult. The gimmicks, gadgets, and propaganda have changed since the days of its illustrious founder, but the basic philosophy and practice remain much the same.

The foreword to an earlier version of Altman's book, then titled *The Chiropractic Alternative,* was written by Mary Jane Newcomb, D.C., Dean of Student Affairs at Cleveland Chiropractic College. She stated that good health results from a nervous system free of the burden of spinal subluxations and that chiropractors are primary-care physicians. Altman also wrote *The Palmistry Workbook.*

Another revealing book is *Essential Principles of Chiropractic, by* Virgil V. Strang, D.C., Dean of Philosophy and Director of Professional Ethics at Palmer College of Chiropractic. Published in 1984 by Palmer College, the book is intended as a text for both chiropractors and students. The foreword was written by Jerome F. McAndrews, D.C., then president of Palmer College. Like most chiropractic propagandists, Strang begins by bashing medical doctors. On the very first page, he states that the "allopaths" (a derisive term for M.D.'s) just give "lip service to the importance of preventive health care" and mistakenly put "most of their eggs in the germ-theory basket." Yes, folks, medical doctors just *imagine* that germs make people sick. All those vaccines and antibiotics claimed to save lives are just hoaxes.

Luckily for humanity, says Strang, "Dr." Palmer discovered that spinal misalignments lead to most pain, illness, disability, and death. Strang concedes that some zealous D.C.'s have oversold the theory by claiming that subluxations are the *only* cause of disease. Modern chiropractors, he says, realize that in some cases the subluxations merely leave the body susceptible to disease instead of causing them directly. Of course, patients still need the ministrations of a chiropractor. People who get regular preventive adjustments will keep their resistance to disease at the highest level.

Now, how's that for a racket? Chiropractors needn't learn the complexities of treating mangled bodies, heart attacks, glaucoma, brain infections, kidney failure, uncontrollable asthma, epilepsy, diabetes, severe high blood pressure, severe depression, or any of the hundreds of other serious problems that medical doctors must sweat over. Chiropractors just manipulate spines. Let the M.D.'s be exposed to AIDS and get called upon to make life-and-death decisions. But give chiropractors equal status and income—all the privileges but none of the responsibilities of physicians.

Strang states that only regular chiropractic adjustments can allow the body's "Innate Intelligence" to sustain health by flowing freely from the brain to every cell. He quotes prominent chiropractor Chester Wilk as supporting chiropractic for the treatment of such things as colds, gastrointestinal disorders, arthritis, sinusitis, hypertension, heart problems, and other potentially lethal diseases. Strang adds deafness, menstrual problems, gastritis, diarrhea, constipation, bed-wetting, and asthma as symptoms calling for chiropractic treatment. He insists that D.C.'s are general practitioners—every bit as much as M.D.'s—because chiropractic "is able to influence biochemical and functional mechanisms throughout the body."

Expressing typical chiropractic philosophy, Strang says:

> The chiropractor offers one service—and only one—which is not duplicated by any other branch of the healing arts. That most distinctive, valuable and potent service is the detection and removal of subluxations which are causing abnormal functioning of the nervous system. . . . The chiropractor stands and falls by the vertebral subluxation.

Strang is partially correct. Without the subluxation, chiropractors have nothing distinctive, nothing to justify their claim to doctoral status and obscene incomes. Yet, incredible as it may seem, a century after the birth of the dogma and decades after its acceptance by state and federal government, chiropractic "subluxations" have not been proved to exist.

"Modern" Chiropractic

Some chiropractors may object that I have quoted mostly those belonging to the "straight" or fundamentalist school of chiropractic. Most chiropractors are not straights, but are "mixers" who do many things besides adjust the spine and who tend to downplay chiropractic theory in public. Most mixers, however, have never really disavowed chiropractic's basic theory. Most still believe that spinal abnormalities are an important underlying cause of human disease. Whereas the straights have tended to confine themselves to spinal manipulation, mixers have rushed headlong into every kind of quackery imaginable.

Anyone who doubts that quackery is rampant among chiropractors need only peruse *The American Chiropractor*, which claims a readership of a majority of America's forty-five thousand or so D.C.'s. This magazine regularly carries ads for homeopathic remedies, glandulars, nutrient concoctions, and dubious diagnostic devices. Many of the articles look like thinly disguised ads for nostrums advertised in the magazine. *The American Chiropractor* has also run ads for a chiropractic practice-building firm, which claimed that its average client's income was $235,000 per year. Fred Barge is on the magazine's editorial board.

One of the brightest of "modern" chiropractors is Louis Sportelli, D.C., a former chairman of the American Chiropractic Association's board of governors. Like most chiropractors, he sees himself as a primary-care physician with a philosophy and methods superior to those of medical doctors. Sportelli is the author and publisher of a widely distributed booklet titled *Introduction to Chiropractic: A Natural Method of Health Care*. This glossy tract—now in its ninth edition—suggests that chiropractic adjustment is not just for backaches, but is the treatment of choice for a wide range of serious diseases, as well as an important preventive measure for everyone from infancy to old age.

In December 1981, during a debate on the "David Susskind Show," Sportelli said, "We manipulate the spine very specifically and very delicately and, I would say, with the kind of skill that a neurosurgeon utilizes in his surgical techniques. It is not by any chance a whimsical crack on the back." When asked about pamphlets suggesting chiropractic adjustments for colds, pneumonia, ulcers, kidney disease, and jaundice, Sportelli replied, "The underlying promise of those health tracts does have as its basis some sound substance," because the nervous system controls most of the organs. When asked whether ten chiropractors looking at the same x-ray would see the same subluxation, he replied, "Depending on what their emphasis was and where they were—I mean the location—they may not come up with the same thing. Absolutely not."

On this same Susskind show, Chester Wilk, D.C., said that a subluxation (which, he asserts, can cause problems throughout the body) might consist of a spinal bone (vertebra) rotating out of place by just one millionth of a millimeter. This is less than the diameter of most protein molecules. Only a madman, a moron, or a chiropractor could believe such nonsense. It clearly illustrates the fanciful nature of chiropractic theory.

In his self-published book, *Chiropractic Speaks Out: A Reply to Medical Propaganda, Bigotry & Ignorance* [1973], Wilk suggests that chiropractic treatment may be a logical choice for a long list of ailments including digestive disorders, arthritis, asthma, colds, dysmenorrhea, sinusitis, neurological diseases, emotional problems, hypertension, and neurological disease. He also recommends "periodic spinal tune-ups as preventive maintenance care."

More Religion Than Science

Chiropractic resembles religion much more than science. Many chiropractors believe in a force or power they call Innate Intelligence (usually capitalized). This is the Life Force or God Within, which controls the functions and activities of all the tissues, glands, and organs of the body, including intellectual functions. It is, they say, inherently unmeasurable, but chiropractors are nevertheless certain that their manipulations and adjustments facilitate its flow and thereby enhance health.

This is similar to the acupuncturists' claim that, with their needles, they can manipulate and balance Qi (Ki), or the Life Force, and thereby promote healing. Other cultists claim to have discovered still other immeasurable and inscrutable forces and energies and to possess unique knowledge and abilities to channel, manipulate, and otherwise affect the Mysterious Forces for healing purposes. Such claims originated with shamans thousands of years ago and have no place in modern scientific health care.

Since the alleged Innate Intelligence cannot be detected or measured, accepting that it exists is an act of faith. Belief that chiropractors can improve its flow and thereby improve health takes another leap of faith. Like other cultists, chiropractors gain converts not by logic but by endless repetition of their nonrational claims. Mr. Altman's book repeats at least a hundred times that chiropractic manipulations and adjustments restore normal energy flow to organs and tissues and thereby promote healing and optimal health. The claim is false, and no amount of repetition can make it true.

Chiropractors don't even know whether their manipulations increase or decrease impulses in the nerves they claim to be helping. Dogma would seem to dictate that adjustments always increase impulses, since the purpose is to free up blockages. But in cases in which manipulation does appear to reduce chronic pain, impulses may be reduced, not increased.[5]

Sects and Subsects

Like all irrational cults based on dogma instead of science, chiropractic is plagued by subdogmas and subsects. The profession puts on a brave united front. Actually, however, it is splintered into several groups that express different degrees of straight and mixer philosophy and dozens of subschools that advocate their own special techniques and gadgets and have various degrees of concern for science and ethics.

Some chiropractors contend that subluxations cause the body to be susceptible to infectious agents, poisons, and malnutrition, whereas other chiropractors insist that these things cause subluxations, which then cause disease. Chiropractors have not clearly defined their "subluxations" or shown how they can be reliably detected and treated. Some educational materials depict everyday subluxations as major displacements of the vertebrae, an impossibility in the absence of severe trauma or wasting disease. Another theory says the problem lies in the facet joints that join the ribs and vertebrae. These are the joints that make the popping sounds that chiropractors find so satisfying. Popping these joints usually has no more significance than popping knuckles, though it sometimes increases mobility and decreases pain in the area. In any case, some chiropractors and patients become regular facet-joint poppers, much as some children become habitual knuckle-poppers.

Many chiropractors now say that subluxations are "functional," not structural. This is an attempt to softpedal chiropractic theory to avoid criticism from real scientists who peer into the body in ever more detail and find no subluxations as described by chiropractors. These alleged lesions are just figments of chiropractic imagination whose location and nature depend on the chiropractor, not the patient.

The main chiropractic organizations are the American Chiropractic Association (ACA), the straighter International Chiropractors Association (ICA) , and the even-straighter Federation of Straight Chiropractic Organizations (FSCO) and World Chiropractic Alliance (WCA). They all promote chiropractic mythology and self-serving propaganda to the public and to legislatures. The ACA is by far the largest of the groups. In a recent poll, 65 percent of WCA members who responded said that their patient education material referred to subluxations as the "silent killer."

While most chiropractors continue to promote the dogma that their manipulations can help in systemic ailments, there is no credible research to support the claim. A reformist group, the National Association for Chiropractic Medicine (NACM), requires applicants to a pledge to "openly renounce the historical chiropractic philosophical concept that subluxation is the cause of disease." Its members limit their practice to musculoskeletal problems and have denounced unscientific methods used by many of their colleagues. Unfortunately, NACM has only three hundred members.

X-rays—A Chiropractic Sacrament

The chiropractor's "subluxation" gives chiropractic its reason to exist, for only chiropractors have the ability to diagnose, evaluate, treat, and prevent subluxations. They claim to be able to detect misalignments using various devices and tests, the most common of which is the x-ray.

During the early 1960s, when the National Association of Letter Carriers included chiropractic in its insurance plan, it received claims for treatment of cancer, heart disease, mumps, mental retardation, and many other questionable conditions. When asked to justify such claims by sending x-ray evidence of spinal problems, they submitted hundreds of x-ray films that supposedly contained subluxations. However, when chiropractic officials were assembled to review twenty selected sets, they were unable to point out a single one.

There is no evidence that subluxations as defined by chiropractors exist or have any clinical significance, or that chiropractors can agree on what x-ray features signify a subluxation. Yet Medicare covers chiropractic patients only for treatment of "subluxations demonstrated by x-rays to exist." In other words, while dentists, physicians, and other health professionals are trying to minimize patient exposure to x-rays, the Medicare law encourages the radiation of millions of people so chiropractors can "document" their alleged subluxations. This is a national disgrace. Exposure to x-rays increases the risk of contracting cancer. An x-ray film should never be obtained unless the potential benefit outweighs the risks. No one knows how many cases of cancer are caused by unnecessary radiation by chiropractors, but any number is too many because there is no benefit to justify any risk.

The x-ray in the hands of some chiropractors is like a horoscope in the hands of an astrologer, but at least astrologers don't dose clients with radiation. *I believe that the use of x-rays to detect "subluxations" is a dangerous fraud and should be stopped. Instead, it is required by law in Medicare cases and encouraged by the chiropractic profession in most others.*

Chiropractic's War on Science

Daniel David Palmer was born in Ontario, Canada, in 1845 and settled in Davenport, Iowa, as a young adult. For a few years he worked as a grocer, but his heart was elsewhere; he was fascinated by the psychic and medical cults popular in his day.

Palmer set up a "magnetic healing" studio in 1886 and practiced the art of personal magnetism for nine years. During this time he became convinced that there was one cause of all disease and became obsessed with finding it. In 1895 his theory gelled. It had long been common practice to apply leeches, hot irons, and other irritants to the spine for various ailments. Palmer tried a certain type of manipulation of the spine. Based on two cases, one of deafness and one of heart disease, which, he claimed, responded to spinal manipulation, Palmer concluded that subluxated (displaced) vertebrae are the cause of 95 percent of all disease. The misaligned vertebral bone, he explained, presses against a nerve, pulling it taut, creating heat in it, and altering nerve impulses through it. Organs served by the nerve become diseased.

The cure is to push the misaligned bone back into place. An acquaintance labeled Palmer's approach "chiropractic," from the Greek "done by hand." In 1895 D. D. Palmer founded the Palmer School of Chiropractic in Davenport. By 1902 the school's influence was spreading nationwide, thanks largely to Palmer's aggressive twenty-year-old son, "B. J." In 1906 the father went to jail for practicing medicine without a license. When he was released, B. J. bought him out of the business for about $2,000. Shortly thereafter, when B. J. published the world's first book on chiropractic, Daniel claimed his son had stolen the work from him. Daniel later set up a rival chiropractic college in Davenport, but it failed and he left town.

B. J.'s school continued to thrive. The course was increased to nine months, and a correspondence course was made available. Graduates received a Doctor of Chiropractic degree, and B. J. became a multimillionaire. Such success was naturally widely imitated. Hundreds of chiropractic schools, including some mail-order diploma mills, set up business. Rather than fight with them, Palmer sold them adjustment tables and other paraphernalia.

Although B. J. always said he agreed with his father that chiropractic would cure all diseases, he went to see medical doctors when he was ill. When he died of colon cancer in 1961, his son David Daniel toned down the flamboyant image of the Palmer School, renamed it the Palmer College of Chiropractic, and worked hard to improve chiropractic's professional image. Today's chiropractic colleges have four-year curricula leading to the Doctor of Chiropractic (D.C.) degree. By upgrading their image and lobbying relentlessly, chiropractors have managed to get themselves licensed in all fifty states, and their services are now reimbursable through Medicare, Medicaid, and most private health insurance plans. Their schools even have an accrediting agency recognized since 1974 by the U. S. Secretary of Education.

Disaster in Court

Having succeeded in the political arena, the chiropractors then went to court. In 1976 Chester Wilk and four other D.C.'s charged that the American Medical Association (AMA) and more than a dozen other organizations had violated the Sherman Antitrust Act by trying to eliminate their profession. In 1981 a jury sided with the AMA, but an appeals court overturned the decision on procedural grounds. Before the retrial, the chiropractors waived their claim for damages, and the parties agreed to have the case decided by a judge.

Under antitrust law, it turned out, scientific truth had little relevance. In 1987 federal judge Susan Getzendanner ruled that the AMA had engaged in an illegal boycott. Although she concluded that the dominant reason for the AMA's antichiropractic campaign was the belief that chiropractic was not in the best interests of patients, she ruled that the AMA had gone too far.

Chiropractors trumpet this case as an endorsement of their methods. But it was not. Close reading of the judge's opinion shows that she had little regard for chiropractic itself. She noted, for example, that during the 1960s "there was a lot of material available to the AMA Committee on Quackery that supported its belief that all chiropractic was unscientific and deleterious." She also noted that chiropractors still take too many x-rays. In a dubious exercise of judicial logic, she ruled that chiropractic's shortcomings did not justify attempting to contain and eliminate an entire licensed profession without first demonstrating that a less restrictive campaign could not succeed in protecting the public.[6]

Like the U. S. Secretary of Education who granted recognition to a chiropractic accrediting agency without judging the validity and value of chiropractic itself, Judge Getzendanner and other judges who upheld her decision discounted the AMA's defense that its actions had been justified by the nature of chiropractic during the years of the boycott. The Court of Appeals said, "Neither the district court, nor this court is equipped to determine whether chiropractic is scientific or not. So the AMA's argument must fail." The U.S. Supreme Court declined to consider the case further.

In other words, the defendants were deprived of their main defense because the judges refused to judge the merits of their argument. Our society may pay dearly for the courts' self-imposed scientific illiteracy. Moreover, other dubious healers may be free to follow in the chiropractors' footsteps. For example, if state legislatures legitimize astrological medicine because of pressure from local astrologers (and don't dismiss the possibility!), antitrust laws could make it difficult for medical organizations to prevent astrologers from participating in insurance programs and gaining hospital privileges. This is essentially what happened with chiropractic.

The AMA has been so cowed by Judge Getzendanner's decision that it is afraid to publish anything remotely critical of chiropractic. Its 1988 annotated bibliography, titled *Alternative Therapies, Unproven Methods, and Health Fraud,* includes entries on a wide range of phony and dangerous remedies but not one word on the preposterous claims made by chiropractors that their manipulations can help in systemic diseases. The book does not mention the 1975 *Consumer Reports* article that exposed chiropractic quackery in all its forms or even the landmark 1975 HEW report, *The Research Status of Spinal Manipulative Therapy*, which concluded that there is no evidence to support the claims that chiropractic manipulations can affect systemic diseases.

"Educational Equivalence"

Chiropractors like to claim they are trained as well as, or better than, medical doctors and are qualified to practice as primary-care providers. This is false and misleading, for the following reasons.

First, chiropractic colleges have lower standards of admission and are much easier for mediocre students to get into. Most medical students have graduated from good colleges with good grades. They are generally better educated than chiropractic students to begin with.

Second, medical students spend far more time studying their art and science before being unleashed on the public as healers and health experts. After four years of largely undergraduate-level study, chiropractic students are free to go out and play doctor. On the other hand, after four years of intensive graduate-level studies and clinical work, medical students are awarded an M.D. degree, but are still far from hanging up a shingle. The vast majority spend several more years in closely supervised postgraduate programs.

Third—and most important—chiropractic colleges teach a lot of bunk. Chiropractic students are exposed to microbiology, physiology, and other basic sciences, but these have little application to their eventual work with patients. (Dr. William Jarvis calls these courses "conversational medicine"—learned for the purpose of sounding well informed.) Much of their time is spent learning chiropractic dogma, adjustment techniques, and marketing techniques, not the scientific approach to diagnosis and treatment. The operating philosophy of most chiropractic colleges is still based on chiropractic dogma. Consider the following statements made in 1990 catalogs and brochures from chiropractic colleges:

• Palmer College of Chiropractic says, "No part of the body escapes the dominance of the nervous system. Spinal biomechanical dysfunction . . . may cause a state of poor health in an area of the body far removed from the spine. . . . The lightest pressure by a vertebra may interrupt the regular transmission of nerve impulses, preventing that portion of the body from responding with its full inherent capacity to demands for proper function." It describes the chiropractor as a primary-care physician, as do all or nearly all chiropractic colleges.

• Los Angeles College of Chiropractic—reputed to be the most scientific of chiropractic's eighteen American colleges—portrays chiropractic as superior to conventional medicine because it is "holistic" and "enhances the body's natural recuperative powers." In reality, it is spine-centered rather than holistic.

• Life Chiropractic College emphasizes that its graduates become primary health-care providers. They do not prescribe drugs or perform surgery, however, because they have a superior tool—spinal adjustment to correct subluxations and thereby "restore proper nerve function so that the body can heal itself naturally." Its president, Sid Williams, D.C., says that spinal manipulations help the body overcome diseases and prevent premature death. A television commercial for his school shows an adolescent boy receiving a neck manipulation as Williams says, "Nearly all children respond well to chiropractic. It helps them stay healthy and be happy. If you would like to help children reach their full potential, consider becoming a chiropractor."

• Sherman College of Straight Chiropractic, a fundamentalist chiropractic school, puts out promotional literature that could have been written by D. D. Palmer himself. One brochure says that the health of all organs depends on the absence of subluxations. "A subluxation is always a terrible condition because it interferes with a person's health," says the brochure. "It is even more terrible because it is not readily noticeable. Since a spinal subluxation cannot be felt by the victim, it is important that every member of the family have periodic spinal examinations by a chiropractor skilled in detecting subluxations." This expresses chiropractic philosophy very well: *create paranoia about a phantom lesion, and make people think it can kill them so they will pay for regular examination and treatment.*

It should be clear that the chiropractic education is still based mainly on century-old nonsense. Yet, these colleges have the full blessings of state and federal governments, and the financial benefits that go with them. Taxpayers and health-insurance buyers pay not only for worthless chiropractic treatments that their gullible neighbors get through workers' compensation programs, Medicare, and the like; they also subsidize the education of the chiropractors who run the racket.

Students Are Victimized

The United States Department of Labor's *Occupational Handbook* lists chiropractic as one of the best career opportunities. *The Jobs Rated Almanac* rates chiropractic tenth best among 250 jobs. The ratings were based on salary, stress, work environment, security, and other factors. It's no wonder that enrollment in chiropractic colleges is growing. But there is another side to the story. Tuition alone averages $10,000 per year. Many rookie chiropractors are deeply in debt when they hang up their shingle. In many communities competition among chiropractors is intense. To make a living, they may have to market aggressively, take lots of x-rays, and find subluxations in everyone they see.

Graduates who realize that what they learned in school is a lot of nonsense can find themselves in a real pickle. Michael Dunn has written about his experiences at a chiropractic college and later as a young D.C. looking for work. The only job offers he got from chiropractors were from practice-management profiteers. In a poignant report, he said:

> One told me I would have to use a verbatim sales pitch to convince all patients that they needed thirty initial visits followed by weekly maintenance adjustments. He also told me that I would have to treat patients within three minutes each, and that he reserved the right to inflict pain upon any of his doctors who failed to comply.[7]

Another D.C. told him that x-ray films of each client were to be obtained every ten visits. Dr. Dunn says he feels victimized by the gigantic lie that chiropractic is a legitimate part of the nation's health-care system. Instead, "Chiropractic biotheology and antiscience attitudes perpetuate its isolation from mainstream health care." Having been taught pseudoscience for four years, D.C.'s are alienated from other professionals. Dunn blames the government in part. The federal government grants recognition and accreditation to chiropractic colleges, lends students money to attend the colleges, and reimburses chiropractors through Medicare. States license D.C.'s. School counselors and federal publications steer students into chiropractic colleges.

Perhaps the biggest mistake made by government, the one that gave chiropractic its greatest boost, was the action of the United States Office of Education granting recognition to a chiropractic accrediting agency in 1974. Students are misled by this accreditation. They should heed the words of the Office legal counsel: *"The Commissioner is not called upon to express his opinion as to the legitimacy or social usefulness of the field of training of the agency seeking listing.*[8] By this reasoning, colleges of flat-earth science, creation science, astrology, numerology, and necromancy can be accredited if their finances and paperwork are in order. Within the past few years, the Secretary of Education has recognized accreditation agencies for naturopathic and acupuncture schools—in effect lending credibility to dozens of quack diagnostic and healing methods. An education official told the National Council Against Health Fraud's attorney, Michael Botts, that astrology schools could acquire accreditation by meeting the agency's requirements.[9] The official was not kidding.

Students considering going into chiropractic should understand that, contrary to chiropractic propaganda, the profession is not generally held in high regard by other health professionals. Nor is it necessarily out of the legal woods. There are lots of clever and hungry lawyers. Some day they are going to find chiropractic malpractice is a mother lode waiting to be mined. Chiropractic abuses and malpractice are rampant, ripe, and ready for discovery (investigative questioning) of the legal kind. If legislators exhausted and corrupted by relentless lobbying can't reign in the chiropractic monster, sensible American juries might do the job. One already ruled against chiropractors in the landmark *Wilk* v. *AMA* case discussed above.

"Drugless Healing"

Chiropractic propaganda emphasizes that D.C.'s don't use drugs. This, supposedly, makes them superior. These promotions are fraudulent on two counts. First, there are no chiropractic treatments that can adequately substitute for the drugs commonly prescribed by M.D.'s for scores of systemic ailments such as ulcers, hypertension, infections, cancers, and asthma. Nor is there evidence that chiropractic treatments can relieve pain as well as the commonly used pharmaceuticals (though for some chronic pain, the risk of using drugs may outweigh the benefit).

Second, many chiropractors recommend their own versions of "drugs" and even sell them to their clients—typically at twice their cost. Although chiropractors are not permitted to write prescriptions for approved drugs, many prescribe and sell megavitamins, assorted pseudonutrients, amino acids, homeopathic remedies, herbal extracts, oral enzymes, raw animal gland products, and an endless array of other unproven concoctions. Some chiropractic journals are full of ads for nostrums of this type, some of whose manufacturers conduct all or most of their business with chiropractors. Some of the products are even alleged to help chiropractic adjustments to "hold" longer. Can you imagine how such a claim could be tested?

Nutrition Quackery and Fraud

In early 1990 an article on spirulina appeared in a small newspaper, a community shopper serving rural Oahu. The writer gushed over the wonders of the miracle algae, especially its alleged ability to enhance the immune system, even against cancer, and to increase energy levels and stamina. She was not identified, but turned out to be a spirulina peddler. I wrote a letter disputing her claims and referring to spirulina as foul-tasting and sometimes toxic pond scum. The next issue of the paper carried a long letter from a local chiropractor attacking me personally and praising the algae. He did not say so in the letter, but I later learned that he is the leader of the local spirulina-peddling ring, the head honcho on top of the pyramid. Advertisements for his clinic identify him as a "nutrition specialist."

Many chiropractors are deeply involved in nutrition quackery. Through their journals, and from their offices, they huckster vast amounts of supplements, "miracle foods," and pseudonutrients that are unnecessary, worthless, and sometimes dangerous. Some have the labels of the products customized so a whole line carries the name of "Dr. Doe." Supplement manufacturers who provide this service promise that the personalized labels will increase the chiropractor's prestige, boost referrals, and provide generous profits from the products themselves.

Standard chiropractic propaganda holds that D.C.'s are more prevention-oriented than M.D.'s and more knowledgeable about nutrition. For example, an article in *The American Chiropractor* describes chiropractors as "the world's foremost authoritative nutritionists" and claims that they "practice a new type of preventive medicine that has hurled them decades ahead of other practitioners."[10] These are flat-out lies. Chiropractic colleges have few real nutritionists on their staffs, and many chiropractors know little more about clinical nutrition than how to peddle worthless supplements. But, since nutrition is "in," claiming expertise in it is a potent marketing tactic.

One chiropractic school that uses this technique to advantage is Life Chiropractic College in Marietta, Georgia. Its promotional literature hypes its program that leads to a B.S. degree in nutrition, as well as a D.C. degree. It is "specifically geared toward students who will go on to earn the D.C. degree and offer nutritional counseling as part of their practice as chiropractors. If you choose to specialize in nutrition rather than chiropractic, Life's program will leave you well prepared for jobs in industry or government where specialized knowledge in nutrition is an asset."

Posing as a prospective student interested in the nutrition program, I have repeatedly written and phoned the college asking for more details, especially on the nutrition program and the credentials of the nutrition instructors. The response was the same every time: they just sent me another general catalogue without the details I requested. I'm a little leery of a college that does not routinely provide information on the credentials of its instructors. I'm downright suspicious of one that ignores repeated requests for the information.

Berman Chiropractic Supply (BCS) of Warwick, New York, sells an assortment of instruments to chiropractors. It also distributes supplements made by Nutri-West of Douglas, Wyoming. BCS has sponsored seminars for chiropractors that focus on nutrition treatments for dozens of serious diseases, including diabetes, infections, kidney failure, whooping cough, and epilepsy. The events of one such seminar were laid bare by a consumer reporter who attended by posing as a chiropractor. The attendees were given a manual titled *Silver Bullets: A Clinician's Guide to Therapeutic Nutrition,* which lists over 140 ailments and the Nutri-West products recommended for each one. The featured speaker was the book's author, naturopath Robert Cass, who had helped Nutri-West president Paul White, D.C., develop some of the company's formulas. The foreword to the manual was written by chiropractor George Goodheart, inventor of the absurd diagnostic system known as applied kinesiology (see Chapter 5).

At the seminar, Cass asked those who had brought tape recorders not to use them. "We'll get into some sensitive material later on," he said. With nothing recorded, "I'll deny everything that I say."

The manual recommends up to eight Nutri-West products for each ailment. For example, for epilepsy the prescription is eight tablets of Pit-Lyph-Whole, said to regulate endocrine balance; eight tablets of RNA-DNA-Plus, referred to as a specific cell activator (whatever that means); nine tablets of Liva-Lyph-Plus to help liver metabolism; eight tablets of Chlorophyll-Plus, said to detoxify the liver; and four tablets of niacin to "nourish nerve supply." That's thirty-seven pills each day. None of the products has been shown to have any effect whatsoever on epilepsy. Similar regimens are prescribed for scores of conditions, some not even recognized by the medical profession but diagnosed by chiropractors.

Chiropractors love to dabble in phony nutrition therapies, but they have long complained that insurance companies won't compensate them for these services. According to the investigative reporter, Cass proposed a solution for this problem: "Creative insurance billing is the way to go." Cass suggested that blood could be sent to him, and that he would forward it to a lab for "nutritional analysis." The inevitable result is that the patient is found to be in dire need of a host of Nutri-West products costing up to a couple thousand dollars per year. The patient must pay for these, but insurance companies and Medicare can be billed for the office call, the blood drawing, and the blood analysis. The take for these "could come to $200 when all is said and done—very easily," according to Cass.[11]

Sleazy Marketing

The founder and president of Life Chiropractic College, Sid Williams, D.C., once appeared on CBS-TV's "60 Minutes," adjusting the neck of a three-day-old infant girl. The treatments were supposedly a general preventive measure. Williams also has been involved in the practice-building business. His programs have taught chiropractors how to make up to a half-million dollars per year. His textbook on practice-building describes how to convince patients that they have spinal weaknesses that could lead to serious diseases if they don't get chiropractic adjustments on a regular basis for the rest of their life. The chiropractor is cautioned to never tell patients they are well or cured, lest they stop coming for adjustments. Tell patients they are "better," but not that they are well. Williams is not a fringe chiropractor, but a leader. He has been president of the International Chiropractors Association, and his chiropractic school is the largest in the world.[12]

Chiropractors won their antitrust suit by pretending to have abandoned old dogma and adopted scientific methods. But literature in most chiropractors' offices continues to make preposterous claims. Here's a sampling from the scores of pamphlets I have collected during the past few years:

• Chiropractic is an excellent treatment for arthritis, hay fever, high blood pressure, colds, asthma, gastric ulcers, angina, impotence, and much more.

• Subluxation is a disease occurring worldwide in epidemic proportions, and it causes dysfunction in every organ of the body.

• Almost all infants have one or more subluxations that require chiropractic care if serious consequences are to be avoided.

• All children need regular chiropractic adjustments to help prevent childhood diseases.

• Regular chiropractic adjustments throughout pregnancy are essential to normal birth and development of the child.

Perhaps the best evidence that chiropractic is still an irrational cult is ACA's eight-page advertisement in *Readers Digest* in March 1988. The lavish color insert cost $800,000. Do you think this massive promotional campaign emphasized what chiropractors said to Judge Getzendanner in court? Of course not. Once the plaintiffs had half-convinced the judge that chiropractors no longer believe the old dogma and are as scientific as M.D.'s, the ACA set out to convince the public that their old dogma is true and that their training and methods are superior to those of M.D.'s.

This ACA promotion emphasizes that chiropractors are really family doctors qualified as general physicians, because "the spine and nerves can affect many different parts of the body" and "doctors of chiropractic have comprehensive training in diagnosis." Moreover, we are told, "chiropractic is used extensively by families as a *preventive method* of health care." And "chiropractic is different in that it emphasizes the body's ability to heal itself," implying that M.D.'s don't believe the body has self-healing powers! The insert goes on to say that people of all ages and occupations need chiropractic care for optimal health. Parents are told that if their children experience changes in energy level, mood, habits, or other unusual signs, they should be immediately taken for a comprehensive examination—not to a medical doctor, but to a chiropractor. This is dangerous advice because chiropractors are not trained to diagnose or treat the serious conditions that can cause these symptoms.

Doubletalk

Chiropractors are masters of doubletalk and weasel wording. Confront them with pamphlets claiming that chiropractic adjustments help prevent childhood disease or are useful for asthma, ulcers, diabetes, and other systemic disorders, and they will say something like, "the nervous system controls all the organs and tissues, and if nerve flow is blocked health will suffer. Our spinal adjustments can help, but we don't claim to cure. Only the body can heal itself." The doubletalk is even written into a contract many chiropractic patients in Hawaii are asked to sign before receiving treatment:

> Chiropractic has only one goal. . . . The purpose of chiropractic is to restore and maintain the mechanical integrity of the spinal cord and its nerve roots. . . . Tiny misalignments of the vertebrae, which interfere with the function of these nerve pathways, are called subluxations. They come from many causes and prevent various organs and glands from working properly. . . . By means of a chiropractic adjustment, subluxations are corrected, thus restoring normal nerve function. . . . This allows that innate healing ability of the body to work at maximum efficiency. . . . With a proper nerve supply, health improves. . . . Regardless of what the disease is called, the chiropractor does not offer to heal or even treat it. . . . His only goal is to allow the body to do its job.

The patient's signature simultaneously indicates acceptance of a lie and absolves the chiropractor of responsibility for the lie.

Doubletalk is an integral part of the profession's activities and is necessary to justify its special status in the health-care system. Chiropractors don't have to justify their treatments with objective evidence that they are necessary or that they help. Since their manipulations normalize the flow of nerve impulses (or Innate Intelligence) and thereby prevent illness and promote healing, it's obvious that everyone needs them. No further research and study is needed. Case closed. Do you disagree? Well, if you speak out vigorously enough, you just might be accused of restraint of trade, unfair monopoly practices, libel, slander, and conspiracy.

Chiropractic Atrocities

Chiropractic has a long history of killing and crippling people, even children, with its fraudulent and delusion-based practices.[1,13] Cancer patients, diabetics, epileptics, and asthmatics have been told to stop using their medications because spinal adjustments would lead to rapid healing, and this has resulted in life-threatening emergencies and even deaths. Healthy young adults have been killed or paralyzed by strokes due to chiropractic manipulations that damaged arteries or veins in the neck. Backs and necks have been broken. The modern chiropractor wants us to believe that these kinds of events are rare and that the profession is now strictly scientific, but this is false.

Consider, for example, the head-squeezing torture of children in Crescent City, California, in 1987.[14-16] (For details see Cranial Osteopathy in Chapter 5.) This case became quite a scandal. A lawsuit alleging such things as fraud, battery, and malpractice resulted in a $565,000 verdict against one chiropractor plus additional out-of-court settlements totaling $207,000 with two others.[17] Some chiropractors say this was fringe stuff and is uncommon. But hundreds, perhaps thousands, of chiropractors have been taught the cult technique. What has become of their thousands of hapless clients? Will they be compensated? Will their payments for the treatments, which generally ran about $3,500, be refunded? Will those who invented, refined, and promoted the technique be disciplined? Will the chiropractors who paid to learn the method be reimbursed and told not to use what they learned? And isn't the chiropractic profession itself responsible for this and similar episodes because it tolerates and encourages nutty theories and practices? Are its journals not full of articles and ads promoting endlessly proliferating fringe techniques and snake oils?

This kind of crackpot treatment is not at all unusual. A variation of the cranial adjustment technique discussed above is called Bilateral Nasal Specific (BNS), invented by J. Richard Stober, D.C. (Chiropractors love to invent manipulative techniques and give them capitalized names as if they were respectable.) The theory of BNS is that by sticking balloons up the nose into the nasal cavities the skull bones can be properly realigned. This helps cure blindness, deafness, paralysis, mental retardation, dwarfism, and other severe problems. Hundreds of chiropractors and other fringe practitioners across the country have been taught the technique. In 1983 a baby died of asphyxiation after a balloon got stuck in her windpipe. The practitioner was found guilty of manslaughter, fined $1,000, and forbidden to practice BNS.[18] Why shouldn't all chiropractors and other fringe practitioners be forbidden to use this invasive and dangerous procedure?

Frightening Studies

A few years ago I learned that a friend of mine was getting chiropractic adjustments once a week for chronic back pain. Her sister, a woman about twenty-five years old who enjoyed generally good health, would drive her to the clinic. She happened to have a marble-sized lump on her shoulder, already diagnosed as a harmless lipoma (fatty tumor) by a physician. I asked her to do an experiment for me. Next time she took her sister to the chiropractor she should ask him whether spinal manipulations could get rid of the tumor. Sure enough, he assured her that if she faithfully came to him once a week it would gradually go away.

This inspired me to take a closer look at chiropractors in Hawaii. In 1988 and 1989, I surveyed chiropractors chosen at random on Oahu. These were successful mainstream practitioners with nice offices and plenty of patients in clean, pleasant waiting rooms. I looked at three factors: advertising, frequency of adverse findings on preliminary examination, and referral practices for serious symptoms.

I stopped sampling ads and promotional literature after twenty-odd examples convinced me that practically all chiropractors on the island use false or misleading marketing techniques. These include free or cheap x-rays, distribution of propaganda tracts, and false and misleading newspaper, television, and radio ads regarding their scope of practice. Many offer free screening examinations, which almost always are followed by recommendations for more tests (not free) or for immediate treatments.

The most disturbing results, which even I didn't anticipate, were my findings about chiropractic referral practices on Oahu. In 1989 I selected ten chiropractors who had advertised free screening and consultation. I told each chiropractor that I had two symptoms: a longstanding gnawing pain in the pit of my stomach that seemed to be relieved by eating and was frequently severe enough to awaken me in the early morning; and attacks of chest pain and severe difficulty breathing especially during exercise, but sometimes at night in bed. I said that I occasionally treated myself with nonprescription remedies and herbs but got only mild relief. I said that I didn't know much about chiropractic or whether it was good for these kinds of problems, but I prefer natural healing to drugs and surgery, so I thought I should find out.

I believe that any competent health professional and even most laypersons would recognize the symptoms I described as very serious and requiring evaluation by a medical doctor. The gnawing pain could signify the presence of an ulcer, and the chest pain could signify either asthma or a heart condition. Although the symptoms I described could represent an illness that could be fatal without proper treatment, not one of these "modern, scientific" Doctors of Chiropractic suggested that I consult a medical doctor! Instead, they assured me that chiropractors often help with such symptoms because spinal subluxations can impair nerve flow to the stomach, lungs, diaphragm, chest muscles, and all of the body's organs. Most showed me models and/or posters of the spine illustrating the process. Most supported my apparent distrust of medical doctors and their drugs, and my preference for natural remedies, and they assured me that chiropractic was truly natural and wholistic.

I believe that the chiropractors' use of the title "Doctor" and their claim to be primary-care physicians is dangerous. Most chiropractors are confused about subluxations and/or the limitations of their manipulations and adjustments. Most cannot be relied on to make appropriate referrals to medical doctors. Moreover, chiropractic manipulations can injure patients. Peter Modde, a reformist who finally gave up practicing chiropractic, wrote a telling article called "Malpractice Is An Inevitable Result of Chiropractic Philosophy and Training"[4] and later published a large book on the subject.[19] Here are some examples he reported:

• A man in his thirties was treated for low back pain by two chiropractors over several months. The pain persisted, so he finally went to a medical doctor. Swollen lymph nodes were found and tests led to a diagnosis of Hodgkin's disease. Proper treatment had been delayed, but it was nonetheless successful, no thanks to the chiropractors.

• A man in his fifties was given spinal manipulations for back pain. Unfortunately, his spine had been weakened by metastatic bladder cancer, and the adjustments broke his back and left him paralyzed from the waist down.

• A woman in her sixties received chiropractic manipulations for neck pain, headaches, nausea, and dizziness (symptoms chiropractors frequently advertise). She died of a brain hemorrhage. It turns out her symptoms were caused by severe hypertension, and she urgently needed medical care.

Some people who go to chiropractors for back, chest, and shoulder pain, as they are encouraged to by advertisements, are actually suffering from heart attacks and require immediate hospitalization. Harm has been documented due to chiropractic treatment of patients with osteoporosis, rheumatoid arthritis, degenerative disease of verterbral discs, infections, and other conditions that require medical care.[20]

Disasters are inevitable as long as chiropractors pretend to be primary-care physicians while they lack diagnostic training and scientifically justified treatments. Chiropractic colleges, which pretend to be medical school equivalents, and state governments, which negligently allow chiropractors to make false claims, share responsibility for the inevitable chiropractic malpractice.

The Big Lie

Many chiropractors claim they are prevention specialists who care about the whole person, while medical doctors mindlessly suppress symptoms with no regard for the cause and prevention of disease. Chiropractors also say that M.D.'s use inferior methods of healing, such as drugs and surgery, whereas D.C.'s use the natural method of spinal adjustment that gets to the real cause of problems. All this is utter nonsense. While medical science has elucidated the causes of hundreds of disorders and developed vaccines, antibiotics, antiseizure drugs, appendix removal, and many other life-saving medications, surgeries, preventive strategies, and nutritional therapies, chiropractic has kept itself secluded in a dark basement of ignorance and dogma and added nothing to the understanding of health and disease. While medical science has shed light on the workings of every cell of the body, every kind of tissue and every organ, D.C.'s have remained hunched over the object of their obsessive devotion, the spine, and learned next to nothing in a hundred years. Their fetish has cost the profession and the public dearly.

D.C.'s don't use approved drugs and surgery, not because they have superior methods, but because they are not qualified to diagnose or treat conditions that require drugs or surgery. Instead of quietly accepting the shortcomings of their training, they claim that their lack of education is an asset that makes them superior to M.D.'s. They allege that they choose not to use drugs and surgery because they have a better method of healing. Their ad campaigns encourage people to see a chiropractor *rather than* a medical doctor when they are sick or injured, as well as for regular checkups and general health maintenance.

"But It Works" (Or Does It?)

Chiropractors frequently produce testimonials from satisfied clients to buttress their claims to legitimacy. Many people who believe chiropractors have helped them will say so. Chiropractic lobbyists trot these people out to tell legislators that D.C.'s are better than M.D.'s and that they deserve full equivalence with M.D.'s in every respect, including hospital privileges. Millions of people swear by astrology, palmistry, psychic readings, faith healing, and past-life regression. Should all of these be legitimized? Should their practitioners be compensated with Medicare and health insurance dollars? Should they have hospital privileges? I don't think so.

People swear by assorted mumbo-jumbo for several reasons. In most cases, it's a matter of natural healing coinciding with or quickly following the treatment. Simply coincidence. Most people don't realize that the vast majority of human aches, pains, and miscellaneous disorders resolve by themselves with no treatment whatsoever.

Of course, chiropractors sometimes do help people, but not by doing anything unique. For example, for chronic low back pain, chiropractors may give good advice about choosing a mattress, lifting heavy objects, back exercises, and so on. They may also crack your back because that's what chiropractors do, not because manipulation is helpful. Without spinal manipulation, chiropractic might not survive.

There is evidence that some of the spinal manipulations done by chiropractors (and some medical doctors, osteopaths, and physical therapists) might be beneficial in some painful conditions, especially those involving the lower back.[21] The evidence is not overwhelming, but let's give them the benefit of the doubt here. Let's suppose that in their one hundred years of cracking, twisting, pulling, pushing, and otherwise manipulating (and sometimes bruising and breaking) the body, particularly the spine, they have come up with some maneuvers that are marginally more effective than the methods used by most physicians or physical therapists for a few back pain syndromes. Would this justify their claims to full equivalence with M.D.'s? Would this be proof that their theory about subluxations causing diseases is correct? Although preposterous, that is their position.

Tremendous Cost

America's annual tab for chiropractic treatment is approaching three billion dollars per year,[12] most of which is wasted. Chiropractors love anecdotes, so they might appreciate one presented at a Hawaii State Senate committee hearing by neurologist Calvin Kam, M.D. A patient was treated for back pain and muscle spasms by three chiropractors in succession. The first did 185 spinal manipulations for alleged misaligned vertebrae over twenty months at a cost (to an insurance company through a workers' compensation program) of $4,000. The second chiropractor diagnosed hyperlordosis and rotational problems in the lower cervical and lumbar areas. He gave 207 treatments at a cost of $5,000. The third chiropractor diagnosed "chronic thoracic and lumbar instability" and gave 267 treatments for $18,000. Despite 650+ treatments costing about $27,000 over a ten-year period, the patient got steadily worse and never returned to work. These figures go up to 1987. As I write this in 1991, he continues to receive chiropractic treatments.

Steady customers like this one can be a chiropractor's bread and butter for a lifetime. With forty or fifty, a chiropractor can live like a king, working one or two days a week. The treatments take about five minutes. No wonder chiropractors drool at the prospect of convincing us all that we need regular spinal examinations and adjustments from cradle to grave. No wonder they lobby relentlessly in state legislatures for an ever-increasing scope of practice and wider coverage by private and government insurance programs. In many states they have gained passage of "insurance equality" laws forcing insurance companies to cover their services whether they wish to do so or not. (And, as far as I know, most do not.)

Sacred Cows?

Many chiropractors bad-mouth scientific medicine every day as a matter of course. Exaggerating its imperfections, misrepresenting its theories, and lying about its results are integral aspects of chiropractic promotion. But let anyone hint that chiropractic is less than heaven-sent and all hell breaks loose. Threats of lawsuits are among the chiropractors' favorite forms of intimidation. For example, when a dentist scheduled a lecture on "Chiropractic in the Light of Scientific Method" for his adult education class on quackery at a college, chiropractors threatened a lawsuit and administrators asked the dentist to soft-pedal any comments on chiropractic. Local D.C.'s attended the lecture with tape recorders, and the dentist was intimidated enough to alter his planned lecture.[22]

Frivolous suits by chiropractors are not common. But the costs of defending against such a suit is high enough that some critics and administrators knuckle under. This is an outrageous state of affairs and should be fought by all who care about the First Amendment and about quality health care. Chiropractors and their attorneys who use such tactics should be taken to court for interfering with business relationships and for abuse of legal process.

Another example of chiropractors' use of intimidation followed a 1986 article on arthritis in *Modern Maturity*, published by the American Association for the Advancement of Retired People. The article mentioned chiropractic methods and devices as among the quack remedies to be avoided. Chiropractors howled in protest. Rather than provide evidence that chiropractors have a safe and effective treatment for arthritis, they threatened to boycott and sue AARP.

When a Hawaii newspaper published a letter in which I took D.C.'s to task for claiming in ads and pamphlets that they prevent and treat ulcers, allergies, asthma, emotional problems, and childhood diseases, the result was a flurry of venomous letters, some to me and some to the paper. They all thoroughly vilified me, but not one seriously addressed the issues I had raised. Some angrily insisted that chiropractors don't claim they can treat such ailments, while others just as angrily insisted that chiropractors can help in systemic ailments.

One chiropractor's wife wrote, "I strongly disagree with Kurt Butler's letter. . . . I was particularly offended by his accusation that any chiropractor would send his family to an M.D. while advising patients otherwise. For the record, our son has never been to an M.D. . . . and never had injections of any kind."

Let me take this opportunity to apologize. For the record, I stand corrected. I hereby admit that some family members and patients of some D.C.'s are deprived of vaccinations and other medical care and thereby endangered by chiropractic dogma.

Clearly, chiropractic has become a sacred cow. There are dozens of books on the shortcomings of the medical profession, and M.D.'s are regularly raked over the coals on talk shows for real and imagined sins. Doctor-bashing has become a national sport, and chiropractors are among the biggest bashers. When was the last time you saw a book or article critical of chiropractic, or heard any discussion of its shortcomings?

Radical Surgery Is Needed

It is abundantly clear that there must be fundamental and far-reaching reforms of the chiropractic profession and its legal status. An effort for rational reform is being led by the National Association of Chiropractic Medicine (NACM)[23] and the National Council Against Health Fraud.[24] Their suggestions include:

• Disavow the pseudoscientific subluxation theory and stop claiming that chiropractors can treat or prevent systemic disorders.

• Stop claiming to be primary-care physicians who should be consulted instead of medical doctors for basic health care needs, obstetrics, pediatrics, or psychologic care.

• Stop using unscientific diagnostic methods such as iridology and applied kinesiology.

• Stop prescribing and peddling megavitamins, herbs, laetrile, homeo-pathic drugs, glandulars, spirulina, and other assorted snake oils.

• Limit the scope of practice to musculoskeletal problems and refer clients to physicians when reasonable and prudent.

• Avoid unnecessary x-radiation of patients.

• Speak out against quackery in the profession and help prosecute chiropractic malpractice cases.

• Stop propagandizing in favor of unscientific chiropractic theory and methods and against medical doctors and public health measures.

• Support and get involved in scientific research on manipulative therapies.

A more far-reaching suggestion is to radically revamp chiropractic education and the profession itself. Shut down all the chiropractic colleges as such, but give them the option of participating in the reform program. All of the students and current D.C.'s would switch to a program, lasting six months to three years, to qualify as a physical therapist, physician's assistant, massage therapist or medical doctor. The profession of chiropractic would disappear.

Another possibility would be to combine the various manual manipu-lative arts (chiropractic, physical therapy, massage, etc.) into one comprehen-sive program that takes the best of the different methods. The credentials awarded, which would determine the permissible scope of practice, would include certificates (earned in one or two years of study) and bachelor's, and master's degrees.

This plan would also include a science-based doctoral program with an emphasis on working with physicians and integrating manipulative therapy into scientific medicine as far as possible. The Doctor of Manipulative Therapy (D.M.T.) would be similar in status to a dentist, podiatrist, or clinical Ph.D. psychologist. Physicians have no objections to competent, ethical practitioners in these fields. These professionals don't falsely claim to have diagnostic, preventive, or therapeutic methods for systemic ailments, nor do they claim to be primary-care physicians, family doctors, or general practitioners. Unlike many chiropractors, podiatrists and dentists don't claim that their treatments will help asthma, ulcers, hypertension, or immune status.

Of course, dental disease, unlike the chiropractic subluxation, is real and can cause serious systemic consequences, including an occasional death. Dentists and their services really are important to our health, but rarely do dentists exaggerate their role or fail to refer when appropriate. Nor do many dentists distribute false and misleading propaganda leaflets in their offices, opposing public health measures and slandering medical doctors.

Similarly, medical doctors gladly refer back patients to physical therapists because they often help and they don't spread bizarre, misleading, and false notions about health and disease. Nor do they claim doctorate-level expertise or the title "Dr." on dubious grounds like chiropractors do. Chiropractic has set itself apart from and above scientific medicine while demanding respect and equality as a scientific health profession. However, respect must be earned. It cannot be mandated.

Should Medical Doctors Refer to Chiropractors?

In most cases, rational health-care professionals should shun chiropractors and counsel against their services. The only exceptions should be D.C.'s who have embraced the reformist principles (above) and preferably belong to NACM. Medical doctors should not view the court's decision in *Wilk v. AMA* as depriving them of their First Amendment rights or their professional responsibility to counsel their patients truthfully.

The law frowns on medical groups and societies organizing boycotts that are binding on their members. But it certainly does not prevent enlightened individual physicians from simply declining to recommend chiropractic treatment or refer patients to deluded practitioners. Nor does it prevent them from publicly declaring that they don't make such referrals because they think chiropractic theory is mumbo-jumbo. In fact, it doesn't stop medical groups from issuing blistering critiques of chiropractic and *recommending* that their members avoid referring to chiropractors until the profession cleans up its act. As long as the organizations don't attempt to *force* their members to boycott or shun chiropractors, they are within their rights.

If this were not so—if physicians were forbidden to tell their colleagues, their patients, and the public at large that chiropractic is an irrational cult that imposes needless risks and costs on its clients and on the public—then the First Amendment would be dead. It is most unfortunate that most rational health-care professionals and their organizations behave as though free speech is already dead and that criticizing the pseudoscientific cult of chiropractic is risky.

References

1. Chiropractors—Healers or quacks? *Consumer Reports* 40:542–547, 606–610, 1975.
2. E. Crelin: A scientific test of the chiropractic theory. *American Scientist* 61:574–580, 1973.
3. E. Crelin: Chiropractic. In *Examining Holistic Medicine* (D. Stalker and C. Glymour, eds.). Buffalo, Prometheus Books, 1985.
4. P.J. Modde: Malpractice is an inevitable result of chiropractic philosophy and training. *Legal Aspects of Medical Practice,* Feb. 1979.
5. *The Research Status of Spinal Manipulative Therapy.* National Instiute of Neurological and Communicative Disease and Stroke Monograph #15, U.S. Dept. of Health, Education, and Welfare, 1975.
6. S. Getzendanner: Memorandum opinion and order in *Wilk et al. v AMA et al.,* No. 76 C 3777, U.S. District Court for the Northern District of Illinois, Eastern Division, 27 August 1987.
7. M. Dunn: Out of the frying pan and into the fire: the chiropractic student reformer graduates. *NCAHF Newsletter,* Sept./Oct. 1985.
8. Federal recognition of chiropractic: a double standard. *Annals of Internal Medicine* 82:712, 1975.
9. Is the bureaucracy mooning science? *NCAHF Newsletter,* May/June 1990.
10. A.J. Lipchultz: The fifth function of water. *The American Chiropractor,* Dec. 1985, pp. 23, 25.
11. Nutrition against disease: a close look at a chiropractic seminar. *Nutrition Forum* 5:25-28, 1988.
12. A study of chiropractic worldwide. Facts Bulletin, vol. 4. Arlington, Va., Foundation for the Advancement of Chiropractic Tenets and Science, 1992.
13. S. Barrett: The spine salesmen. In *The Health Robbers* (S. Barrett, ed.). Philadelphia, George F. Stickley Co., 1980.
14. P. Cooke: The Crescent City cure. *Hippocrates* 2(6):60–70, 1988.
15. Unorthodox "cure for kids spawns lawsuits, outrage. *San Francisco Examiner,* 6 March 1988.
16. L.B. Silver: "Magic cure": a review of the current controversial approaches for treating learning disabilities. *Journal of Learning Disabilities* 20:498–512, 1987.
17. K. Frazier: Jury awards $565,000 in a suit against Ferreri technique. *Skeptical Inquirer* 16(2):124, 1991.
18. *NCAHF Newsletter,* Jan./Feb. 1985.
19. P.J. Modde: *Chiropractic Malpractice.* Columbia, Md., Hanlow Press, 1985.

20. P. Schwartzman and A. Abelson: Complications of chiropractic treatment for back pain. *Postgraduate Medicine* 83:57–61, 1988.

21. P.G. Shekelle et al.: *The Appropriateness of Spinal Manipulation for Low-Back Pain. Part I: Project Overview and Literature Review.* RAND, Santa Monica, Calif., 1991. Note: Although chiropractors have promoted the RAND study as an endorsement of chiropractic, it is not. It merely supports the use of manipulation for carefully selected patients. Only a few of the reports identified by the RAND panel involved manipulations done by chiropractors; most were done by medical doctors.

22. Confronting chiropractic in the classroom. *NCAHF Newsletter,* Nov./Dec. 1989.

23. C.E. Duvall, Sr., and C.E. Duvall, Jr.: Rational chiropractic practice. *Occupational Medicine and Legal Sourcebook,* Sept. 1985.

24. NCAHF position paper on chiropractic, 1985.

4

Acupuncture, Naturopathy, and Other "Health-Care" Wanna-Bes

Practicing medicine is serious business because it has a major impact on people's quality of life and, at times, deals directly with life or death. To practice medicine in a competent manner, it usually is necessary to acquire a college education, attend medical school for four years, take one or more years of full-time postgraduate training, pass a licensing examination, and then participate in continuing education throughout one's entire professional career. Some medical doctors manage to deliver substandard, incompetent, or unethical care. But the large majority of consumers who seek medical care in an intelligent and responsible manner will obtain what they need.

This chapter is about people who want (or actually have) the privilege of diagnosing and/or treating others without the responsibility of knowing what they are doing. They are a mixed bag:

• Acupuncturists are free to make diagnoses and administer treatment that has no scientific basis. Those who lack medical training are permitted to practice independently in some states and under medical supervision in others.

• Astrologers are permitted to give people all sorts of advice about physical and emotional problems.

• Ayurvedic medicine is traditional Hindu folk medicine. It is vigorously promoted in the United States and other western countries by Maharishi Mahesh Yogi's transcendental meditation (TM) movement. Physicians and lay followers of the guru market a line of products as well as services.

• Christian Science practitioners claim that they can cure anything through the use of prayer and "correct thinking." They rarely are held accountable for their actions, even when death results from medical neglect.

• Evangelical "healers" don't bother to make diagnoses but claim to be able to help whatever ails people. They collect money and make promises they can't keep, with virtually no legal restraint.

• Homeopaths claim that the full range of human ailments can be cured by highly diluted remedies. Some practitioners are physicians or other health professionals who are licensed to practice their profession; other practitioners are unlicensed laypersons. Homeopathy also is promoted on a do-it-yourself basis through the sale of products in "health food" stores and a few drugstores.

• Multilevel marketing involves person-to-person sales of products and distributorships. About forty companies are marketing vitamins, minerals, herbs, homeopathic remedies, weight-loss products, and/or other health-related items. A few of their distributors are licensed health professionals, but most are laypersons who are neither qualified nor legally allowed to advise people on health problems. Yet most of them get away with doing so.

• Naturopaths are licensed in a few states, where they are permitted to function as primary-care providers, make diagnoses, and administer a wide range of treatments that have no scientific basis.

Acupuncture and Related Practices

Westerners have always been fascinated with the marvels and mysteries of the Orient, and they have been easy marks for mystical flimflam and hocus-pocus from that part of the world. The story of acupuncture illustrates this well.

The ancient Chinese practice of sticking needles into the body to influence the flow of so-called "vital energy" (also called "Qi" or "Ki") has changed little over several thousand years except that the number of acupuncture points (where Qi supposedly can be influenced) has grown from about 365 to over 2,000. The West has discovered, embraced, rejected, and rediscovered acupuncture several times in the last few centuries. Even electroacupuncture was used in France more than 150 years ago. The latest rediscovery was tied in with political events that gave acupuncture powerful momentum that will last into the twenty-first century.

America Falls for Mao's Hoax

Ironically, the Chinese themselves have rejected acupuncture as worthless several times in their long history, only to see it resurrected. Ancient superstitions often are hard to shake. When President Nixon and other Americans visited China in the early 1970s, acupuncture happened to be in favor. This was because Chairman Mao, unable to provide rational health care to the hundreds of millions of Chinese with only thirty to forty thousand real doctors, had reversed a twenty-year-old Kuomintang policy and declared acupuncture and other ancient practices to be valid. This provided at least an illusion of health care. Suddenly, by acknowledging its "barefoot doctors," China had no doctor shortage after all. Long live Chairman Mao and his great wisdom!

It was important to sell this illusion to the West in order to show that China, under the leadership of Chairman Mao and the Party, could fend for itself and take care of its people without undue Western influence. More than that, thanks to the brilliance of the Fearless Helmsman, the wisdom of China was to be shared with the West. Both acupuncture and independence were sources of great pride to the Chinese. It became politically correct (and therefore definitely beneficial to one's health) to believe in acupuncture. It is not surprising that Chinese doctors and patients put on a spectacular show for visiting American journalists and politicians.[1] The featured attraction was acupuncture anesthesia for major surgery. Patients chatted, snacked, and praised Chairman Mao while having a brain tumor or goiter removed. A film of brain surgery was even shown at a convention of the American Medical Association.

The sensation these claims created was enough to catapult acupuncture into the limelight in the West. Unfortunately, it was all a hoax. The patients had been carefully selected and indoctrinated, and the demonstrations staged. Many if not all of the patients had been given a tranquilizer, local anesthetic, and/or painkiller in addition to the acupuncture. Even at the peak of its popularity in China, acupuncture anesthesia was used in no more than 5 percent of the operations because it usually doesn't work.[1] Reliable chemical anesthesia is now back in favor in China.

During the 1970s, American entrepreneurs, both medical and non-medical, used Madison Avenue techniques to promote clinics, "quickie" seminars, demonstrations, books, correspondence courses, and do-it-yourself kits. Today, acupuncturists are treating psychoses, cancer, AIDS, infections, diabetes, hypertension, heart disease, vision and hearing loss, drug addiction, obesity, arthritis, appendicitis, and virtually anything else they please. Some health insurance carriers pay for acupuncture treatment, but so far neither Medicare nor Medicaid does so. Acupuncturists are working hard to change this and may succeed.

Most states still restrict the use of acupuncture to physicians or persons operating under the direct supervision of physicians. In some states, however, it is permitted without medical supervision. Some individuals who perform acupuncture prescribe herbs and call their approach "Chinese medicine."

A Closer Look

The theories and practices of traditional acupuncture have been handed down largely unchanged from ancient Taoist China. As in all primitive animism, unseen vital forces and spirits are believed to control everything. The basic theory is that the human organs are subject to disease when there are imbalances in the Qi or vital energy flow, which has two components: yin and yang, or feminine and masculine. "Balance" between these forces can be restored by using extremely fine needles or other means to stimulate various points said to be located along fourteen (some say twelve) "meridians" running the length of the body. Each point corresponds to an organ and its functions. The needles are inserted into the skin and twirled to move the Qi into or out of different organs as deemed necessary. Then they may be left in for several minutes. In a variation called moxibustion, small piles of moxa, the leaves of the Chinese wormwood tree, are burned at the ends of the needles or directly on the acupuncture points.

The points chosen for stimulation depend on the symptoms, the season and weather, the patient's gender, the time of day, and, above all, the results of taking the pulse at the wrist. Pulse-taking requires several minutes, but it can take much longer because it is believed that each wrist has six pulses, corresponding to twelve different organs, and that each pulse has about twenty-five qualities. So some three hundred distinct characteristics in a patient's pulse must be evaluated to make a diagnosis and commence treatment. Expert pulse-readers supposedly can detect illnesses long before there are any symptoms and cure them with acupuncture treatments. The needles are inserted rapidly or slowly, twirled clockwise or counterclockwise, used hot or cold, left in for longer or shorter periods, and removed rapidly or slowly, according to their postulated effects on yin or yang to the liver, lungs, heart, or other organ.

Using these methods, thousands of acupuncturists are now practicing throughout the United States and claiming to have effective treatments for obesity, hypertension, ulcers, neurological disorders, and many other health problems. "Colleges" (some just storefronts and office suites) of acupuncture and "oriental medicine" are training thousands more such "experts." These schools can appeal to people who want to play doctor without going to medical school or even to college. Their programs are cheaper, shorter, and easier. While medical students must train for some six to ten years after college, in some states acupuncturists can hang up their shingle two or three years after high school and treat the same diseases as medical doctors.

Many "oriental medicine" practitioners use not only acupuncture, but herbal drugs and radical diets. Some prescribe animal parts as aphrodisiacs, youth potions, and remedies for serious diseases. Their fetishes for rhino horns, black bear gallbladders, tiger penis, and the like support the slaughter of these endangered animals. Even the beloved and heavily protected panda high in the rugged and isolated mountains of West China is not safe from profiteers. Increasing numbers are being caught and killed in traps illegally set by poachers for musk deer. These little deer have scent glands which produce an oil that superstitious humans believe is a miraculous medicine and aphrodisiac. The deer—and accidentally the pandas—are slaughtered because of an ancient superstition that has spread to major Western cities.

Not surprisingly, non-M.D. acupuncturists have had some serious turf disputes with M.D.'s and are bound to have more as they demand separate-but-equal status, including control over who can do acupuncture. Incredibly, the traditional acupuncturists seem to be slowly winning this battle. In some states they even set the requirements for M.D.'s who want to practice acupuncture for the treatment of pain.

Acupuncturists Declare War on Modern Medicine

Many acupuncturists are at war with modern medicine and make no secret of it. In 1981 the keynote speaker at a meeting of the American Association of Acupuncture and Oriental Medicine likened scientific medicine to death and decay and acupuncture to full liberation. "Acupuncture is part of a New Age which facilitates integral health and the flowering of our humanity," he said. His messianic address laid out a plan for advancing acupuncture while undermining the public's faith in modern medicine and educating people that they need alternative medicine.[2]

Some state laws authorizing acupuncture accept ancient oriental animist dogma at face value. Hawaii, for example, defines acupuncture as the art of controlling and regulating the flow and balance of the body's energy, "the most important single factor in maintaining the well-being of the organism." Training requirements emphasize learning traditional Chinese physiology "including the five elements organ theory," traditional Chinese diagnosis "including pulse diagnosis," and traditional pathology "including the six Yin and seven Chin." Other state laws have similar language.

Do you think these are flowery words that don't mean much? Do you suppose that acupuncturists aren't really practicing medicine but just treating pain syndromes? Think again. A few years ago an acupuncture clinic opened in a small town on Oahu. This "Holistic Healing Center" has no medical doctor on its staff, just an acupuncturist and a couple of massage therapists. Their ads in the local shopper claimed they have effective treatments for respiratory ailments, circulatory problems, gastrointestinal disorders, urinary tract diseases, sexual problems, obesity, and more. In an interview in the paper, the acupuncturist said:

> I want to emphasize that acupuncture and herbal medicine can successfully treat a variety of ailments. Many people focus on the idea of pain management. But actually the science of acupuncture covers everything from pain control to internal disorders, from chronic illnesses to gynecological problems, respiratory disorders to skin problems. . . . The list can go on and on.

A slick brochure published by the Hawaii Association of Certified Acupuncturists lists "conditions and disorders treatable by acupuncture." These include acute sinusitis, the common cold, tonsillitis, asthma, cataract, gingivitis, duodenal ulcers, diarrhea, acute and chronic colitis, osteoarthritis, and bed-wetting, as well as many pain syndromes. When I asked the Hawaii State Regulated Industries Complaints Office whether the claims made by the clinic and the association were legitimate, I was told that acupuncture can be used in any condition, including cancer, and that practitioners can advertise that they treat any disease as long as they don't promise cures. Nonmedical acupuncturists can't do surgery or prescribe prescription drugs, but they appear to be free to claim that their treatments are equal or superior to surgery or drugs.

Oriental medicine and acupuncture schools aren't content to teach ancient Chinese quackery; they teach "modern" quackery as well. For example, the Oriental Medical Institute of Hawaii, a clinic by day and school by night, has included Kirlian photography, iridology, and electroacupuncture (see below) in both its treatment programs and its curriculum. This school is approved by the Hawaii State Department of Education.

I wrote to the Superintendent of Education, suggesting that the approval be withdrawn because, by teaching quackery as legitimate health care and by huckstering it to the public, the school was fostering fraud. In addition, I warned, by endorsing fraudulent practices, the Department of Education leaves the state vulnerable to massive liability because patients harmed by the school's graduates could sue the state. I was told that the department is looking into my complaint, but I doubt if any action will be taken. My subsequent inquiries have gone unanswered.

Beware of M.D.'s Who Convert to Traditional Acupuncture

A growing number of medical doctors may be incorporating traditional acupuncture into their medical practice. Despite the fact that acupuncture is based on mystical notions of the human body, a program sponsored by the

American Academy of Medical Acupuncture (AAMA) has been available through the extension division of the University of California, Los Angeles. The program has taught hundreds of M.D.'s to use the needles not just for pain relief, but for the treatment of disease in the Chinese tradition.[3]

AAMA's founding president, Joseph M. Helms, M.D., is vice president of the World Health Organization's World Federation of Acupuncture-Moxibustion Society, which establishes training guidelines for the AAMA. The World Health Organization has stated that acupuncture is effective against acute bacillary dysentery, shock, cataract, myopia, acute sinusitis, tonsillitis, asthma, gingivitis, peptic ulcers, and osteoarthritis. Since there is no scientific evidence to support this position, I assume it involves political shenanigans.

According to Helms, most graduates of the UCLA program go on to use acupuncture on perhaps 80 percent of their patients with great success for such problems as "recurrent respiratory infections, irritable bowel syndrome, certain kinds of headaches and sexual dysfunctions, problems with fatigue, minor depression, and recurrent urinary tract infections." Dr. Helms says that an M.D. who completes the course can treat "a broader range of problems than he can strictly with his allopathic training."

Do you believe that a 220-hour acupuncture course can prepare its graduates to offer better treatment than they learned during four years of medical school plus years of additional postgraduate training and experience? To 80 percent of their patients? Do you think medical schools have been negligent in overlooking a miracle of healing while leaving their graduates helpless to treat 80 percent of their patients? Can you guess why Helms's course is in the department of continuing education rather than the main medical school curriculum?

Another example of an M.D. who practices traditional Chinese medicine is Dr. Cyrus Loo of Honolulu. A graduate of the University of Cincinnati Medical School, Loo practiced dermatology until the years following Chairman Mao's acupuncture anesthesia hoax. Loo says acupuncture can not only cure a cold, the flu, dizziness, acne, hair loss, epilepsy, gallbladder disease, gout, and many other common problems, but can also help in AIDS. In diagnosis, he uses a "neurometer," a galvanometer similar to the EAV device described later in this chapter. It is an unproved device but plays a key role in Loo's practice.

Loo claims to have discovered an acupuncture point, which he calls the Loo point.[4] "Discovering the Loo Point was like Christopher Columbus discovering America," he says modestly. He says that needling this point, which is near the ankle, can cure a variety of aches and pains as well as herpes zoster (shingles), psoriasis and many other skin conditions, postpolio weakness, hepatitis, macular degeneration (loss of central vision, usually with aging), and even cancer. He claims to have treated thousands of cases using the Loo Point and claims a 95 percent success rate "regardless of the type of disease or injury." No peer-reviewed journal has published evidence to support these claims.

Loo is not regarded as a fringe practitioner by the general public. On the contrary, he often is lionized by the press and is proud of his involvement in the community. I once criticized Loo's public claims about acupuncture in a letter to a Honolulu newspaper. In his reply he accused me of "European chauvinism tantamount to discrediting China and her people" and insisted that acupuncture is not a placebo but a physiological remedy for all the ills he mentioned before, including AIDS. Now there's one for the books. Criticizing wild claims about acupuncture makes me a racist. During all those years acupuncture was out of fashion in China, were the Chinese discriminating against themselves?

Ancient Magic, Not Science

Acupuncture originated in China some four thousand years ago, long before there was any real understanding of human physiology and anatomy or even physics and chemistry. Bodies were not dissected and studied, and each organ was either yin or yang and was likened to one of the "basic five elements": water, metal, earth, fire, or wood. No one knew what the body's actual organs do or how they do it. The network of meridians and points, claimed by the traditionalists to function independently of the nervous and circulatory systems, has never been proven to exist. The concept of twelve pulses for twelve organs is sheer fantasy.

Acupuncturists speak of moving yin and yang energies along the meridians to and from yin and yang organs, guided by scores of superstitious principles. They say, for example, that the spleen is the center of thought, the liver produces tears, and the kidneys are the seat of willpower and fear. Perhaps the height of absurdity is reached with homuncular acupuncture. This concept, which has become dogma in some circles, holds that each ear has acupuncture points for the entire body arranged in the form of an inverted dwarf curled up in the outer ear. The feet, hands, and face are also said to have points for all the organs. But not all the schools agree on these points, or even on the total number of points, which is put at anywhere from 35 to 2,500.

A Powerful Placebo, Not a Panacea

Acupuncture does appear to afford significant relief in some cases of chronic and recurrent pain. It may also ease the symptoms of withdrawal from addicting drugs. This has led to speculation that the pain relief is mediated by endorphins, and further speculation that if acupuncture can affect endorphins it might affect other hormones and enzymes and thereby exert systemic effects. Acupuncture promoters take these hypotheses as established fact and use them to mislead the public. At best, however, acupuncture is nothing more than a potent placebo.

The trappings of acupuncture include a "learned clinician" armed with the wisdom of the ancient East in a room with impressive (and fanciful) posters and models of the human form with all its meridians and acupuncture points. And the needles! In the hands of the Master, they are the magic tools that access, adjust, and balance the cosmic forces that give life. The treatment itself originated as a magico-religious ceremony, and it remains a compelling Eastern healing ritual to this day. Moreover, it's wonderfully simple and nonpolluting. There are no pills to take, no side effects to worry about, and no plastic wrappers or bottles to throw away.

The Hazards of Acupuncture

Students of traditional acupuncture are warned that a slightly misplaced needle can cause more harm than the disease they are trying to cure by moving the Qi the wrong way or by damaging a blood vessel or nerve. The needles used in the old days were more like slender knives and did pose severe risks. But most of today's needles are hardly thicker than a human hair and carry only a small risk of causing injury. Still, cases have been reported of hepatitis, AIDS, and a variety of severe bacterial infections that were contracted from improperly sterilized needles. Perhaps the greatest danger comes from relying on acupuncture instead of scientific diagnosis and treatment. It should be obvious that inhibiting pain without diagnosing the cause can be very dangerous.

We all know better than to take aspirin to, say, relieve a toothache without getting a dentist to clean out the infection and repair the tooth. It is similarly unwise to rely on an acupuncturist without consulting a medical doctor to determine the cause of the problem. Acupuncturists who are deluded about the powers of their art cannot be relied on to refer patients to real doctors in an appropriate and timely manner.

The Bizarre Case of EAV

Electroacupuncture according to Voll (EAV), which Reinhold Voll, M.D., of West Germany named after himself, is based on traditional acupuncture but goes even further off the deep end. During the 1970s, Voll developed a device that he claimed could measure "energy" flow along "acupuncture meridians." He claims that his techniques can determine the cause of any disease, immediately and precisely, without reference to any other test or to the patient's history or medical records. He simply detects the "energy imbalance" causing the problem.

Voll claims to be able to pinpoint the site of a lesion in an organ, such as the precise location of a peptic ulcer. He even claims that arthritis, diabetes, heart disease, and other ailments can be traced to tuberculosis, venereal disease, or other infection in ancestors several generations ago. In one alleged case, Voll traced the cause of a stroke to smallpox vaccination decades earlier. This man was paralyzed on one side, but Voll's diagnosis and homeopathic medication had the man jogging within an hour. He was, we are told, permanently cured.

Voll's original device has undergone many modifications, but its basic make-up has not changed. It is simply a galvanometer, a device that measures changes in the electrical resistance of the patient's skin. One wire from the device goes to a brass cylinder covered by moist gauze, which the patient holds in one hand. A second wire is connected to a probe, which the doctor touches to "acupuncture points" on the patient's other hand or foot. This completes a low-voltage circuit and the device registers the flow of current. The information is then relayed to a gauge that provides a numerical readout. More recent versions make sounds and provide the readout on a computer screen. The treatment selected depends on the scope of the practitioner's practice and may include acupuncture, diet, homeopathic remedies, and/or surgery. In the United States, EAV devices are most popular among homeopaths.

Not long ago, I attended a conference of true believers in "electrodiagnosis" (or "electrodermal screening" or "EDS," as it was called at the conference). The conference brought together chiropractors, naturopaths, acupuncturists, competing gadget peddlers, and marketers of all sorts of nutritional, herbal, and homeopathic remedies claimed to help correct the "imbalances" detected by the devices.

"Modern" Acupuncture: Needling Trigger Points

Many acupuncturists are medical doctors who have abandoned the fanciful ancient theories, the meridians, and most of the acupuncture points themselves. For example, Felix Mann, M.D., a British physician who studied acupuncture for many years and helped popularize it in the West, now says that acupuncture points and meridians do not exist. He notes that if all the acupuncture texts are to be believed, "there is no skin left which is not an acupuncture point."[5] He also experimented with acupuncture anesthesia and concluded that it was barely adequate in about 10 percent of cases, and, in these, "something allied to hypnosis may be taking place."[1]

Modern medical acupuncturists use fewer points and believe these are nerve-muscle junctions rather than mystical windows to vital energy flow. Instead of twirling the needles, the doctors usually send tiny electrical currents through them. The treatments appear to be helpful against certain types of chronic pain, but the results are usually not dramatic and treatment sometimes must continue daily for months. In fact, studies involving patients with trigeminal neuralgia and miscellaneous musculoskeletal aches and pains suggest that even modern acupuncture is no more than a very good placebo.[1]

Another type of needle therapy for chronic pain is the so-called dry needling of "trigger points." These are thought to be little knots of damaged and degenerating muscle fibers that are tender to pressure and, by their effects on surrounding nerve and muscle tissue, may cause pain some distance away. Sticking a hypodermic needle into a trigger point, either dry or with injection of a little salt water, is said to speed resolution of the problem, though the mechanism is not clear. Western physicians have been experimenting with this type of needle therapy for almost a century. One theory is that needling stimulates pressure and stretch receptors in the muscles, which send impulses along sensory nerves to the brain, where they interfere with and overwhelm incoming pain impulses. But this would hardly explain long-term pain relief from ten-minute treatments.

In any case, this type of therapy has nothing to do with traditional acupuncture, though it is possible that acupuncturists sometimes unknowingly needle trigger points. Such needling might provide pain relief and lead to exaggerated testimonials and general support for acupuncture's claims. In fact, for all we know, acupuncture was originated on the strength of success in needling trigger points.

Acupressure and Reflexology

Traditional acupressure, also known as *do-in* or shiatsu, is similar to traditional acupuncture, but the acupuncture points are stimulated by hand rather than with needles. With a few months of training, practitioners can set themselves up as quasi-physicians and practice their brand of acupressure. In Hawaii, shiatsu therapists are eligible for payment from workers' compensation funds. A typical advertisement or business card says, "specializing in sports injuries, stress reduction, back problems, headaches, blood circulation, automobile accidents. Workers' compensation." Many also prescribe and peddle vitamins, herbs, and other assorted snake oils.

The Acupressure Institute in Berkeley, California, has trained thousands of practitioners and is approved for continuing education credit by the California Board of Registered Nurses (CBRN). Founder Michael Reed Gach, who conducts many of the institute's workshops, claims his techniques are useful for treating arthritis, PMS, and obesity, as well as a myriad of aches and pains. He also says his techniques can improve circulation and enhance alertness and productivity. CBRN also gives credits for attending seminars on crystal healing and visiting Mexican cancer clinics that dispense quack remedies that are illegal in California.

Reflexology is an offshoot of acupressure that was developed by an American physician at the beginning of this century. Also called "zone therapy," it involves pressure on areas of the hands and feet said to correspond to the body's internal organs. Using thumbs and fingers, the reflexologist rubs, massages, slaps, and applies prolonged deep pressure to specific areas, which supposedly alleviates symptoms and tones the body's organs. Books and articles on reflexology make fantastic claims about curing and preventing all manner of ailments and even injuries and poisonings. Reflexologists claim that their treatments can help prevent ulcers, migraines, and viral infections, as well as improve circulation, reasoning, and productivity, and cleanse the body of toxins. The toxins are not named, but one "registered certified reflexologist" in New York City recommends bathing after a session in order to "wash away released impurities." Her treatments cost about a dollar per minute.

As far as I know, the claims made for acupressure and reflexology have never been scientifically studied, much less proven. Anyone with persistent pain or other symptoms should consult a physician. Like ordinary foot massage, reflexology treatments can be pleasant and relaxing, and there are no potentially contaminated needles to worry about. It should also be noted, however, that acupressure treatments are sometimes painful.

Astrology

Astrology is a booming business in the United States, grossing billions of dollars each year. There are thousands of professional astrologers in the country, some making six-figure incomes, a few even more. Almost 1,500 newspapers and magazines publish astrology columns. Thousands of books and several magazines are devoted entirely to the subject, and scores of television and radio stations dispense advice based on astrology. Even telephone astrology using 900 numbers is proliferating. Some astrologers use computers to derive their advice.

From the 1920s to the 1960s, about 15 to 20 percent of Americans believed in astrology. Since the sixties, astrology's popularity has grown steadily, especially with young people. Now about 50 to 60 percent of American teenagers are believers.[6] Nobody knows how many millions of people base important decisions about relationships, work, travel, investments, health, and hiring and firing (an outrageous form of bigotry and discrimination) on astrological considerations. The thought that a true believer might have a finger on the trigger of a nuclear weapon or poison-gas launcher is not comforting to me.

Astrological Quackery

Astrologers have always maintained that horoscopes are important to health. "Cancers" are said to be prone to stomach disorders, "Leos" to heart disease, "Libras" to migraine headaches, and so on. Details of the horoscope allegedly provide precise information on a person's physical and mental health. None of the claims is supported by scientific evidence, yet prescriptions for diets, herbs, medicines, exercise, sex, and love are based on the horoscope and the current state of the heavens.

Psychiatrist Carl Jung, popular with today's mystical psychologists, used the horoscopes of his patients to help in diagnosis and treatment. Some Jungians and other mystically oriented psychologists still use this practice. Astrologer Joan Quigley, who counseled former president Reagan and his wife says a horoscope can tell more about a person than a psychiatrist can tell after many hours of consultations. She predicts that astrology will eventually be taught in schools and colleges and will have as much professional prestige as medicine.

Astrological advice sometimes appears in places you might not expect. A few years ago, *Weight Watchers* magazine carried a "horoscope" column that contained tips and encouragement for dieters. Its words of wisdom included: "try a wild new recipe" (Taurus); "tempt your taste buds with low-calorie seafood dishes" (Pisces); "join an exercise class and learn new tricks" (Gemini); "let your mate help with your diet—it's easier with support" (Libra); "incorporate an exotic food into your menu" (Aquarius); "vitamin-rich veggies get you through the flu season sniffle-free" (Sagittarius); "the planets bring you an energy boost—use it constructively to reach fitness goals" (Aries); and "though you feel others haven't noticed your weight-loss achievements, a good friend has been singing your praises" (Aries).

If astrology were valid and could perform as advertised, it would be a marvelous tool for health professionals of all kinds. But astrology is 100 percent rubbish, and basing decisions regarding health on any false doctrine is inherently dangerous. Astrological nutrition and medicine are quackery.

Astrology Disproved

Astrology was devised thousands of years ago when humans imagined the earth and the people on it were the center of a caring universe. Stars and planets were thought to be gods and goddesses not very far away. Human fantasies attributed powers in various spheres of life to these gods. Mars governed physical energy, Mercury ruled mental energy, Venus determined love and beauty, and so on. But rational people have known better for hundreds of years. The stars and planets are not gods, and they don't care about us. They are billions of miles away. From such a distance, there is no force, energy, or mechanism by which they could possibly affect humans at the moment of birth or at any other time. The gravitational and electromagnetic effects of the earth, trees, rocks, buildings, lights, furniture, and other people are millions of times greater than those of the distant stars. Earthly forces don't affect our personality or fate, so how could distant ones?

Not only is there no theoretical basis for astrology, there is no factual basis either.[7] If astrology were valid, some hard evidence should have accumulated after thousands of years. Instead, astrology has failed every scientific analysis or test to which it has been subjected.

According to astrology, the sun sign affects the personality, which affects every aspect of life, including career choice. If this were true, various professions should attract clusters of people with the same sign, but they don't. Ministers, athletes, politicians, doctors, lawyers, musicians, carpenters, police officers, research scientists, and others show a random distribution of sun signs.[8]

According to astrology, certain signs are said to be most compatible with each other. If this were true, this should be reflected in marriage and divorce statistics. Again, there are no data to support the superstition. Given the widespread belief in astrology, we might expect to find at least a small effect caused by the belief itself. That is, some people might avoid considering a potential partner with the "wrong" sign. But so far even this effect has not been demonstrated in the United States.

If astrology were valid, astrologers should be able to match personality profiles with natal charts. They can't do this, not even slightly better than just guessing.[9] One astrologer who accepted a $100,000 challenge to determine the sun signs of twelve subjects whom he interviewed to his satisfaction, embarrassed himself on national television. He was positive he could get the sun signs of all twelve subjects right on James Randi's paranormal special on the Fox network in 1989. The odds favored his getting one of the twelve correct if he just guessed. But he failed to get even one.

If astrology were valid, people should be able to recognize expert interpretations of their horoscopes. That is, if an astrologer constructs charts for several people, then writes his interpretation of each, subjects should be able to recognize themselves and pick out the commentary that goes with their chart. But this doesn't happen. In actual tests, most people have been satisfied with whatever horoscope interpretation they have been given. In one study, approximately 150 people who responded to an ad from "Astral Electronics" were given a free "ultra-personal horoscope" interpretation. More than 90 percent were happy with the interpretation and said they recognized themselves. The horoscope was that of mass murderer Dr. Marcel Petiot.[10]

Don't Blame the Moon

Even the moon, the closest and most likely heavenly body to exert an influence, has none of the effects long claimed by astrologers.[11] Some people not generally inclined to believe in astrology give the "lunacy" concept some credence. They reason that if the moon can affect the ocean tides, surely it can affect humans, who are about 60 percent water. Actually the moon—and the sun—affect the tides only of unbounded oceans, not small containers of water. There are no tidal shifts in glasses, buckets, tubs, swimming pools, or small lakes. Nor do they occur in humans. Even if they did, astrologers have never explained how this would affect one's personality or fate. It seems to me this would just make us look and feel funny. Moreover, standard calculations for the gravitational pull on humans show that, for example, a mother holding her child exerts about twelve million times as much tidal force on her child as the moon. Thus, it is not surprising that no evidence supports the idea that the phases of the moon affect human behavior.

Because the media so frequently repeat the myth that people are more likely to do nutty things during a full moon, some police officers believe there is a correlation between the full moon and criminal behavior. This could lead them to be more vigilant and to make more arrests on full-moon nights, which would tend to perpetuate the illusion. Moreover, some people may be more likely to go outdoors when the moon is bright, and this could lead to more crimes. Even these factors, however, have not been strong enough to make a significant difference. Actual tabulations have acquitted the full moon of all charges of responsibility for murder and other criminal behavior.[12]

"Psychic Astrology"

Would you like to "hit it big" and accrue "up to millions"? Cope better with important personal relationships? Have everything mapped out so you can "fulfill your dream of living the good life"? About a year ago, a reporter I know received this solicitation in the mail with an invitation to complete a "psychic interview form" and send it with $19.95 for his "Personal Forecast and Life Development Chart"—guaranteed to provide "full Good Luck/Money instructions" for the next year or his money would be returned.

This sales pitch—in an envelope marked "absolutely confidential"—was mailed by "psychic astrologer" Irene Hughes. "Dear Tom," the letter said:

> Your name got on my special list. The moment I saw it there I had a hunch: a psychic "gut feeling." I knew I should contact you. I said to myself "things are not right with this friend. I must help my new friend."
>
> Now I happen to be famous for spotting people in trouble, and helping them.... Even officials of the Church and Government call on my services. Being able to "receive" psychic impressions from anywhere in the world . . . I've been nearly 100% successful assisting important world figures in ways that amaze authorities.
>
> Right this minute I'm concentrating on you. On how Irene Hughes should and must help you. What my gut feeling tells me is this. You have a serious personal problem. *It is eating away at you*. . . .
>
> There is no shortage of so-called psychics or astrologers out there willing to help you. . . . They will take your money and not actually *do* anything for you or tell you anything you didn't already know.... You don't know how lucky you are that a truly qualified psychic counseling expert – someone known to be "right" as a psychic 74 out of 75 times – is now on to your problem. . . . Normally my consultation services cost a client $500.00 or more, plus expenses.

I don't know whether Ms. Hughes's ability to help people has been scientifically tested. But I do know that her selection of "Tom" was not psychic because *he doesn't exist*. "Tom" is just one of many assumed names the reporter uses to obtain offbeat publications and inquire about get-rich-quick schemes. He receives a steady stream of mail from entrepreneurs who have acquired his name for their "sucker lists."

The Media Love Astrology

Astrologers churn out hundreds of forecasts regarding the fate of scores of movie and television stars, athletes, and politicians. Their predictions are almost always wrong. So are their predictions for earthquakes and other catastrophes. In spite of this, many publishers keep printing the predictions without ever comparing the previous ones with the facts. Talk-show hosts are equally unfair to their audiences. For example, in May 1988 Geraldo Rivera hosted five well-known astrologers. No skeptics were on the show.

Geraldo's illustrious stargazers were asked to predict whether, based on their horoscopes, George Bush or Michael Dukakis would be elected President of the United States. At this time Dukakis was ahead in the polls. Four of the astrologers were positive he would win—on the basis of his horoscope, of course. No one mentioned the opinion polls. The fifth, Arch Crawford, declined to make such a prediction because, he said, he specialized in financial astrology. He went on to predict a stock market crash on November 13, 1989, with the Dow Jones Industrial Average "in the area of 400 to 800." Needless to say, Geraldo didn't remind his audience of these predictions when they turned out to be incorrect.

Religion or Fraud?

Should astrology be considered a religion, a massive fraud, or something else? Some skeptics consider it a religion, but most astrologers don't consider themselves ministers; in fact, many belong to mainstream churches. Besides, astrology does not provide a coherent, comprehensive set of beliefs regarding the origins and purpose of human life, or the nature of the hereafter, if any. Nor does it provide a code of ethics and morals by which people should abide. And even people who believe in astrology rarely have astrologers preside at weddings or funerals.

Many astrologers promote themselves as professionals with knowledge of a great science and the skill to apply it to humans, institutions, corporations, and even animals. Since no evidence supports these contentions, it seems reasonable to conclude that the entire multibillion-dollar industry is based on lies. People who profit from astrology, including astrologers and all their pandering publishers and promoters, are perpetrating a fraud for the purpose of making money.

The First Amendment gives Americans the right to promote any set of beliefs no matter how thoroughly discredited they may be. The law protects Flat Earth Society members as well as astrologers and their publishers. The First Amendment, however, offers only limited protection to commercial speech, so some astrologers could be charged with fraud. In practice, though, astrologers are never prosecuted, no matter how outrageous their claims.

Is Astrology All Bad?

Do astrologers perform any useful function? What about those who use the trappings of astrology to provide advice and moral support to individual clients? Are they really practicing psychology while hiding behind the easier-to-obtain title of astrologer? Can they function appropriately as marriage, family, and career counselors? Can they help people to understand their options, clarify goals, and deal with grief?

Many astrologers who do counseling are nice, sensitive, caring people who give reasonable advice and an ego boost to confused clients. The popularity of this astropsychology may also reflect the limited availability and high cost of good psychotherapy, as well as the stigma attached to seeing a psychiatrist or psychologist. All kinds of people consult astrologers; it's chic. But popular belief says that only people with "mental problems" should consult highly trained health professionals.

Astrologers undoubtedly make matters worse in situations that call for more skilled therapists, but their form of counseling seems relatively harmless for clients who otherwise might not discuss their concerns with anyone. The danger arises when astrologers are consulted by people who need expert care. Persons who are manic-depressive, schizophrenic, or anxiety-prone and those who have sleep disorders or any kind of serious physical problem should seek the best medical care available. Using astrology as a substitute for proper therapy in such situations is akin to playing Russian roulette. However, as astrology and quackery continue to flourish, we will see more astrological quackery, including the dangerous varieties.

Astrology also harms society in a more general way. It promotes widespread superstitious, irrational, and magical thinking, which can't be good for any society. America desperately needs more scientists and a scientifically literate work force and voting public, not to mention leaders. It is ironic that as America has approached the twenty-first century, its appetite for astrology and other pseudoscience and quackery has grown faster than its appetite for astronomy and other real sciences.

Ayurvedic Medicine

Ayurvedic medicine is Indian folk medicine with roots going back about two thousand years. It is promoted in America by disciples of Maharishi Mahesh Yogi, the transcendental meditation (TM) guru. By far the most publicized practitioner is Deepak Chopra, M.D., a Western-educated Indian physician who turned to Ayurvedic medicine after converting to the TM religion.

Chopra's books include *Creating Health: Beyond Prevention, Toward Perfection* [Houghton Mifflin, 1987], *Return of the Rishi: A Doctor's Search for the Ultimate Healer* [Houghton Mifflin, 1988], *Quantum Healing: Exploring the Frontiers of Mind/Body Medicine* [Bantam, 1989], and *Perfect Health* [Crown Publishers, 1990]. All are dedicated to the Maharishi, whose "extraordinary insight" and "timeless knowledge" enabled Chopra to restructure his reality.

The beliefs and practices of Ayurvedic medicine fall into three categories: (1) some that are obvious, well established, and widely accepted even by people who have never heard of Ayurveda; (2) a few that proper research may eventually prove valid and useful; and (3) absurd ideas, some of which are dangerous.

The first category includes such advice as don't overeat or overexercise, get adequate rest and sleep, don't let your job stress you to the point of making you miserable, take time to relax in silence, and take joy in the simple things in life. In other words, moderation and happiness can help people be healthy.

The second category includes the hundreds of medicinal herbs codified in Ayurvedic texts. These are used alone and in combinations for scores of ailments. While some of these substances may be safe and effective for certain conditions, it is foolish to accept Ayurvedic dogma about them unless scientific studies have shown benefit. This is illustrated by the case of *Rauwolfia serpentina*, one of the few Indian medicinal herbs to find its way into Western medicine. Beginning in the 1950s, the main active component of the herb, reserpine, was used to treat psychosis and high blood pressure. Careful studies since then have shown that the drug can cause depression, headaches, nightmares, irregular heartbeat, diminished libido, aggravation of ulcers, and a variety of other adverse effects. At the same time, safer and more effective drugs were developed for treating psychosis and hypertension. The turnaround took place over a decade or two. Ayurvedic physicians, on the other hand, have used the herb for hundreds of years without a thorough understanding of its dangers and limitations. Because they don't evaluate the effects of their prescriptions in a systematic, scientific manner, the same is probably true for most of the herbs they use.

The third category of Ayurvedic medicines includes Dr. Chopra's advice for preventing and reversing cataracts.[13] Each day, he advises, brush your teeth, scrape your tongue, spit into a cup of water, and wash your eyes for a few minutes with this mixture. This is about as rational as the old folk remedy for a dog bite: rubbing saliva from the dog into the wound. Both practices can induce dangerous infections. Chopra also says that a savage beating can cure epilepsy, though he doesn't say whether he recommends this.

Since Ayurveda attributes many diseases to demons and astrological influences, it is not surprising that incantations, amulets, spells, and mantras are commonly used remedies. Goat feces washed with urine is prescribed for alcoholism and indigestion, milk mixed with urine for constipation. Enemas of animal blood are recommended for hemorrhage. Enemas of urine and peacock testicles are used to treat impotence. Hundreds of such remedies are codified in Ayurvedic texts such as *Caraka Samhita,* translated and edited by P. V. Sharma. Other examples of Ayurvedic absurdities are discussed below.

Dubious Psychosomatics

A key aspect of Ayurvedic medicine is the determination of the patient's "body type," the combination of physical and psychological traits that supposedly indicates which of three alleged fundamental forces is predominant. Prescriptions for herbs, diet, and exercise are based on this determination. The three forces are called *vata, pitta,* and *kapha.* Vata types are said to be restless, high-strung, and prone to insomnia and hypertension. Pitta types are said to be smart, quick to anger, and prone to rashes and ulcers. Kapha types are said to be strong, even-tempered, and prone to obesity.

The traits used to determine one's type include hair color, hair oiliness, skin color, body-frame size, weight, eye size, muscle strength, preferred temperature of food, resting pulse rate, voice pitch, sex drive, and speed of eating and walking. For example, a vata type is indicated by dry hair, dark skin, small eyes, a restless mind, muscle weakness, a preference for warm food, a weak or irregular sex drive, a high-pitched voice, a fast walk, and fast eating. A kapha type is indicated by oily hair, light skin, large eyes, a calm mind, strong muscles, strong libido, a low voice, slow walking and eating, and a tendency to gain weight easily.

This system of evaluating the body is so simplistic and absurd that I see no point in attempting to catalog its weaknesses.

Chopra Chooses Ayurvedic Mysticism

Chopra's own words show how he has given up critical thinking in favor of ancient dogma. He says that a good Ayurvedic physician can tell a meditator from a nonmeditator, diagnose illness, and prescribe appropriate remedies, all by feeling the patient's pulse.

Chapter 8 of *Return of the Rishi* describes the work of "master Ayurvedic physician" Brihaspati Dev Triguna. Chopra says he visited Triguna accompanied by a friend named Farouk, who introduced Chopra as a "beacon of wisdom" at the great medical center in Boston. After feeling Farouk's pulse for a few seconds, Triguna concluded, "You are too thin. You don't eat. You are weak." He advised him to take time to eat regular meals, to eat more slowly, and to get adequate rest. Chopra thought this was brilliant and noted, "I had always thought Farouk had a starved, sickly body myself."

Then Triguna took Chopra's pulse and concluded, "You are always trying to beat a deadline. . . . You have a healthy body, but your life is moving too fast." He advised Chopra to slow down, watch a sunset, spend more time with his wife and children, and move his bowels at the same time every day. Again, Chopra thought this was brilliant. "It was a pivotal moment for me," he says. "I felt as if Dr. Triguna read me well, very well. . . . I felt that his simplicity of speech was wise. Yes, if I did these things I would be all right. . . . I was deeply affected."

The chapter also notes that in seminars with corporate executives and politicians, Triguna feels their pulse and tells them to slow down, don't worry so much, chew slowly, and move their bowels at the same time every day. He also prescribes herbs as his "chief method of actually curing illness." Chopra provides no details or follow-up information by which a reader could judge whether anything useful takes place during Dr. Triguna's consultations. But he concludes that "Dr. Triguna has peered into the whole man. . . . He has perfected his intuition and made one human instinct a tool of medicine."

Chopra espouses Ayurveda's mystical medicine the way one might believe in a religion:

Ayurveda's approach to physical disorders is not basically physical at all. . . . Faced with any illness, the vaidya [Ayurvedic physician] turns directly to Nature's intelligence, where he finds the real cure. The herbs, minerals and metals that he uses think the way we do. For every part of our bodies, Nature provides a substance to complement it. Medicine then consists of letting like speak to like. Take the remedy whole, as Nature provides it, and through its similarity to ourselves, it can restore health. Ayurveda works because it corrects a distortion in consciousness—a wrong wiggle goes back into line.

Does Chopra actually believe that herbs, minerals, and metals think in the same sense that humans do?

Chopra repeatedly asserts that "for every thought there is a corresponding molecule. If you have happy thoughts, then you have happy molecules." I wonder what a happy molecule looks like under a microscope. Chopra also asserts that masters of Ayurvedic medicine can determine an herb's medicinal qualities by simply looking at it. Scientific study is therefore unnecessary.

Chopra promotes the Ayurvedic claim that certain exercises and asanas (yogic positions) can stimulate endocrine glands to excrete their hormones. Since he is an endocrinologist, he should not find it difficult to perform studies to test this concept. For example, he could take blood before, during, and after these exercises and check the levels of the hormones in question. The results could be published and the exercises tested in a variety of metabolic disorders. As far as I know, he has never conducted any such study.

Transcendental Miracles

Chopra claims that "TM scientists" have proved that group meditation, or even just the presence of regular meditators in a town or city, can cause crime rates to drop dramatically, decrease illness even among nonmeditators, and protect whole populations from falling bombs. This is called the "Maharishi effect." The most dramatic example of this effect supposedly occurred in the winter of 1983 when seven thousand TM-ers meditated together in Fairfield, Iowa, the site of Maharishi International University (MIU). The result, Chopra claims, was a worldwide decrease in crime rates and international hostilities and an increase in stock market indices across the globe. He says that meditation can be used for national defense and to end war forever. According to Fairfield police reports, however, the crime rate in the county has increased through the 1980s and is comparable to that in comparable cities. Even MIU campus is a frequent target of burglars and other criminals.[14]

Chapter 13 of *Return of the Rishi* repeats without questioning the claim made by the Maharishi and TM-ers that they can levitate by practicing meditation. Chopra says that the Maharishi began teaching "yogic flying" in 1975, but the technique was not publicly demonstrated for about ten years. On August 15, 1986 (India's Independence Day), the guru arranged for demonstrations in major cities around the country and abroad. The media were informed and dutifully showed up. Chopra attended the event in Cambridge, Massachusetts.

Even Chopra uses the word "hopping" to describe the crosslegged TM-ers moving across the stage, which was covered with six-inch-thick foam padding. "One after another, the six flyers bounded across the stage; the plopping sound as they landed sounded convincingly soft." (Why people who can "levitate" need foam padding to descend from an elevation of one or two feet is unstated.)

After describing how one "flyer" had hopped 150 feet in 22.5 seconds at a previously held event, Chopra says, "By comparison the Wright brothers flew 120 feet at Kitty Hawk for 12 seconds." Of course, TM-ers remain airborne for about a second and travel at most six feet per hop, while the Wrights actually flew nonstop, but this distinction seems to have escaped Chopra. He even claims that 15,000 American TM-ers (including himself) have learned yogic flying by applying "the science of consciousness . . . India's legacy to human knowledge." He says that the "technology" behind yogic flying could "make the work of Galileo, Newton, and Einstein pale by comparison" and that "the evidence and proof are there in abundance." In fact, it is so easy for TM-ers that for them "flying is simply a habit."

Large publishers appear to have no qualms about publishing Chopra's ideas, and major talk-show hosts have yet to challenge him on any of them. None has asked him for a demonstration of levitation or flying ability.

A Challenge to Deepak Chopra

Dr. Chopra acts as though his mission in life is to bring to America the wisdom of ancient India, as perceived by Maharishi Mahesh Yogi and the TM cult, especially as it relates to health and disease. Since I suspect he could use a little reality testing, I have a challenge to him and all the others who perpetrate the concept of "yogic flying." *Show me one person who can levitate, and I will donate the royalties from this book to Maharishi International University or the American Association for Ayurvedic Medicine.* Should this challenge be met, I promise to surrender the full amount of each royalty check within one week of receiving it.

I'll even make it easy. The demonstrator needn't fly, or even levitate. All he has to do is sit on an industrial-type or veterinary scale and decrease his body weight by 5 percent for fifteen seconds, using mental power alone. He will have one full hour to accomplish the feat under the observation of a panel of scientists and magicians (to rule out trickery) as well as video cameras. All I am asking is that one yogi do 5 percent of what Chopra says thousands can do, make themselves weightless by the power of mind alone.

If the chosen yogi fails, two others of Chopra's choice will be given the same opportunity. To be eligible for the prize, Chopra must first agree that, if all three yogis fail the challenge, he will publicly admit that he has been mistaken, he will advise the public to stop paying money for flying lessons, and he will ask the Maharishi to return all the money would-be flyers have paid TM organizations for levitation or flying lessons since 1975, plus 5 percent per annum interest.

Chopra's Messianic Mission

The Maharishi and his disciples have described big plans. They hope to set up Ayurvedic medical centers throughout the U. S. and to train more Ayurvedic physicians. "The potential is there," Chopra says, "for transforming the face of medicine entirely, and not just in India." Since Maharishi ceremoniously dubbed Chopra "Dhanvantari (Lord of Immortality), the keeper of perfect health for the world," he has been Ayurveda's number one evangelist and propagandist in this drive. He calls Ayurveda "a medicine for mankind."

Maharishi's Heaven on Earth Development Corporation has said it would create at least fifty "Cities of the Immortals" with homes built according to ancient Ayurvedic laws. Chopra will supervise their health clinics. Therapies will include meditation, primordial sound therapy (silent chanting), warm-oil enemas, herbal-oil massages, special baths, specific exercises that allegedly stimulate certain endocrine glands, and scores of herbal medicines. The homes planned for the Los Angeles area are expected to range from $750,000 to $2,000,000.[13]

Chopra is the ideal propagandist for Ayurveda because, as a medical doctor, he can give it a respectable scientific aura. He occasionally gives therapeutic drugs and surgery their due for infections, cancers, and heart conditions. Yet at other times he says that "the direct nondrug cures (especially TM) are more effective because they exhibit more complete, holistic knowledge and more pervasive correlation." On a "Sonya Live" program, he said that antibiotics and anticancer drugs don't work. He blamed chemotherapy and radiation for "an epidemic of immuno-compromised disease," which is pure poppycock.

In *Return of the Rishi,* Chopra criticizes Western treatment of asthma and claims to have an antiasthma diet. He says that the diet, along with a daily routine of positive thinking, meditation, exercise, and herbs, can not only minimize attacks, but can "readjust" and bring back body physiology from "the specific imbalance that causes asthma." He fails to mention the one natural measure that is by far the most important for most asthmatics: avoidance of allergens such as animal hair and house dust, which contains allergenic insect waste and body parts. Most asthma is caused by allergies to inhaled substances. Vacuuming up dust mites may not seem very exotic, but it is far more effective than meditation and positive thinking. Desensitizing shots sometimes help, and allergies often clear up by themselves, but there is no certain cure.

Chopra also exaggerates the importance of positive thinking in cancer therapy. He says, "Physicians who regularly treat cancer patients know very well that the ones who have a strong, positive attitude do much better than those who have a negative attitude, who face their cancer feeling only helplessness and despair. . . . The difference between positive and negative attitudes is like having two different diseases. One we pronounce curable, the other incurable." This is not correct. Although a positive attitude may help a cancer patient feel better, comply with treatment, and have a better quality of life, no scientific study has demonstrated an effect upon the cancer itself.

Oncologist Dr. Saul Silverman has been treating cancer patients for about twenty-five years. Among the six thousand-odd people he has cared for, he has seen about a dozen cases of spontaneous remission from "terminal cancer." In these "miraculous" cases the disease was so extensive that, according to the odds, the patients should have died within months. Instead, they recovered and lived for many years without evidence of recurrence. Dr. Silverman studied these cases to determine what might account for the patients' unexpected recovery. He concluded that positive thinking had nothing to do with it; nor did prayer, meditation, or visualization.

Dr. Silverman has seen many patients whose disease progressed relentlessly, even though they expressed great determination to live.[15] He has also seen some patients who had just the opposite course. One man in his sixties, for example, had an incurable, usually lethal cancer and no optimism whatsoever. His attitude was, "Why bother treating me at all? I'm going to be dead in a month or two." Although the man remained depressed, his cancer remitted. Six years later, long after total recovery, he was just starting to cheer up and admit that maybe he was going to be okay.

It may make people feel good to believe that positive thinking and positive emotions prevent cancer deaths, but that doesn't make it true. If optimism and cheerfulness were important in the prevention or cure of cancer, large-scale studies would surely find evidence that people who are depressed have a higher incidence of cancer. But no such association has been found.[16]

Telling patients they can recover if only they have the right attitude and imagine the cancer receding can increase their sense of failure and inadequacy. Besides, if confidence in recovery is so important, why do people who take laetrile and other snake oils and submit to psychic-surgery hokum, with complete confidence in these quack remedies, die just the same? If faith is a powerful medicine, why would modern medicine have developed at all? The shamans and faith-healing priests and evangelicals would have obviated the need for doctors. Churches and healing temples would exist where hospitals now stand.

Chopra mentions a few patients who got better after practicing visualization techniques and positive thinking. But they also underwent conventional cancer therapy and probably would have died without it. Yet Chopra insists they were cured by mere desire. In *Creating Health* he states that "Disease and aging persist because of myths and prejudices that propel people into decline. Our current belief system grew through centuries of cultural conditioning and indoctrination." Yes, friends, we only get sick and die because these are cultural traditions. Funny how thousands of cultures all have these same traditions.

A Money-Making Machine

If you think modern scientific medicine with its high-tech diagnostic machinery and sophisticated drugs is expensive, wait until you see what Ayurveda can do for your bank account.[17] A "detoxifying" massage can cost $130 or more; a week in an Ayurvedic center can set you back $4,000; a year's worth of the recommended "purification" treatments and herbs can easily exceed $5,000; the introductory seven-session TM course costs about $400; a crowded seminar with Chopra can cost about $100 per person. A yagya, a sacrificial ceremony to please Vedic gods, costs between $3,000 and $12,000. Such ceremonies are recommended for a wide variety of illnesses. I have seen no prices for the ass-urine treatment of epilepsy, the elephant-urine treatment of constipation, or the bloodletting treatment for impotence.

Believers who are serious about staying healthy and retarding the aging process could spend $10,000 or more per year. Many movie stars and other celebrities espouse Ayurveda, spend a great deal of money on it, and help publicize it. At age forty-six, ex-pop star Mike Love of the Beachboys claimed to have the body of an eighteen-year-old Adonis, thanks to Ayurvedic medicine. Sure, Mike.

Victims Fight Back

Not everyone who gets involved with TM and Ayurveda takes the ripoffs lying down. Some are fighting back. Several hundred former participants have formed a group called TM-EX. They say that long-term meditation has caused memory loss, confused thinking, and anxiety. Others have complained about the cultlike atmosphere at Maharishi International University, mass meditation to ward off tornadoes, and breach of contract for failing to teach them to fly as promised.

One founder of TM-EX, who taught TM for eight years, accused the movement's leadership of negligently failing to warn newcomers about possible harm, even though they were fully aware of TM's dangers. Another former TM teacher sued MIU for fraud and negligence and was awarded

$139,000 by a jury.[18] He testified that prolonged meditation had caused headaches, anxiety, violent impulses, hallucinations, confusion, memory loss, paranoia, and other symptoms that kept him from living a normal life. For information on TM-EX and its newsletter, write TM-EX, P.O. Box 7565, Arlington, VA 22207.

MIU promises to confer a competitive edge in the business world and used to point to alumnus Ed Beckley, the "Millionaire Maker," as an example of what they could achieve. But Beckley's Credit Card Millionaire System and No Down-Payment Real Estate schemes got him in trouble with Iowa's Attorney General, and he had to repay customers some $2.4 million. He had to lay off most of his 560 employees and declare bankruptcy. Despite all this, MIU is not only accredited (by the North Central Association of Colleges and Schools) but is one of the biggest private-school recipients of state and federal education funds. This shows what a religion can get away with by posing as a science.

Christian Science

Christian Science has its roots in faith healing and continues to function as both a system of healing and a system of worship. The Christian Science Church categorically rejects all the findings of modern scientific medicine, as well as the scientific method itself.[19] Although opposed to the use of all medicines, surgery, and modern diagnostic techniques, it presents itself as an effective alternative to modern medicine. There is no limit to the diseases claimed to be treatable through Christian Science.

Christian Scientists view illness as an illusion that can be dissolved by mind. This is because matter derives from mind, not vice versa. Its founder, Mary Baker Eddy, was a product of New England in the 1800s, the heyday of bohemian Boston's transcendentalist movement with its Brahmins and mystics. She was also heavily influenced by mesmerism and spiritualism, which were popular then.

Eddy's own guru for a time was Phineas Quimby, a mesmerist healer. He coined the term "Christian Science," and his writings apparently formed the basis of Mrs. Eddy's chapter on training healers in her "sacred text," *Science and Health*. Critics have accused her of outright plagiarism by copying into her book some thirty pages verbatim and one hundred pages in substance from *The Metaphysical Religion of Hegel*, by Francis Leiber. In any case, Eddy regarded disease as a manifestation of disturbed thinking that could be corrected by metaphysical means, primarily the prayers of Christian Scientists. When things went wrong, when recoveries did not take place and people died, she blamed demonic influences.

The church trains Christian Science "practitioners" who accept "patients" and administer "treatments." Mrs. Eddy promoted her religion as a system of medicine, and believers still see it as such. She advertised an "opportunity to acquire a profession by which you can accumulate a fortune" and urged her practitioners to base their fees on those of local physicians. She was a strong believer in homeopathy. She felt her system was the wave of the future, while regular medicine belonged in the dustbin of history.

Despite such claims, Christian Science remains exempt from medical licensing laws, provided its practitioners don't take up "agencies of the flesh," that is, material or physical remedies of any kind. Christian Science training deliberately omits anatomy, physiology, symptomatology, and pathology. Their practitioners are instructed not to diagnose, take a patient's temperature, or use any physical means of treatment. Yet Christian Science claims to be far superior to modern medicine. The church even discourages practitioners from reporting suspected communicable diseases to health departments. This ensures that the practitioners aren't accused of attempting to diagnose, which could lead to charges of practicing medicine without a license.[20]

Even though Christian Science practitioners do not diagnose, treat, administer or prescribe drugs, take pulses or temperatures, or even relieve pain and discomfort with ice packs, hot packs, and massage, their services are covered by hundreds of insurance companies, including Blue Cross/Blue Shield and many plans for government employees. What services? Singing, reading Eddy's writings to patients, and praying in their behalf! Practitioners don't even have to see their patients, but can do "absent treatments" after telephone consultations. Just as remarkable, the practitioners can sign certificates for sick leave and disability payments, even though they cannot diagnose. They need only certify that the person is "under my professional care." The IRS recognizes practitioners' charges as "medical expenses" that may be deductible for persons who itemize deductions. Medicare and Medicaid reimburse for Christian Science nursing care.

The church's most dangerous aspect is its opposition to medical care for seriously ill children. Its practitioners are not duty-bound to refer to physicians when their treatments don't work. Nor are they trained to recognize what symptoms require expert care. This ignorance, as well as the belief that symptoms are worsened by thinking about them, has led parents and practitioners to disregard or try to pray away such serious symptoms in children as high fevers, convulsions, vomiting, delirium, and severe coughing. Not surprisingly, many Christian Science children have died unnecessarily from pneumonia, meningitis, diabetes, ruptured appendix, bowel obstruction, and other diseases and complications. Nevertheless, Christian Scientists have carved out large exemptions from negligent homicide and child-neglect laws for both themselves and other antimedical sects.

In many states, Christian Scientists have achieved exemptions from metabolic testing for newborn infants, prophylactic eyedrops for newborn infants (to prevent blindness from gonorrhea), premarital and prenatal blood tests for adults, tuberculosis testing for public school teachers, and immunizations for school children.

For nearly a century American courts have held that parents have a duty to care for their children in health and sickness. They must provide the necessities of life, of which appropriate medical care is one. Failure to do so can result in charges of negligent homicide and manslaughter. As early as 1903, courts ruled that parents can be held criminally responsible for not obtaining proper medical care for their sick children. Faith healing has not been considered proper care, and religion is not usually a lawful excuse for negligence. The courts have also consistently held that mandatory vaccination for school children is not a violation of the Constitution, even if their family's religion frowns on immunizations.

Nevertheless, state legislatures continue to bow to pressure from the wealthy, sophisticated church. Almost all states provide religious exemptions from immunization requirements. And almost all states have exemptions in their criminal code, juvenile code, or both, that provide religious immunity from abuse and neglect laws. If a parent sees that a child is suffering severe pain, has convulsions, or is vomiting blood, the law in most states requires the parent to either obtain proper medical care for the child or to pray (or hire someone to pray) for the child. The two are considered morally, medically and legally equivalent. In one of the few challenges to immunization exemptions, the Mississippi Supreme Court ruled that the state's religious exemption law violated the Fourteenth Amendment because it denied some children the right to equal protection from disease.

The federal government has an interesting role in this strange state of affairs. In 1974, at the urging of the Christian Science Church, the Department of Health, Education, and Welfare (HEW) placed a provision in the Code of Federal Regulations to the effect that parents who use prayer or faith healing instead of medical treatment cannot be considered negligent. This was a federal mandate, which means that states had to pass a version of it or risk losing federal funding for child-protection programs.

Critics believe these laws have contributed to many unnecessary and agonizing deaths of children. The laws also discourage others who might suspect child abuse and neglect from reporting it. If your Christian Science neighbors are exempt from neglect laws, you may believe it is pointless to report to health authorities that their little girl has had major seizures several times a day for months and has never been seen by a doctor. Teachers and child-protection agencies may draw similar conclusions. If the child dies, the coroner may assume that the death need not be reported to a prosecutor, or the latter may assume the case is not criminal.

The federal government reversed itself in 1983 when the Department of Health and Human Services (HHS), HEW's successor, removed the religious immunity provisions from the federal mandate. States are now required to define failure to provide necessary medical care as child neglect. However, HHS has not enforced this mandate as vigorously as it did the earlier policy. Today most states are still out of compliance because they have religious exemptions in their criminal and juvenile codes, but only a few have been challenged by HHS. In other states, prayer is considered fully equivalent to medical care. In most cases where a sick child is deprived of medical care and dies of a generally curable illness, his parents cannot be charged with negligence as long as they prayed for the child or hired someone else to do so.

The church continues to insist that its treatments are effective and to demand privileges and rights not accorded to others, including the right to endanger children and injure them by failing to provide necessary medical care. Christian Science children are second-class citizens since they do not have the same right to health care, both preventive and therapeutic, that other children have. And Christian Science healers continue to enjoy special privileges others do not enjoy in blatant violation of the doctrine of separation of church and state. The church still believes its healers are superior to physicians and forbids Christian Science treatments for those undergoing medical treatment. This uncompromising attitude encourages avoidance of medical care, and it will continue to kill children until the laws are changed.

Prospects for the future of Christian Science are mixed. While membership numbers are a secret, the number of congregations in the United States has declined about 2 percent a year for the past twenty years. Nevertheless, there are still several thousand churches in at least fifty countries, and the mother church in Boston remains wealthy and politically influential. Moreover, the laws it has inspired are still on the books, ready for other faith healers to exploit. Just as chiropractic's success with the legislatures opens the gates for naturopathy, homeopathy, acupuncture, and other pseudosciences, Christian Science has established precedents for other varieties of cults that advocate avoidance of medical care. It would not surprise me if many Protestant, Catholic, and New Age cults demand full legal equality with Christian Scientists.

Evangelical Healing

The idea that some people can magically cure illnesses in others by merely touching them, praying for them, or performing magical rituals goes back to primitive shamanism. Christian evangelical healing originated in America and Europe in the 1800s. The characteristic fire-and-brimstone preaching sprinkled with outrageous claims and promises of miracles seems to have started with the Reverend William Branham from Indiana. His great financial success inspired scores of imitators to hit the road, fleecing local sheep throughout the country.

Evangelical healing hasn't changed much since then, except that most of the traveling is now done through the airwaves. Rex Humbard and Oral Roberts set the format and style used by most of today's televangelists, some of whom have become wealthy by peddling little more than cheap tricks. In *The Faith Healers* [Prometheus Books, 1987], James Randi provides most of the following information.

• W.V. Grant has used mnemonics, crib sheets, hand signals from confederates in the audience, and other gimmicks to lead people to believe he is receiving information about them from a divine source.[21] He credits Holy Spirit Power, the Gifts of the Spirit. He proclaims that he uses no trickery, only divine power, but he actually does mentalist tricks known to magicians for many decades. He has been observed putting healthy people in wheelchairs and ordering them to walk (miraculously) after his Gift heals them. He does dramatic individual healings as well as mass healings that supposedly cure hundreds at once of arthritis, heart disease, cancer, blindness, deafness, paralysis, and everything else.

These demonstrations loosen wallets in a hurry and donations pour in. Not one of his thousands of alleged healings has ever been medically documented. On the contrary, many of those allegedly cured call him a liar and a fake who should not be allowed to steal from the public. Grant also makes money through mail-order sales of a wide variety of publications, tapes, courses, worthless diplomas, and holy knickknacks. He has even marketed herbs and supplements alleged to cure AIDS and other diseases.

• Peter Popoff has grossed tens of millions of tax-free dollars through televised performances in which he called out people in the audience, named their ailment, and performed miraculous healings with the power of Jeeezzus.[21] It turned out he was using a tiny radio receiver, hidden in his ear, to get the information broadcast by his wife backstage. After this was exposed by James Randi on Johnny Carson's "Tonight Show," Popoff's syndicated program was dropped by the eighty or so metropolitan stations that had carried it for years and thus aided and abetted the swindle.

Popoff has also made millions working a huge mailing list, peddling prayer cloths, sacred gloves, holy ribbons, sacred handkerchiefs said to be imbued with Popoff's sweat, and other charms and gimmicks. Randi's book describes in exquisite detail how, in 1985, Popoff staged a claim that "satanists and secular humanists" had broken into his headquarters and destroyed 100,000 Bibles he was planning to send to Russia. During his video production he used a cut onion to produce real tears as he appealed for donations to cover the cost of the allegedly damaged Bibles. What he actually showed, according to Randi's investigation, was not 100,000 ruined Bibles, but remains of 10,000 pamphlets that had been hosed down by Popoff's own agents.

• Oral Roberts is the founder of the Evangelistic Association in Tulsa, Oklahoma. His conglomerate employs some three thousand people, brings in hundreds of thousands of tourists each year, and is a major factor in the Tulsa economy. It consists of Oral Roberts University, a nursing home, a retirement center, condominiums, banks, and a variety of other businesses. Roberts has claimed to have divine visions and miraculous powers by which he can heal the sick, cast out demons, and raise the dead. His organization has declined challenges to produce evidence to support any of these claims. Roberts's success is not based on scientific evidence, but on his ability to attract donations.

In 1981 Roberts opened the City of Faith, a $250,000,000 medical complex where "prayer and scientific medicine can be merged." The complex included a medical school, a research center, and a 777-bed hospital opposed by community leaders who said that Tulsa already had enough hospitals. In 1989 Roberts announced that unfilled beds—a problem from the beginning—had forced him to close the school and shut down his hospital. At its peak, the facility had only 148 inpatients. Along the way, Roberts attracted notoriety with broadcasts portraying God as a terrorist holding him hostage and demanding millions of dollars be paid lest the dedicated evangelist be snuffed.

• Pat Robertson, director and host of the Christian Broadcasting Network's "700 Club," claims to have Word of Knowledge (direct messages from God) about people with diseases and the ability to direct God's healing power. Robertson claims to be able to heal broken bones, make the crippled walk, and banish advanced diseases of all kinds, including AIDS. He works in a shotgun manner so the results cannot be ascertained. For example, he'll say something like: "There's a woman in Cincinnati with undiagnosed lymph cancer that's been making her feel unwell lately. God is now healing it. There! You'll be better now." Robertson even asserts that he can move hurricanes away from populated areas and speak to throngs of Chinese in English while they miraculously hear his words in their own regional dialects.

As far as I know, he is the only current evangelist-healer who campaigned for the U. S. Presidency (for the 1988 election) and was probably the first to do so since William Jennings Bryant. I shudder to think about the impact a faith-healer President might have on America's health-care system.

• Robert Tilton, also known as Pastor Bob, grosses an estimated one million dollars per week through his televised ministry, which is carried by nearly one hundred stations across the country. His main gimmick is the ultimate in simplicity. During the healing frenzy he puts a hand up to the camera and invites viewers to put their hands on the image of his hands on their television screens. By this means, the Spirit of God goes through his hands and into them where it cures whatever might ail them, including AIDS.

Evangelicals versus Christian Scientists

While Christian Scientists deny the very existence of disease and pray for the elimination of the illusion, evangelical healers claim to cure real diseases caused by Satan. While Christian Science healers quietly and earnestly pray for friends and neighbors, and make a moderate but steady income, the modern-day Elmer Gantrys typically use trickery to make mountains of money from gullible audiences. While Christian Scientists have formal classes and credentials, work within our legal system, and lobby for greater privileges, evangelicals don't bother much with credentials, formalities, and legalities. Evangelists do pretty much what they please. Most maintain enough of a religious facade to keep tax collectors, bunko squads, and politicians far away. They sell bogus miracles and delusional frenzy to desperate and gullible people. Since they do it in the name of Jeeezzus, however, the donations they rake in are rarely reportable to the IRS or otherwise accountable.

Despite recent scandals, many evangelicals are still doing well financially. They don't seem inclined to lobby for inclusion in health insurance programs, which might invite unwanted scrutiny. If they did, who would stop them? Legislators who consider chiropractic, naturopathy, acupuncture, Christian Science, and scientific medicine to be separate-but-equal professions? Governors and Presidents who wear religiosity on their sleeves?

Psychic Diagnosis and Healing

From time immemorial some people have claimed to be able to see, understand, and cure diseases by using psychic powers.

• Edgar Cayce's disciples and imitators claim to psychically see inside the body, even from thousands of miles away, to locate, diagnose, and treat any lesion, abnormality, or sickness that is present. During the first half of the twentieth century, Cayce, originally a professional photographer, devoted several hours each day to going into a trancelike state and doing "readings," some 14,000 of which were recorded by a stenographer.[22,23]

No scientific study of the results of Cayce's treatments has ever been undertaken; his followers simply take Cayce's words as gospel. The transcripts have been preserved, edited, and published in various forms by the Association for Research and Enlightenment in Virginia Beach. A.R.E. does a brisk business selling pamphlets, books, and tapes on such disorders as diabetes, allergies, obesity arthritis, multiple sclerosis, mental illness, and baldness. Even a few medical doctors are convinced Cayce was a genuine psychic who revealed important healing techniques. For example, Norman Shealy, M.D., first president of the American Holistic Medical Association, credits A.R.E. with his own "transformation towards holistic health."

It is not clear how Cayce derived his (mis)information. Supporters say he probably gleaned it telepathically from osteopaths and other "natural healers" and their texts. Skeptics suspect he was a fantasy-prone personality and a victim of self-delusion. His most common prescriptions were for manipulations, massage, baths, castor-oil packs, enemas, and various poultices.[24,25] Cayce's readings state that smoking tobacco is not only harmless, but is positively beneficial in moderation for most people.[25] (I wonder how he divined that.) While Cayce may have been honest and sincere, though deluded, some contemporary "psychic" diagnosticians and healers are just con artists who make a living exploiting the gullible.

• Psychic surgery is not a case of delusion, but of deceit.[26,27] The scam is often promoted by film or videotape. In a typical production, a woman with inoperable spinal tumors lies on her stomach, fully conscious. The "surgeon" holds his hands just above the flesh of her lower back and then kneads the flesh with his fingers. Suddenly, blood appears as his fingers seem to sink into the flesh. They quickly withdraw with stringy bits of bloody material said to be tumors. The wound then appears to close spontaneously as the assistants sponge up the blood. The patient reports no pain.

Many patients have been shown undergoing "surgery" for tumors, heart disease, and other disorders. The pattern is always the same, from the kneading to the appearance of blood, to the pulling out of tissue, to the mopping up. Some of the patients are interviewed; all say they feel better. Some patients flew from the United States to the Philippines in a chartered jet liner and paid up to several thousand dollars each for psychic surgery treatments. The genius at work, who explained his talent in terms of mental power and cosmic vibrations, was the late Tony Agpaoa, an ex-magician who probably became one of the wealthiest men in the Philippines.[28] Many of his imitators have also done well for themselves.

At a screening I attended, most of the two hundred or so members of the audience appeared favorably impressed. Many felt they had witnessed a miracle. Few spotted the sleight-of-hand, the subtle pressing down of the flesh to create a little pool to hold the "blood" (typically betel nut juice) that was sneaked in, probably from capsules in the cotton, and the palming of bits of animal tissue. Most people in the audience were not desperately ill, yet they were taken in by the scam. It's not surprising that cancer patients are easily victimized.

Psychic surgery has been debunked and exposed as a fraud many times. With a supply of "blood" and chicken guts, some sleight-of-hand and a lot of gall, any good magician could make a fortune with the racket. Randi has demonstrated the procedure on the "Tonight Show." Fortunately, few magicians are such scoundrels. Unfortunately, the exposés have not put much of a dent in the business. The power of suggestion—the placebo effect—is no doubt the basis of whatever success, or seeming success, is achieved. All that blood and guts can have a powerful impact on the mind. While the emotional impact of the treatment may be substantial, it is only temporary and cannot alter the course of a serious disease. The danger, of course, is that victims who are convinced they are cured may rely on this belief instead of getting effective medical care.

• Qigong (pronounced "chi-gung") is an ancient Chinese system of healing, both oneself and others, by manipulating alleged mystical energies. Qigong masters can allegedly see into bodies without x-rays, even at a distance like Edgar Cayce, and cure all kinds of serious diseases, including cancer and AIDS. This psychic medicine has waxed and waned in popularity in response to political and cultural circumstances. Maoism, a Chinese version of Marxist materialism, could coexist with acupuncture because, with its purported meridians, points, and energies (Qi), it can at least appear natural rather than supernatural. Like acupuncture, Qigong involves the meridians that allegedly carry Qi. In the internal form of this traditional healing art, the Qi is controlled with relaxation, breathing, and concentration techniques. The external form, however, in which Qigong masters radiate healing Qi from their fingertips to affect miraculous cures, was too mystical for the Maoists, and they suppressed Qigong altogether. Since the late 1980s, Qigong, like many other mystical and superstitious concepts and movements, has experienced a strong revival. The system is used in hospitals and clinics throughout China and has recently arrived in America, Australia, and Europe. Like acupuncture and Ayurveda, it may spread and become entrenched as a part of "holistic healing" and "alternative medicine." Scientific tests of Qigong masters in China have revealed no evidence of any paranormal powers.[29]

Multilevel Quackery

Perhaps the fastest-growing segment of the snake-oil business consists of multilevel companies that recruit thousands (and sometimes even hundreds of thousands) of untrained individuals into the business of playing doctor with their relatives, friends, coworkers, and neighbors. Often they have tried the products, concluded that they work, and become suppliers to spread the word and pick up some cash in the process.

Multilevel marketing (also called network marketing) is a form of direct sales in which independent distributors sell products, typically to their friends and acquaintances. In theory, distributors can make money not only from their own sales but also from those of the people they recruit. To become a distributor they complete a simple application and pay a small fee. This enables them to buy products "wholesale," sell them "retail," and recruit other distributors who can do the same. When enough distributors have been enrolled, the recruiter is eligible to collect a percentage of their sales. Companies suggest that this process provides a great money-making opportunity. However, people who don't join during the first few months of operation or become one of the early distributors in their community are unlikely to build enough of a sales pyramid to do well.

Most multilevel companies that market health products claim that their products can prevent or cure a wide range of diseases. A few companies merely suggest that people will feel better, look better, or have more energy if they supplement their diet with extra nutrients. When clear-cut therapeutic claims are made in product literature, the company is an easy target for government enforcement action. Some companies run this risk, hoping that the government won't take action until their customer base is well established. Other companies make no claims in their literature but rely on testimonials, encouraging people to try their products and credit them for any improvement that occurs.

Most multilevel companies tell distributors not to make claims for the products except for those found in company literature. (That way the company can deny responsibility for what distributors do.) Many companies, however, hold sales meetings and arrange telephone conference calls during which people tell how the products have helped them. Testimonials may also be trumpeted in company magazines, audiotapes, or videotapes.

Government enforcement action against multilevel companies has not been vigorous. These companies are usually left alone unless their promotions become so conspicuous and their sales volume so great that an agency feels compelled to intervene. Even then, few interventions have substantial impact once a company is well established. Here are a few facts about three multilevel companies involved in the sale of herbal remedies.

• During the mid-1980s, Herbalife International, Inc., raked in hundreds of millions of dollars before government agencies intervened. Early in its operation, its various products were claimed to heal some seventy diseases, help attain and maintain a healthy weight, aid digestion, heal and "cleanse the system," increase energy and alertness, improve cardiovascular function, combat aging, and improve mood.[30] At Congressional hearings in 1985, company officials admitted that many of their customers experienced unpleasant side effects, which was not surprising because the products contained laxatives. 1987 Herbalife and its president, Mark Hughes, agreed to pay $850,000 to the state of California for making false medical claims and operating an illegal pyramid-style scheme. Adverse publicity cut sales drastically, but the company still grosses over $100 million a year.

• Another large company, Sunrider International, was not deterred by Herbalife's legal problems. Its literature and distributors suggest that its products can help the body heal itself, "cleanse the body," improve emotional well-being, increase alertness, decrease pain, improve circulation, and enhance immunity, fertility, stamina, and vigor, all by "nourishing" specific organs. The alleged nutrients that accomplish these wonders are not named, and no evidence is provided to support these wild claims.

Sunrider's activities illustrate how law-enforcement agencies are often ineffective in stopping quackery by large corporations. In 1983 the FDA told Sunrider, among other things, to stop claiming that its Calli Tea helps users be "slender, energetic, and full of life." In 1990 the company signed a consent agreement with California authorities to pay $175,000 in penalties for false advertising of its products.[31] Yet in 1991 the company's sales materials still promoted its products for obesity, infections, arthritis, multiple sclerosis, gout, eye problems, diabetes, and more. A distributor told me the products had cured her mother's cholesterol problems, a friend's hypertension, and her cat's cancer. She suggested, as does some Sunrider literature, that the products can allow people to stop using doctor-prescribed drugs for a wide variety of serious disorders. On the strength of such claims, Sunrider has become a major player in the snake-oil industry with sales over $300 million in 1990.

The company's charismatic founder and president is Tei Fu Chen. Allegedly from a family of prominent Chinese herbalists, he claims to be a medical doctor educated in Taiwan and a pharmacist licensed in the United States. In a May 1991 telecast, "Inside Edition" reported that a lawsuit filed against Sunrider revealed that he had no credentials in either medicine or pharmacy. Sunrider literature calls Chen a "world renowned nutritionist," though he has no credentials in nutrition either. He claims his theories are supported by scientific research, but refuses to cite the studies on the grounds that "scientific evidence can always be disputed." Instead, he urges us to have faith in his (apparently bogus) credentials and "the long history of Chinese success" in medicine. He claims he has converted the wisdom of the ancient principles of yin and yang into modern molecular terms. He provides no details, just the end result: everyone needs his pills, powders, potions, teas, and ointments for maximum health. In 1992 the lawsuit described on "Inside Edition" came to trial. After deciding that Sunrider had violated Arizona's racketeering laws, the jury awarded actual and punitive damages totaling $650,000 to the plaintiff.

• Nature's Sunshine Products is another fast-growing company. Its more than four hundred products include many that are claimed to "nourish" or "support" various body organs. Its salespeople, dubbed "Natural Health Counselors," are taught to use iridology, muscle-testing (a type of applied kinesiology), and other dubious methods to convince people that they need the products.[32] The company also markets a "weight-loss and lifetime nutritional program" based on the "glandular body typing" of Dr. Elliot Abravanel described in Chapter 1.

Homeopathy

Homeopathy is a system developed in the late 1700s by Samuel Hahnemann, a German physician. Its basic principle is expressed in the homeopathic law, *similia similibus curentur* ("like cures like"). Hahnemann drew this conclusion after experimenting with cinchona bark, which contains quinine and was known to cure malaria (then called "intermittent fever"). After taking the drug, he experienced palpitations, rapid pulse, prostration, flushing, and thirst, symptoms that he believed were very similar to those of malaria. He generalized from this and asserted that if a substance given to a healthy person causes certain symptoms, small amounts of the substance will cure a person sick with those symptoms.

Based on this simple notion, Hahnemann built an enormous edifice of dogma and promoted it with the zeal of an evangelist. He vented his wrath on followers who did not toe the line exactly: "He who does not walk on exactly the same line with me, who diverges, if it be but the breadth of a straw, to the right or to the left, is an apostate and a traitor."[33]

Hahnemann stated that a drug-induced disease will drive out a preexisting disease if the two are similar. The entire edifice of homeopathy was then constructed by claims of similarities between various substances and diseases. For example, suppose a person is experiencing delirium, hallucinations, dilated pupils, and wild, insane behavior. The proper remedy is a little belladonna, large doses of which cause these symptoms in normal persons. Or, if signs of kidney or liver disease or anemia occur, the proper remedy is a little arsenic, which can produce these problems in healthy persons. Colds and hay fever are treated with homeopathic extracts of onion since normal amounts cause the eyes to run.

A favorite homeopathic remedy is extract of aconite (also known as monkshood, friar's cap, and wolfsbane), a plant so toxic that simply picking the flowers can cause tingling and numbness in the fingers. Just 5 mg of the active alkaloid can kill a person. Homeopathic preparations of aconite are advocated as a first aid for shock, stroke, heart attack, and other very serious conditions. It is also used in preparations for children. The "logic" behind aconite's use is that, like the effects of this extremely lethal chemical, the above-mentioned conditions generally come on suddenly and with great severity. Like cures like, remember. Strychnine is also popular with homeopaths.

How far do homeopaths carry their dogma? Do they treat lead poisoning with more lead? Incredibly, the answer is yes. Bee stings are treated with more bee venom, mercury poisoning with more mercury, and so on for many kinds of poisoning. Fortunately, as described below, homeopathic remedies are so dilute that the amounts of added toxins are insignificant.

Not all homeopathic medicines are derived from toxic substances. Extremely small doses of calcium, iron, magnesium, and other common minerals are used for severe pain and a wide variety of serious diseases and infections. People normally get far more of these minerals from small amounts of food, but the minerals in the homeopathic pills are supposedly made more potent by the methods used to prepare them. Even plain old calcium carbonate, which many people take in doses of hundreds of milligrams as an antacid or calcium supplement, becomes Calcarea carbonica, a wondrous antiviral drug at infinitesimal doses, in the hands of homeopaths.

The Magical World of Homeopathic Pharmacology

Homeopathic lore states that their remedies have been tested by administering them to healthy volunteers who recorded every physical, mental, and emotional effect they perceived over a period of time. These effects are then said to be the symptoms amenable to homeopathic doses of the substances. These tests are called "provings." Homeopaths believe they prove not only what substances do at physiological doses, but also what they do in vanishingly small doses, with the effects increasing as the dose approaches zero. In Hahnemann's guide to provings, subjects attribute every little ache, brief pain, tight muscle, bad mood, erection, and fart to the substance being tested. The provings for most of today's commonly used homeopathic remedies were done more than 150 years ago and recorded in reference books (materia medica) that practitioners use for selecting remedies. A few practitioners, however, use "electrodiagnostic" devices or computer programs to select their remedies.

Do you think that the physiological effects of herbs, minerals, and assorted toxins can be ascertained this way? Most people given a pill and encouraged to attribute all sorts of things to it will do so! This should be obvious to rational people, but homeopaths don't get it. It would be interesting to see whether subjects in a "proving" can distinguish between a substance they have just tested and a placebo. But, as far as I know, no such experiment has been done.

Some homeopaths refer to people and drugs in a manner resembling that of astrology. One textbook, for example, describes "the belladonna" as a violent character prone to "turmoil in the brain," and "the arsenicum," as a "covetous, malicious money-maker with green, putrid excretions."[34] The remedies for these flawed personality traits, of course, are belladonna and arsenic. While homeopathy claims to be a "natural" healing profession, it not only has a pill for *everything,* but claims that thousands of substances are a remedy for something.

Homeopathic Alchemy

The magic of homeopathy lies in the process that embues mundane and lethal substances with miraculous powers during their preparation. Nonsoluble substances are repeatedly crushed and diluted with lactose, a process called trituration. Soluble substances are repeatedly diluted with alcohol or water and shaken vigorously, a process called succussion. According to homeopathic theory, these methods are essential to the activity and assimilation of the remedy, but since there is no detectable difference between substances subjected to pounding and shaking and those not so abused, there is no way to enforce this requirement. It's a question of faith, similar to questions like, "Was the holy water really properly blessed" and "How could one ever be sure?"

An even stranger feature is the assertion that the smaller the dose, the greater the potency. For example, for symptoms resembling arsenic poisoning, the homeopath (or homeopathic manufacturer) dilutes some arsenic in lactose, takes a small amount of the mixture and dilutes it with more lactose, and so on, dozens or hundreds of times. The remedy is supposed to become more potent with each dilution. For maximum potency, dilution continues even after it is mathematically impossible that a single atom of arsenic remains, and the remedy continues to get more potent! The arsenic, chamomile, or calcium carbonate that is no longer present affects the person through "vibrations" it has left behind. That's really what they say.

Homeopaths present themselves to the public as scientific practitioners, but they are really mystical cultists who believe in a "vital force," disturbance of which is the cause of disease. The supposed disturbance can be corrected by the "spiritlike essence" of homeopathic medicines. Obviously, homeopathy resembles alchemy and is absolutely incompatible with modern science. In fact, if homeopathy were true, there could be no chemistry as we know it because there would be no pure substances or recognizable chemical laws. Every substance would imprint its vibes forever on everything it ever came in contact with. Since everything and every substance would have its own unique history, it would have its own unique properties that could not be divined by all the most powerful computers in the world.

Homeopathic theory was thoroughly demolished in 1842 by Oliver Wendell Holmes in his essay, "Homeopathy and Its Kindred Delusions"[35] and has been further refuted many times since. Nevertheless, homeopathic remedies are recognized as drugs by federal law. They were given legal status by the 1938 Federal Food, Drug, and Cosmetic Act, which recognized as drugs all substances included in the *Homeopathic Pharmacopeia of the United States.* The FDA has permitted homeopathic products to be marketed even though they have not been demonstrated to work. Listings in the book are not based on scientific testing but on "provings."

The number of physicians who practice homeopathy is small—at most a few hundred—but many chiropractors, naturopaths, and other fringe practitioners are prescribing and selling homeopathic remedies for the gamut of disease. And "health food" stores and a few pharmacies display scores of homeopathic preparations labeled for use in specific ailments or to strengthen specific organs. An alleged homeopathic aphrodisiac has been huckstered on program-length TV commercials that touted the substance's listing in the *Homeopathic Pharmacopeia* as proof of its legitimacy.

Homeopaths assert that their preparations are so potent that serious harm can come from inappropriate use. Are homeopathic drugs so powerful that they can permanently screw up the vital force? Why aren't homeopaths fighting tooth and nail against the proliferation of over-the-counter homeopathic remedies? As with the other mysteries and paradoxes of homeopathy, only the vital force knows.

Dana Ullman, Master Promoter

Dana Ullman, America's foremost promoter of homeopathy, also peddles books and a variety of products. One is a "homeopathic tranquilizer" containing passion flower, hops, and chamomile. This product violates classical homeopathic principles in several ways. Homeopathic medicines are supposed to be given only after proper "provings" and only one at a time. Here is a combination product that has not been "proved." Moreover, since these herbs are generally recognized as tranquilizers in normal doses, they should be stimulants in homeopathic doses. Yet, the product is sold as a tranquilizer. This illustrates the fact that with homeopathy the potions are whatever their peddlers say they are. Since they usually don't do anything anyway, those who buy them can imagine any effects they want.

Ullman's book, *Homeopathy, Medicine for the 21st Century* [North Atlantic Books, 1988], typifies the combination of fuzzy thinking and messianic attitude characteristic of homeopaths. Ullman claims the book "synthesizes homeopathy, Jungian psychology, alchemy, and the new physics." According to the book's introduction:

> By providing a diagnostic system that assesses the whole organism rather than simply its parts, and by being a therapeutic system that works by stimulating a person's own immune and defense system rather than by simply controlling or suppressing symptoms, homeopathy will inevitably become an integral part of health care in the United States.

The "diagnostic system" used by homeopaths involves compiling all the patient's symptoms, personality traits, and various other attributes and finding the substance(s) that supposedly "fit" them. Homeopathy considers this superior to modern medicine's silly habits of doing a medical history, blood studies, biopsies, and bacterial cultures and assessing such things as the functioning of the heart, lungs, and other organs. Since homeopathy is entirely symptom-oriented, it matters little what the medical diagnosis is. Homeopaths concern themselves with determining what substance has been reported to cause symptoms most closely resembling those of the patient. Homeopathic doses of that substance are then administered. This, we are told again and again (and again), stimulates the immune system, resolves the problem, raises the overall level of health, and prevents recurrence.

For this reason, states Dana Ullman, homeopathic medicines are "likely to become the treatment of choice in viral conditions." He also states that "it is becoming increasingly obvious that homeopathic medicines provide a viable, safer alternative to antibiotic use." He assures us that homeopaths have already enjoyed substantial success in treating AIDS, herpes, influenza, bladder infections, ear infections, chickenpox, meningitis, plague, cholera, scarlet fever, yellow fever, typhoid, and strep throat. He predicts that homeopathic remedies will largely replace antibiotics in the twenty-first century.

Like most homeopathy promoters, Ullman asserts that immunization against infectious diseases is based on the homeopathic "law of similars." There is not a microgram of truth to this statement. Vaccines are not small doses of substances that would cause disease if given in large doses. Nor do they become more potent with decreasing dosage. On the contrary, if the dose is too small, the vaccine has no effect. Nor must they be subjected to succussion to be effective. Vaccines are killed or weakened organisms that are left sufficiently intact to stimulate the formation of specific antibodies so the body's immune system can attack if the intact organisms enter the body. In this respect, their effect is similar to that of large doses of the live microbes, not the opposite.

Homeopathic history-taking includes many questions about symptoms, feelings, likes and dislikes, moods, and behavior. Ullman says that "homeopathy is the science of finding the medicine that is most similar to the person . . . a substance that matches the essence of the person's characteristics." This is called the person's "constitutional medicine." Whatever ails the person, says Ullman, the constitutional medicine is most important, and treatment starts with it. When treating infections in women, Ullman says, "it is not so important to know what *microorganism* has infected the woman as it is to know *what kind of woman* the microorganism has infected."

Another important consideration is how the herb or other substance "grows and acts in nature, and how these characteristics correspond to the person who needs the medicine." For example, "Pulsatilla is a small and delicate flower with a flexible stem that moves with the wind (moody, easily 'taken with the wind'). It grows in clusters (dependence on others) in dry, sandy soil (thirstlessness)." Therefore, "the women who need Pulsatilla are gentle, mild, yielding, agreeable, sensitive, greedy for affection, emotionally dependent, easily brought to tears, especially just prior to menstruation . . . . Pulsatilla women rely on feelings in making decisions . . . are easily led by others and easily hurt . . . dislike warm rooms, and have unstable circulation. They are averse to eating fat and to warm food and drinks."

In contrast, consider the Sepia woman, whose constitutional medicine is homeopathically prepared cuttlefish. They are "often overworked housewives or assertive career women . . . outspoken, direct, industrious." Their "inner irritability creates a bossy and nagging personality." They are "fault-finding, easily offended, disposed to quarrel . . . do not enjoy sex . . . and may become indifferent to their husbands and even to their children, . . . may feel cold in a warm room, . . . tend to have low thyroid hormones, low blood pressure, and adrenal deficiency. . . . common symptoms include weakness in the small of the back and headaches."

The absurdities of homeopathic theory are too voluminous to discuss in this book, but one more—the concept of "miasms"—deserves special mention. Homeopaths believe that people can inherit acquired diseases (or something "similar") from their parents. For example, if one of your parents or even a distant relative had gonorrhea before you were born, you may inherit a gonorrheal "miasm," which means you "tend to manifest symptoms of overgrowth of tissue (enlarged organs, tumors, warts, fibrous growths or cysts, excess weight), accumulation of mucus, and disturbances of the pelvic and sexual organs," and you "may be restless, cross, irritable, absentminded, selfish, and mischievous."[36]

Promotions for Ullman's book claim it presents scientific support for homeopathy. The book claims that scores of homeopathic medicines are effective for practically every disease known, yet it presents only a handful of questionable studies to support the use of a half dozen remedies in a few self-limiting conditions. This is typical of homeopathic logic. Hahnemann developed the whole theory of homeopathy after experimenting with one drug on himself, and he didn't even use a homeopathic dose in that study.

Similarly, Ullman generalizes from half-baked studies of a few medicines and concludes that the entire *Homeopathic Pharmacopeia* has thereby been scientifically proven safe and effective for scores of ailments. As we have seen, homeopathy makes fantastic claims that are completely contrary to very well established principles of physiology, biochemistry, and pharmacology. Extraordinary claims demand extraordinary proof, but all Ullman provides is a smidgen of flimsy evidence. Someone claiming that the earth is flat would have to marshal a mountain of very impressive evidence to outweigh what centuries of contrary evidence have established. Ullman and homeopathy are light-years away from having proved their case.

Throughout the book Ullman uses heads-I-win, tails-you-lose sophistry to support homeopathic dogma. On one page he says, "Homeopaths have found that the correctly prescribed medicine tends to work immediately." Elsewhere in the book he says that patients given homeopathic medicines commonly get worse before they get better. He calls this a "healing crisis" and it too is proof that the medicine is not a placebo, that it really has physiological effects that ultimately lead to recovery.

Further insight into Ullman's reasoning abilities is provided by the following episode. Ullman claims that properly controlled scientific studies have proved the efficacy of homeopathic remedies. A few years ago, a National Council Against Health Fraud Bulletin mailing mentioned that there have been no such studies in which homeopathic medicines have been independently analyzed for adulteration (sneaking known effective drugs into the formulations). Ullman responded that when studies are double-blind and placebo-controlled there is no need for adulteration analysis. This is an inexcusable lapse in logic for someone who claims to be educating America for twenty-first-century medicine. Consider, for example, the report of an asthmatic patient who responded strikingly to Dumcap, a homeopathic remedy manufactured in Pakistan. When the remedy was analyzed, it turned out to contain medications known to be effective against asthma.[37] Even a perfectly controlled study might not detect a fraud involving adulterated pills without analysis of the pills. So much for Ullman's "scientific proof."

A Pandora's Box of Snake Oils

There is no question that homeopathic products are a waste of money. But are they dangerous? If properly manufactured, they will do no direct harm because their "active" ingredient is so dilute that it exerts no effect whatsoever. More important, however, is the danger of a person with a serious health problem being under the care of an irrational practitioner. *Consumer Reports* has concluded:

> Any system of medicine embracing the use of such (homeopathic) remedies involves a potential danger to patients whether the prescribers are M.D.'s, other licensed practitioners, or outright quacks. Ineffective drugs are dangerous drugs when used to treat serious or life-threatening disease. Moreover, even though homeopathic drugs are essentially nontoxic, self-medication can still be hazardous. Using them for a serious illness or undiagnosed pain instead of obtaining proper medical attention could prove harmful or even fatal.[38]

Naturopathy

During the late 1970s, the wife of a naturopath in Hawaii died at the age of twenty-six. The "official" cause of death was Hodgkin's disease, but it would be more accurate to say that she was killed by her husband's belief system. When her disease became apparent, he was sure he could cure her with baths, herbal teas, homeopathic remedies, and laetrile. Since these remedies are worthless against cancer, her disease progressed. By the time she had lost confidence in naturopathy, it was too late. The physicians who examined her were sickened by what they found. They advised that the therapy they had to offer (massive radiation) at this late stage would make her miserable and was unlikely to cure her. She chose to forego the treatment and died a few months later.

The naturopath was not an unlicensed quack posing as a doctor. He was licensed and practicing within the scope permitted by his license. He was not investigated, sued, prosecuted, or even reprimanded. In the states where naturopaths are permitted to practice, they are permitted to call themselves doctors and represent themselves to be family physicians. About a year after the woman's death, driven by intense curiosity, I visited the naturopath at his home. After we discussed the weather and real-estate prices, I nervously brought up the subject of his wife's illness and death. To my surprise, he discussed the matter calmly and voiced no regrets about his efforts to help her the "natural" way.

Naturopathic Notions

Naturopathy is based on the notion that diseases are caused by the accumulation of toxins in the body and should be treated by natural methods that rid the body of these toxins. The toxins are not named, and "natural" is not defined, so anything goes except what state law prohibits, which isn't much.

Since states have written naturopathic concepts into their laws, it behooves us to examine these concepts (better late than never). The laws generally say something to the effect that naturopaths use "natural" medicines and healing methods. Does this mean that there are "unnatural" medicines and healing methods? What might they be? Can anything that improves your health or saves your life be unnatural?

Naturopathic treatment may include enemas, starvation, doses of vitamin C equivalent to a hundred oranges a day, doses of vitamin A equivalent to fifty carrots, foul-tasting and toxic herbal teas, and raw beef gland pills. Do these seem "natural" to you? Medical doctors administer vaccines, antibiotics (which are extracted and derived from a wide variety of "natural and organic" microbes), morphine (from opium poppies), and digitalis (originally extracted from foxglove plants, but now synthesized in more potent forms in laboratories). Would you consider them "unnatural"?

Immunizations against a dozen killer diseases have significantly extended human life expectancy. Vaccinations work by stimulating the immune system to make antibodies to specific viruses and bacteria, so if the organisms enter the body they will be destroyed before they can multiply. Rather than support this triumph of modern scientific preventive medicine, that is also as "natural and organic" as anything could be, naturopaths propagandize against it. Never mind that it saves lives; it doesn't fit with their dogma about toxins.

Worse yet, some naturopaths espouse an "immunization kit" containing homeopathic solutions and pills that supposedly protect against polio, measles, pertussis, tetanus, and other lethal diseases. Parents led to believe that these kits will protect their children are being fleeced, and their children are being placed at risk. This hoax is not limited to the far fringes of the cult. The Academic Dean of the National College of Naturopathic Medicine, Jared Zeff, N.D., said, in reference to such products, that some naturopaths give conventional vaccines and some give homeopathic pills that "stimulate the immune system."

Common Naturopathic Methods

Naturopaths who get a foot in the door may milk the health-care system for everything they can get. For example, as I write this, a Hawaii naturopath has been treating a man with low back pain for some four years. He has been using homeopathic pills and acupuncture and charging $1,200 per month for them. He also has been treating this same man with chelation therapy for alleged lead poisoning. This costs another several hundred per month. The naturopath has been making about $1,200 to $1,500 per month from one patient for years, with no improvement to show for it, and he persists with no serious challenge from government authorities.

Although there is no evidence to support the toxin theory, there is no end to the crackpot methods naturopaths use to get rid of the alleged toxins. Their favorites include high colonics, fasting, an assortment of bizarre dietary regimens, megavitamins, pangamic acid and other pseudonutrients, many unproven and toxic herbal medicines, homeopathy, acupuncture, reflexology, chelation therapy, and a wide assortment of quack cancer and AIDS drugs such as laetrile, hydrogen peroxide, and miscellaneous herbs and herbal extracts. Quack diagnostic methods popular with naturopaths include iridology, applied kinesiology, Electroacupuncture according to Voll and other electronic gadgetry, hair analysis, cytotoxic testing, and live cell analysis. Chapters 1 and 5 cover most of these methods.

These worthless procedures and nostrums are the stock-in-trade of naturopathy. There are a great many of them because naturopathy is among the most eclectic of the quack systems. In this respect they are much like the majority of chiropractors, who don't confine their treatments to manipulating the spine. The use of these methods could get medical doctors sued, fired, and/ or delicensed, but in the hands of naturopaths they are "natural healing methods." Americans are wasting billions of health-care dollars on them.

Naturopathy's War on Rational Medicine and Public Health

Like chiropractic, naturopathy was born around the turn of the century. The term seems to have been coined by John H. Scheel, a German homeopath. Early practitioners were mostly European emigrants who used hydrotherapy, herbal medicines, and manipulations. Like homeopaths and chiropractors, naturopaths see themselves as superior to medical doctors because they understand special secrets of health that M.D.'s don't. Therefore, they are not only fully qualified family physicians and primary-care providers, but they also feel free to treat cancer and AIDS patients and other seriously ill people whom even the best family doctors would refer to specialists. The National College of Naturopathic Medicine catalog suggests that naturopathic techniques will lead to "a revolution in health care."

Like chiropractors, naturopaths try to poison the public's mind against M.D.'s. They claim that naturopaths look to the real cause of disease (toxin accumulation), while M.D.'s only cover up the symptoms. They are holistic and really care, while M.D.'s just want to keep you sick so they can keep taking your money. It follows that naturopathic alternatives are superior, even in cases of infections, cancers, and AIDS, for which they claim to have superior treatments. Many naturopaths oppose important public-health measures such as milk pasteurization and vaccinations.

Convergence with Chiropractic

Naturopaths and mixer D.C.'s have become almost indistinguishable in their fraudulent promotion methods, in their slander of rational medicine, and in the plethora of quack methods common to their trades. It is hard to think of a snake oil commonly used by one but not the other. They both prescribe and peddle megavitamins, various pseudonutrients, homeopathic remedies, unproven herbal remedies, and raw gland extracts. Much of what is said in Chapter 3 about chiropractic either already applies to naturopathy or probably will in the future. Predictably, naturopathy is imitating the strategy used by chiropractic and may eventually be legalized through the U.S.

Both chiropractors and naturopaths indulge in irrational and dangerous gadgeteering. A monument to their convergence came in 1983 when Scot Olsen, a licensed naturopath in Alberta, Canada, used a chiropractic technique.[39] He inserted a balloon up the nose of a twenty-month-old girl, purportedly to enlarge her small skull. The balloon lodged in the girl's throat and she strangled. While a judge did find the naturopath guilty of criminal negligence and called the treatment "outright quackery," he sentenced Olsen to only one day in jail and a $1,000 fine.

Naturopaths and chiropractors both administer high colonics, acupuncture, and spinal and cranial manipulations for the treatment and prevention of serious diseases. They both use preposterous diagnostic techniques such as iridology and applied kinesiology. And they both wax mystical about "energy flow." The only serious difference between them is that chiropractors say they treat spinal subluxations so "nerve energy" can flow efficiently, while naturopaths say all those same treatments are necessary to cure and prevent toxin accumulation. Chiropractors have a spine fetish, while naturopaths have a colon fetish.

Naturopathic Education

There are only two full-time naturopathic schools in the United States: Bastyr College in Seattle, Washington, and the National College of Naturopathic Medicine (NCNM) in Portland, Oregon. Each has a four-year curriculum leading to the Doctor of Naturopathy (N.D.) degree. The cost is about $10,000 per year. The federal government will help pick up the tab through guaranteed student loans and other assistance. Thus, the taxpayers subsidize the training of quacks who may later defraud, sicken, or kill some of them and work to undermine tax-supported public-health measures. Some of the tab is also picked up by companies that market snake oils that the naturopaths later prescribe and peddle. For example, in 1988 John Bastyr College received about $20,000 in money and laboratory equipment from American Biologics, a company once described as the major laetrile distributor of the world.[40] The college has also received large donations from dozens of manufacturers of homeopathic and food-supplement products.

But I digress. Naturopathic colleges are similar to chiropractic colleges in that they present a pseudoscientific facade while they train students to practice cult medicine. Their curricula contain courses in basic sciences (anatomy, physiology, and biochemistry), as well as several disease-related courses with names similar to those given at medical schools. But most of the clinical courses involve pseudoscientific practices. (At Bastyr College, for example, the course on oncology includes "alternative therapies for cancer.")

Their libraries are poor in scientific journals and rich in self-serving cult periodicals, trade publications that promote quack remedies, and antiscience cult propaganda tracts. They carry many quackery-promoting books but few scientific rebuttals to them. NCNM's library carries several books detailing the use of laetrile for cancer.

Naturopathy and the Law

The catalogs of both naturopathic colleges say that naturopaths practice in every state under various legal provisions. Seven states, the District of Columbia, and several Canadian provinces have specific licensure laws. Several other states and provinces have right-to-practice laws. In other states, N.D.'s are tolerated but not officially permitted to practice. Naturopaths and their associations are working hard for full national legalization.

   Both naturopathic colleges claim to train fully capable primary-care physicians. The NCNM catalog, for example, says, "Naturopathic physicians as primary care providers are trained to be the doctor first seen by a patient for general health advice, preventive care and diagnosis and treatment of various acute and chronic conditions." The law and the highest education officials in the nation are increasingly going along with this. The United States Department of Education (USDE) recognized the Council on Naturopathic Medical Education (CNME) on an interim basis as an accrediting agency, even though it is recognized by only a few states. Recognition was not made permanent, not because of opposition from organized medicine, but because naturopaths with lesser credentials (such as a correspondence-school diploma) fear restrictions on their practices.

   As licensure spreads, critics of naturopathy may be at increasing risk for antitrust actions. There will probably not be a naturopathic parallel to the *Wilk* v. *AMA* chiropractic case discussed in Chapter 3. Organized medicine has learned its lesson and is unlikely to attempt to eliminate naturopathy or any other nonscientific type of health care that achieves licensure. A nation that condones astrology in the White House and Reaganesque antiregulation mania in all branches of government is unlikely to tolerate "monopolistic" practices by scientific medicine. So the public will have little protection by either the government or responsible professional and scientific associations.

   Naturopathy is a pseudoscientific healing cult and a hazard to the public's health. It has a symbiotic and unethical relationship with the "health food and natural therapeutics" industry, the makers and wholesalers of the snake oils they use. But this doesn't matter to the USDE. In 1974 (when it was called the U.S. Office of Education), it recognized an accrediting agency for chiropractic education—even though in 1968 the U.S. Department of Health, Education, and Welfare had concluded that "chiropractic education does not prepare its practitioners to make an adequate diagnosis and provide appropriate treatment."[41] At that time, the Commissioner of Education said that his actions have nothing to do with the scientific validity or the usefulness of the field of training in question. The important factors are widespread acceptance and facilities, assets, and paperwork that are up to par. Although this received little publicity, the 1968 HEW report drew the same conclusion about naturopathy as it did about chiropractic.

It is frighteningly clear that as America approaches the twenty-first century, any quack healing system, and perhaps any bogus and fraudulent profession of any kind, can legitimize its scam and the teaching of its scam if it can organize itself properly and get its paperwork together sufficiently to please USDE. The mistaken dogmas of chiropractic and naturopathy can maim and kill people. If they, can gain USDE recognition without scientific support, is there any reason that crystal healing, past-life therapy, astrology, palmistry, necromancy, and dozens of other cults based on dogma and superstition can't do the same? In fact, a USDE official has stated that the department would probably recognize an accreditation agency for schools that train astrologers if one were to meet current USDE criteria.[42]

How about schools to teach securities and jewelry fraud? Does it make sense to outlaw selling fake stocks, gold, and diamonds while we have government-sanctioned and subsidized schools promoting bogus cancer and arthritis remedies? What are fancy certificates, metals, and stones compared to human health and life? If we're really going to deregulate to the point of madness, let's at least be consistent. Do not stock swindlers have as much right to their jobs as naturopaths have to theirs? Don't students of jewelry fraud have as much right to loans and scholarships as students of health fraud?

Why do state legislators swallow naturopathic propaganda and allow naturopaths to practice? I don't doubt that the main cause is ignorance. After all, our lawmakers were treated to the same mind-numbing and science-poor education as most Americans. Political corruption, however, may also play a role. After I testified at a Hawaii state legislative hearing regarding a bill on naturopathy, I received an anonymous phone call from a man who claimed to be a good friend of a local naturopath. He said he saw his friend and two other naturopaths each give cash to a key legislator at a campaign fundraising party. He said that his naturopathic friend later told him that the naturopaths had been told how much they had to come up with to secure the lawmaker's vote. They met and agreed on how much each would pay. It was several hundred dollars, depending on the size of the practice. This caller seemed very sincere and genuinely disgusted by the corruption he had witnessed. But I can't rule out the possibility that it may have been a dirty trick, that a naturopath was trying to goad me into libel or slander so I could be sued, discredited, and silenced. If this was the case, it seems equally corrupt.

Corrupt or not, like chiropractic before it, naturopathy has succeeded in writing some of its mystical dogma into state laws. For example, Hawaiian law defines naturopathy as:

> the practice of natural medicine, natural therapeutics, and natural procedures, for the purpose of removing toxic conditions from the body and improving the quality, quantity, harmony, balance, and flow of the vital fluids, vital tissues, and vital energy; and the practice of diagnosing, treating, and caring for patients using a system of practice that bases its treatment of physiological functions and abnormal conditions on natural laws governing the human body."

This is the language of *religion,* not science. "Natural," "toxic," "harmony," "balance," "vital," "abnormal condition," and "natural laws" have special meanings to naturopaths—meanings rooted in their dogma rather than science. Other states that license naturopaths have similar laws.

Another frightening development is a law passed recently in Oregon that allows naturopaths to prescribe a wide variety of antibiotics, hormones, and other potent drugs for the treatment of infections, endocrine disorders, heart disease, hypertension, and other serious diseases. Even cocaine and opium are included on the list. The use of prescription drugs goes against naturopathic dogma and tradition, but it apparently occurred to naturopaths that their scope of practice was too limited. Never mind that naturopaths are not adequately trained in the diagnosis and treatment of conditions calling for the use of the drugs. This preposterous law puts powerful drugs in the hands of unscientific practitioners who now present a greater danger to the public than ever. Will they base their prescriptions of the drugs on such naturopathic diagnostic techniques as applied kinesiology, radionics, and iridology? The Oregon legislature is either corrupt, incredibly gullible, or both.

By legalizing naturopathy, legislatures have written quasi-religious dogma into state laws. It is nonsense to categorize healing methods and professions by their "naturalness." The only attributes that should count are effectiveness and safety as shown by proper studies. Healing methods are either supportable by scientific evidence or they are not. Those that are not should not be supported by public funds, and their practitioners should not be allowed to fraudulently claim that they are scientifically based when, in fact, they are based on cult dogma that is contrary to the facts and hazardous to the health of patients.

References

1. P. Skrabanek: Acupuncture: past, present, and future. In *Examining Holistic Medicine* (D. Stalker and C. Glymour, eds.). Buffalo, Prometheus Books, 1985.
2. National Council Against Health Fraud Bulletin Board. July/Aug, 1989.
3. Acupuncturists cross needles. *Medical Tribune,* Sept. 14, 1989.
4. *Honolulu Star-Bulletin* , Oct. 26, 1987.
5. S.T. Botek: One doctor's acupuncture odyssey. *Medical Tribune,* May 2, 1984.
6. K.T. Frazier: Gallup Poll of beliefs: Astrology up, ESP down. *Skeptical Inquirer* 13:244–245, 1989.
7. The best summaries of the case against astrology are R.B. Culver and P.A. Ianna: *Astrology: True or False? A Scientific Evaluation.* Buffalo, Prometheus Books, 1988; and L.E. Lawrence: *Astrology Disproved,* Prometheus Books, 1977.
8. G.A. Dean et al.: The Guardian Astrology Study: a critique and reanalysis. *Skeptical Inquirer* 9:327–338, 1985.
9. S. Carlson: A double-blind test of astrology. *Nature* 318:419–425, 1985.
10. M. Gauquelin: *Dreams and Illusions of Astrology.* Buffalo, Prometheus Books, 1979, pp 105–107, 119–121.
11. I.W. Kelly et al.: The moon was full and nothing happened: a review of studies on the moon and human behavior and lunar beliefs. *Skeptical Inquirer* 10:129–143, 1985.
12. T. Hines. *Pseudoscience and the Paranormal.* Buffalo, Prometheus Books, 1988.
13. D. Franklin: The Maharishi's medicine man. *In Health,* May/June, 1990.
14. *TM-EX Newsletter,* Spring 1991.
15. S. Silverman: Medical "miracles" still mysterious despite claims of believers. *Psientific American* (Sacramento Skeptics), Sept. 1, 1989.
16. A.B. Zonderman et al.: Depression as a risk for cancer morbidity and mortality in a nationally representative sample. *Journal of the American Medical Association* 262:1191, 1989.
17. Costs are revealed by TX-EX in various publications. See, for example, the essay, History of Ayurveda. Also see reference 26, below.
18. *NCAHF Newsletter,* Jan./Feb., 1991.
19. For an insightful discussion of the philosophy and psychology of Christian Science, see R.J. Brenneman: *Deadly Blessings: Faith Healing on Trial.* Buffalo, Prometheus Books, 1990.
20. The legal situation regarding Christian Science is examined by Rita Swan

in *The Law's Response When Religious Beliefs Against Medical Care Impact on Children,* which is available for $10 from CHILD, P.O. Box 2604, Sioux City, IA 51106.

21. J. Randi: *The Faith Healers.* Buffalo, Prometheus Books, 1987.
22. G. Cerminara: *Many Mansions.* New York, New American Library, 1950.
23. T. Sugru: *There Is a River.* New York, Dell, 1974.
24. M.E. Carter and W.A. McGarey: *Edgar Cayce on Healing.* New York, Paperback Library, 1972.
25. Excerpts from the Edgar Cayce Records. A.R.E., 1957.
26. J. Randi: *Flim-Flam.* Buffalo, Prometheus Books, 1982.
27. W.A. Nolen: *Healing: A Doctor in Search of a Miracle.* New York, Random House, 1974.
28. Dr. Nolen's book (reference 27) reports that a Philippine physician who tracked Agpaoa's activities closely estimated that he saw hundreds of patients each month and collected an average "donation" of at least $200 per patient, giving him an income of over $40,000 a month.
29. P. Kurtz et al.: Testing psi claims in China: visit of CSICOP delegation. *Skeptical Inquirer* 12:364–366, 1988.
30. Herbalife agrees to pay $850,000 penalty. *Nutrition Forum* 4:15, 1987.
31. *NCAHF Newsletter,* July/Aug., 1990.
32. J. Raso: The shady business of Nature's Sunshine. *Nutrition Forum* 9:17–23, 1992.
33. T.L. Bradford: *The Life and Letters of Samuel Hahnemann.* Philadelphia, Broericke and Tafel, 1895, p. 304, as reported in reference 36, below.
34. N. Puddephatt: *The Homeopathic Materia Medica: How It Should Be Studied.* Rustington, England, Health Sciences Press, 1982.
35. O.W. Holmes: Homeopathy. Excerpted in *Examining Holistic Medicine* (D. Stalker and C. Glymour, eds.). Buffalo, Prometheus Books, 1985.
36. D. Ullman: *Homeopathy for the 21st Century.* Berkeley, North Atlantic Books, 1988.
37. Adulterated homeopathic cure for asthma. *Lancet,* April 12, 1986, pp. 862–863.
38. Homeopathic remedies: these 19th century medicines offer safety, even charm, but efficacy is another matter. *Consumer Reports* 52:60–62, 1987.
39. Bilateral nasal specific. *NCAHF Newsletter,* Jan./Feb., 1985.
40. Bastyr College cites Bradford donations. *The Choice* 15(1,2): 33, 1989.
41. *Independent practitioners under Medicare: A Report to Congress.* Washington, D.C., U. S. Department of Health, Education, and Welfare, 1968.
42. Is the bureaucracy mooning science? *NCAHF Newsletter,* May/June 1990.

5

More Snake Oils, Scams, and Wild-Goose Chases

This chapter is a handy guide to "alternative medicine's" bag of tricks. Along with the diets and healing systems discussed in previous chapters, these are the stock-in-trade of the quackery industry. I wish I could say the list is complete, but quacks dream up new ways to steal your money every day. Nevertheless, this chapter should answer your questions about many of today's leading health scams. The following are included, in alphabetical order: "alternative" cancer therapies, amino acids and protein supplements, applied kinesiology, aromatherapy, Bach Flower Remedies, barley green, bee pollen, BHT, biorhythms, blood type → personality type, body wraps and contour creams, carnitine, carnivora, catalyst-altered water, cell salts, cell therapy, chelation therapy, Chinese herbal remedies, chlorophyll, clinical ecology, colonic lavage, colostrum, cranial osteopathy, cryonics, crystal healing, cytotoxic testing, dental-amalgam phobia, diet pills and potions, diet sodas, DMSO, electrical muscle stimulation, fasting, Feingold diet, firewalking, fish oils, fluoride phobia, fructose, germanium, Gerovital, "glandulars," grapefruit, hair analysis, herbs, hydrogen peroxide, "hypoglycemia," ion generators, iridology, Jason Winters products, Kirlian photography, lecithin, live cell analysis, mineral supplements, "organically grown" foods, oxygen inhalation, "pangamic acid," past-life therapy, radionics, raw milk, rebirthing, royal jelly, seawater, snake blood, snake venom, spirulina, sports drinks, subliminal persuasion, superoxide dismutase, tanning pills, therapeutic touch, UFO abduction therapy, vitamin supplements, wheat germ oil, and yeast syndrome.

"Alternative" Cancer Therapies

In *Healing: A Doctor in Search of a Miracle* [Random House, 1973], Dr. William Nolen tells of Mary, a thirty-five-year-old mother of three who had early, treatable cancer of the cervix. Radiation and surgery frightened her, so when she heard that laetrile could cure cancer, she decided to try it. If it didn't work, she reasoned, she could go back for standard therapy. Neither her husband nor Dr. Nolen could dissuade her. She spent about $1,000 per month for the treatment. By the sixth month, she was bleeding every day and losing strength. She returned to Dr. Nolen and requested surgery, but by then the cancer had spread throughout the pelvis. She died a month later. There have been many such cases.

Cancer quackery is among the most widespread and lucrative types of quackery. It is also among the most despicable. Its victims are desperate and vulnerable and, therefore, easy prey for those promising false hope at a high price. There are so many varieties of cancer quackery that a thorough discussion would require a book. Fortunately, two books on the subject have been published within the past two years. *Unconventional Cancer Treatment,* prepared by the U.S. Office of Technology Assessment, is a comprehensive study of dietary, herbal, psychological, pharmacologic, and other approaches to cancer that have become substantial industries despite lack of evidence that they work. *Dubious Cancer Treatment,* published by the Florida Division of the American Cancer Society, is based on a seminar in which experts from all over the country shared the results of their investigations.

Proponents of cancer quackery like to refer to their methods as "alternatives." However, since ineffective methods are not true alternatives to effective ones, the terms "unscientific," "nonscientific," "dubious," "questionable," or "quack" are more appropriate. Regardless of what we call it, the problem of cancer quackery is so serious that the American Cancer Society has a Committee on Questionable Methods and publishes reports on many such methods.

The society defines questionable methods as "lifestyle practices, clinical tests, or therapeutic modalities that are promoted for *general* use for the prevention, diagnosis, or treatment, of cancer and which are, on the basis of careful review by scientists and/or clinicians, not deemed proven nor recommended for current use." Here are a few thoughts about some of the currently used methods the American Cancer Society has evaluated.

Many salves, poultices, and plasters have been applied directly to tumors with the hope of burning them away. The Hoxsey method, available at a clinic in Mexico, includes a product of this type. In recent years scientists have found chemicals that can destroy some superficial skin cancers. Except for that, however, corrosive agents are worthless against cancer.

Pau d'arco tea, sold through "health food" stores and by mail, is said to be an ancient Inca Indian remedy prepared from the inner bark of various species of *Tabebuia*, an evergreen tree native to the West Indies and Central and South America. Proponents claim that pau d'arco tea is effective against cancer and many other ailments. *Tabebuia* woods contains lapachol, a chemical recognized as an antitumor agent. However, human studies have found that as soon as significant blood levels are attained, undesirable effects were severe enough to require that the drug be stopped. Varro E. Tyler, Ph.D., a leading authority on plant medicine, has noted that pau d'arco's "lack of proven effectiveness, potential toxicity, and high cost ($12 to $50 per package) render its use both unwise and extravagant."[1]

Many dietary approaches have been recommended, including fasting, megadoses of nutrients, consumption of raw foods, and various complicated dietary regimens. Proponents of the Gerson diet claim to accomplish "detoxification" by daily enemas and a diet consisting primarily of fresh fruit and vegetable juices. This method was developed by Dr. Max Gerson, a German-born physician who emigrated to the United States in 1936. The treatment, available in Mexico, is still actively promoted by Gerson's daughter, Charlotte Gerson Straus. Although she claims high cure rates, there is no evidence that the clinic actually keeps track of its patients after they leave the clinic.[2]

The macrobiotic diet is a semivegetarian approach claimed to cure cancer and many other health problems. There is no evidence that it works, but there is evidence that it is nutritionally inadequate for cancer patients.[3]

Many questionable promoters treat cancer patients with oxygen-rich compounds (germanium sesquioxide, hydrogen peroxide, and ozone). Their use is based on the erroneous concept that cancer is caused by oxygen deficiency and can be cured by exposing cancer cells to more oxygen than they can tolerate. These compounds have been the subject of legitimate scientific research. However, there is little or no evidence that they are effective for the treatment of any serious disease.[4]

"Antineoplastons" is the name given by Stanislaw R. Burzynski, M.D., to substances that he claims can "normalize" cancer cells that are constantly being produced within the body. He has published many papers in which he claims that antineoplastins extracted from urine or synthesized in his laboratory have proven effective against cancer in laboratory experiments. He also claims to have helped many people with cancer get well. A detailed analysis of Dr. Burzynski's claims has been written by Saul Green, Ph.D., a biochemist who worked for many years at Memorial Sloan-Kettering Hospital doing research into the mechanisms and treatment of cancer. Dr. Green does not believe that any of the substances Dr. Burzynski calls "antineoplastons" has been proven to "normalize" tumor cells.[5]

Cancell is a dark brown liquid said to "digest cancer cells." The FDA states that it is composed of ordinary chemicals, including nitric acid, sodium sulfite, potassium hydroxide, sulfuric acid, and catechol. There is no scientific evidence that Cancell is effective against cancer or any other disease. The FDA has taken its promoters to court to try to stop its distribution.

Laetrile, a drug that achieved great notoriety during the 1970s and early 1980s, is the trade name for a synthetic relative of amygdalin, a cyanide-containing chemical in the kernels of apricot pits, apple seeds, bitter almonds, and some other stone fruits and nuts. Many laetrile promoters have called it "vitamin B_{17}" and claimed that cancer is actually a vitamin deficiency disease that laetrile can cure. The cyanide, they say, is harmless to healthy tissue but deadly to cancer cells. They also claim that laetrile has been suppressed by government and orthodox medicine in order to perpetuate the profits of the cancer research and treatment industries. The facts are otherwise. Many studies in laboratory animals conducted at prestigious laboratories have failed to detect any beneficial effects of laetrile on cancers.[6] Several studies of case reports of patients treated with laetrile have concluded that it didn't work. And a controlled study on cancer patients at the Mayo Clinic found no anticancer effect but found significant blood levels of cyanide in some of the patients.[7]

"Metabolic therapy" is a loosely defined approach whose proponents claim to diagnose abnormalities at the cellular level and correct them by normalizing the patient's metabolism. According to its proponents, cancer and other "degenerative" diseases are the result of metabolic imbalance caused by a buildup of "toxic substances" in the body. (They claim that scientific practitioners merely treat the symptoms of the disease while they treat the cause by removing "toxins" and strengthening the immune system so the body can heal itself. Of course, the "toxins" are neither defined nor objectively measurable.) "Metabolic" treatment regimens include diets, enemas, vitamins, minerals, glandulars, enzymes, and various nostrums that are not legally marketable in the United States. Some regimens include laetrile. No scientific study has ever shown that "metabolic therapy" or any of its components is beneficial against cancer.[8]

Revici Cancer Control (also called lipid therapy) is based on the notion that cancer is caused by an imbalance between constructive (anabolic) and destructive (catabolic) body processes. Its proponent has been Emmanuel Revici, M.D., an elderly physician who practices in New York City. His treatment is said to be based on his interpretation of the specific gravity, pH (acidity), and surface tension of single samples of the patient's urine. Revici also claims success against AIDS. Scientists who have offered to evaluate Revici's methods have never been able to reach an agreement with him on procedures to ensure a valid test. However, his method of urinary interpretation is obviously invalid. The specific gravity of urine reflects the concentration of dissolved substances and depends mainly on the amount of fluid a person consumes. Urine acidity depends mainly on diet, but varies considerably throughout the day. Thus the acidity of a single sample of urine can provide no useful information about a patient's metabolism. The surface tension of urine has no medically recognized diagnostic value.[9]

Immuno-augmentative therapy (IAT) was developed by Lawrence Burton, Ph.D., a zoologist who states that IAT can control cancer by restoring natural immune defenses. He claims to accomplish this by injecting protein extracts isolated with processes he has patented. However, experts believe that the substances he claims to use cannot be produced by these procedures and have not been demonstrated to exist in the human body. He has not published detailed clinical reports, divulged the details of his methods, published meaningful statistics, conducted a controlled trial, or provided independent investigators with specimens of his treatment materials for analysis. During the mid-1980s, several cases were reported of patients of Dr. Burton who developed serious infections following IAT.[10]

Hariton Alivizatos, a Greek physician who died in 1991, claimed to have developed a blood test that could determine the type, location, and severity of any cancers.[11] He also claimed to have developed a "serum" that helped the patient's immune system destroy cancer cells, and helped the body rejuvenate parts destroyed by cancer. Although he did not publicly reveal the contents of his "serum," knowledgeable observers believe that its main ingredient was niacin.

Virginia Livingston, M.D., who died in 1990, postulated that cancer is caused by a bacterium that invades the body when resistance is lowered. She claimed to strengthen the body's immune system with various vaccines (including one made from the patient's urine), a vegetarian diet, vitamin and mineral supplements, visualization, and stress reduction. She claimed to have a very high recovery rate but published no clinical data to support this. Researchers at the University of Pennsylvania Cancer Center who compared seventy-eight patients with advanced cancer treated at the university center with seventy-eight similar patients treated at the Livingston-Wheeler Clinic found no difference between average survival time of the two groups. However, patients in the Livingston-Wheeler program reported more pain and difficulty with their appetite.[12]

O. Carl Simonton, M.D., Bernie Siegel, M.D., and several others claim that meditation and mental imagery techniques can benefit cancer patients. But they have published no controlled studies that support their theories.[13] Simonton theorizes that the brain can stimulate endocrine glands to inspire the immune system to attack cancer cells. His system for motivating "positive attitudes" includes having patients imagine their cancer cells being destroyed by their own immune systems. Basically, the technique involves thinking of benefiting from therapy, enjoying health, standing in a beautiful environment, and other favorable events. Although "positive attitudes" may prolong life if they inspire people to cooperate with recommended treatment regimens, there is no scientific evidence that the progression or regression of tumors is related to the patient's mood. Although meditation and the like may help people relax, people who use imagery *instead* of proven treatment are buying themselves a death sentence. Critics have also blasted the idea that suppression of the immune system is a major cause of cancer. If it were, AIDS patients (whose immune systems certainly fail) would develop the common forms of cancer. But they don't. The cancers they develop are otherwise quite rare.

Amino Acids and Protein Supplements

Amino acids are the nitrogen-containing building blocks of proteins. The body uses them to make muscle, bone, and other tissues and organs, as well as hormones and enzymes. Twenty-two amino acids are used to make the proteins essential to human life. Some can be made from others (plus metabolic scraps of carbohydrates), so only nine are required in the adult diet. These are known as the essential amino acids. All protein-containing foods contain them, even grains and potatoes. Anyone who eats normally gets more than enough amino acids. This simple fact has not prevented the "health food" industry from peddling isolated amino acids in pills, powders, and potions claimed to be wonder cures for herpes, depression, obesity, pain, fatigue, insomnia, aging, small muscles, and dozens of other problems.

None of these claims for amino acid supplements has been proven, but widespread use of the products has led to several tragedies and could well cause more. In 1989, the amino acid L-tryptophan began triggering an epidemic of eosinophilia-myalgia syndrome (EMS), a previously rare disorder character-ized by severe muscle and joint pain, weakness, swelling of the arms and legs, fever, skin rash, and increased numbers of eosinophils in the blood. More than 1,500 people are known to have become seriously ill—some paralyzed—and more than twenty deaths have been reported.[14] L-tryptophan had been illegally promoted as a remedy for insomnia, depression, and several other conditions.

Although it appears that the trouble was caused by a contaminant in the manufacturing process of the leading bulk manufacturer, a few cases have been reported in people who took supplements of lysine, another amino acid.[15]

There is good theoretical reason to be leery of amino acid supplements. Amino acids compete with each other for absorption into the body and into the cells. A large excess of one amino acid can suppress absorption and utilization of others that are just as essential. Our digestive and metabolic mechanisms evolved over millions of years of eating natural foods. Our bodies have a certain wisdom. Why should we monkey around with their efficient mechanisms on the word of some pill peddler? These are theoretical concerns, but animal studies have bolstered these fears enough so that way back in 1972 the FDA warned that isolated amino acids could be dangerous and banned their sale unless they were proven safe. In 1974 the agency officially removed them from its Generally Recognized as Safe (GRAS) list.

Unfortunately, the FDA action had little effect. No one knows how much harm the products may have done. Imbalances of amino acid levels induced by supplements could produce delayed symptoms that would be difficult to trace to the supplements. Accelerated aging of the kidneys, for example, would not have serious consequences for many years.

Excessive intake of whole proteins is also unwise. Bodybuilders and athletes who gorge on meat, fish, and protein powders in an effort to build their muscles are undoubtedly doing themselves more harm than good. Muscle mass is built in response to exercise, not the level of protein in the diet. Grossly excessive intake of protein for prolonged periods may damage the kidneys and have other harmful effects.

The New York City Department of Consumer Affairs has warned consumers to beware of terms like "fat burner," "fat fighter," "fat metabolizer," "energy enhancer," " performance booster," "strength booster," " ergogenic aid," " anabolic optimizer," and "genetic optimizer." Manufacturers surveyed by the department were unable to provide a single published report from a scientific journal to back the claims that their products did any of these things.[16] Calling the bodybuilding supplement industry "an economic hoax with unhealthy consequences," the department issued "Notices of Violation" to six companies and challenged the FDA to clean up the marketplace nationwide.

Applied Kinesiology

Applied kinesiology (AK) is the brainchild of a chiropractor named George Goodheart. According to AK theory, weakness and disease in vital organs can be detected as weakness in muscles allegedly associated with those organs.

Trained applied kinesiologists (AKers) purport to diagnose a wide variety of health problems with muscle-testing techniques. Moreover, they can then treat the diseases with spinal manipulation, acupressure, special diets, dietary supplements, and whatever else they happen to believe in.

One account of the system is the book *MRT* [Marek, 1979], by chiropractor Mark Grinims and acupuncturist Walter Fischman. They promise that their system will determine exactly which nutrients your body requires and which foods, cosmetics, fabrics, and chemicals you are allergic to. All this without testing your blood, analyzing your diet, or having you eat or inhale any substances. They also claim that the "revolutionary" system of "muscle response testing" (MRT) will directly diagnose diseases, even in babies and animals.

Whether called applied kinesiology or muscle response testing, this silly pseudoscience is used by many chiropractors, naturopaths, oriental medicine practitioners, and assorted cranks. The essence of AK is this: a subject to be tested stands erect with one arm relaxed and the other held straight out with the palm down. The tester presses down on the subject's wrist for a second or two and gauges the resistance to the pressure. Now a finger of the subject's free hand is stuck into a bottle of aspirin (for example) so it is in contact with the tablets. The extended arm immediately weakens, we are told, because aspirin is a poison and the body's "aura" somehow senses this.

AK practitioners also claim that nutritional deficiencies, allergies, and other adverse reactions to food substances can be detected by placing substances in the mouth so that the patient salivates. "Good" substances will make specific muscles stronger, whereas "bad" substances will cause specific weaknesses. A series of tests for nutrients can take many hours over a period of days or even weeks. Since our requirements supposedly change often, retesting at least every two months is recommended. As if this were not enough, the procedure is also recommended for a long list of suspected allergens that could cause vague but serious problems without our knowledge. Some AKers even claim that testing can reveal what music and colors we should favor or avoid.

There is not a shred of evidence that muscles can be affected in this magical manner. We are supposed to accept the dogma on faith. The subjective sense of resistance is obviously no measurement. Even if it were, or if accurate measurement were made with instruments, many variables can affect muscle strength from moment to moment, including the subject's or even the tester's knowledge of the substance being tested. Belief in such nonsense can have tragic consequences. Based on AK testing, a Canadian physician assured a mother that her two young children were not allergic to peanut butter. She took them home and gave each a tiny amount on bread. They both collapsed and almost died from anaphylactic shock, a potentially lethal allergic response.[17]

Chiropractors typically invent silly systems of diagnosis and treatment and promote them to the public without the most rudimentary testing for validity, safety, and effectiveness. It would seem that an eighth grader capable of a little critical thinking would realize that a few simple tests could show whether AK has any validity. But chiropractors (and naturopaths) have accepted AK without testing its most fundamental assumptions. This was left to real scientists.

In a study that advocates should have done many years ago, the abilities of experienced AK practitioners were tested. It was determined that (1) AKers don't agree with each other in their diagnoses, (2) AK is not accurate in determining vitamin or mineral status as determined by blood and tissue studies, and (3) AK testing of muscle strength does not give accurate results.[18] In other words, applied kinesiology is a fantasy based on magical thinking typical of chiropractors. Its promotion to the public as a valid diagnostic tool is another in a long list of frauds perpetrated by "alternative" practitioners.

Aromatherapy

Aromatherapy is a semiautonomous branch of herbalism that uses aromatic oils from roots, flowers, barks, leaves, and resins. These are diluted with vegetable oil, and the mixtures are rubbed into the skin, used as inhalants, or (rarely) ingested. The treatments are alleged to prevent and cure scores of ailments including many serious diseases. There is no evidence whatsoever to support these claims. Therapists often determine what oil to use by using a lock of hair or a handwriting sample from the patient in a dowsing (divining) ritual. The application of the chosen remedy is likely to be equally irrational. One favorite method is to massage the oil into the area of the spine that allegedly corresponds to the area of the body allegedly responsible for the symptoms.

Although it is hard to believe that anyone is foolish enough to believe that aromatherapy is effective against serious disorders, the therapy is surely harmless in itself. No doubt it also has placebo power with its "therapists," rituals, and strong aromas, so it might afford pain relief in some cases. However, it should not be used instead of proper medical care. Any severe or persistent symptom should be evaluated by a medical doctor.

The concept of aromatherapy may hold great commercial promise for the cosmetics industry, an industry with a long history of deceiving the public. Major firms are developing and test-marketing colognes, shampoos, aftershave lotions, and the like, allegedly for stimulating, relaxing, or otherwise affecting mood and thereby helping health. Major battles with regulatory agencies and critical health professionals may be looming.

Bach Flower Remedies

Dr. Edward Bach was a British physician who converted to homeopathy as a young man in the 1920s. He soon retreated further into unreason and developed a medical system all his own. He claimed that he could divine or intuit the effects of ingesting a flower by simply holding a hand over the flower. Using this mystical knowledge he came up with thirty-eight remedies, alcohol solutions of the volatile oils of thirty-eight flowers.

Each Bach Flower Remedy is touted for the treatment of a specific negative emotional state such as procrastination, jealousy, guilt, depression, anxiety, loneliness, and shyness. But the medicines are not just for the treatment of unhappiness in its various forms. Bach also believed that all physical disorders have their roots in the mind, and if the basic mental problems can be corrected, any disease can be overcome.

In the United States, Bach remedies are distributed by Ellon Bach, USA, Inc, of Lynbrook, New York. The company's promotional flyers claim that modern medicine has "confirmed Bach's findings"; that the remedies have been proven safe and effective; and that they are widely used by doctors, dentists, nurses, and other health professionals. Promoters even claim that the products are great for animals (including fish) and plants. They apparently believe that animals and plants have the same mental tendencies as humans and can use the same medicines to overcome apathy, grief, resentment, and so on.

Ellon Bach, which also sells wall charts and books promoting the Bach Remedies, claims that the remedies "are a complete system of emotional stress relief" and that "emotions play a major role in the progression of nearly all disease." A 1986 issue of *The Edward Bach Healing Society Newsletter,* which has the same mailing address as Ellon Bach U.S.A., contains an article on the use of Bach Remedies for children. Among other things, the author recommends three remedies for sibling rivalry, three for temper tantrums, and four for children who are bullied.

The claims made for the Bach Remedies are not only unsubstantiated but preposterous. Yet the ingredients in the products are officially recognized as nonprescription drugs and are listed in the *Homeopathic Pharmacopeia of the United States.* They illustrate how the FDA's tolerance of homeopathy is enabling worthless medicines to be marketed to an unsuspecting public. Since the alleged effects of the flowers are based on intuition (fantasy) rather than scientific studies, anyone can play the game. Other companies are now marketing scores of flower essence remedies with claims rivaling those of the Bach Remedies.

Barley Green

"Barley green" is a powder made by squeezing the juice from young barley leaves and letting the water evaporate. The remaining powder is sold as a miracle food that allegedly increases health, vitality, and longevity. The product is sold throughout the United States through a pyramid sales scheme. Promotional literature and sales talks are loaded with false and misleading claims. Barley green is said to be a rich source of important nutrients including sixteen vitamins, eight essential amino acids, vitamin B_{12}, superoxide dismutase (SOD), and chlorophyll, which allegedly helps cure anemia. The vitamin claim is remarkable because there are only thirteen vitamins, and barley green is not a good source of any of them. The product has minimal amounts of amino acids. SOD is an enzyme made in our cells; we do not need to ingest it. If we do, it is simply digested and has no significant effects. Chlorophyll has no role in the human body and also is digested rather than absorbed intact into the body.

Barley green is also marketed as a panacea that can cure many diseases, including arthritis and cancer. There is no evidence whatsoever for the claims. To buttress the phony case for their product, barley green promotional literature falsely claimed that research on the product was done by a "Research Professor" named Dr. Yasuo Hotta at the University of California. As it turns out, Hotta was not a professor and didn't do research on barley green at U.C. He did work in a biology research lab at U.C. San Diego, but the work had nothing to do with either barley green or nutrition.[19]

Bee Pollen

Bee pollen is heavily promoted as a superfood, especially for boosting athletic performance, but with many other health benefits as well. The pollen is gathered by bees and stripped from them by devices placed in the hives. Since the pollen comes from many flowers, its composition and nutritional value vary considerably with location and time of year. Sugar is the main component, accounting for at least 50 percent of the weight. Protein, fat, and water are the other major components. Pollen also contains some vitamins and minerals.

Bee pollen propagandists claim that thrity-two grams of pollen (about three tablespoons) supply all the protein and vitamins one needs daily. A typical batch of pollen contains about 20 percent protein, or about six of the thirty-two grams, a small fraction of the RDA. The DNA, RNA, and enzymes are often cited as "essential biofactors" of great benefit to health, but they have very little nutritional or other value. They are simply digested and used for energy.

Pollen can cause reactions from sniffles to anaphylactic shock in those allergic to it or any of its many contaminants. Besides containing pollen from several types of flowers, the products often are contaminated with insects, their feces and eggs, rodent debris, fungi, and bacteria. Persons allergic to bees are perhaps most at risk since the pollen is mixed with nectar and carried between the insect's legs. Some pollen products feature pollen gathered directly from flowers, so they contain no bee body parts. Nevertheless, allergic reactions to the pollen are still possible.

Pollen promoters claim that pollen improves athletic performance and stamina. They have lots of anecdotes and testimonials, but no scientific studies. In a study at Louisiana State University, half the members of the swimming team took ten pollen tablets a day for six months, one quarter took five pollen and five placebo tablets, and one quarter took ten placebo tablets. No measurable difference in performance was found among the three groups. The study was then repeated with groups of swimmers and high-school cross-country runners. Again, taking bee pollen conferred no measurable benefit.[20]

Some promoters have proclaimed bee pollen a cure for many health problems, including hair loss, failing memory, alcoholism, eye problems, diabetes, and much more. Sometimes they refer to "Russian studies" and "secret documents" to imply that Soviet-affiliated countries have used pollen for many purposes but want to keep it secret because it gives their athletes, and possibly their soldiers, an edge. Such claims are cynical marketing ploys.

BHT

BHT (butylated hydroxytoluene) is an antioxidant widely used as a food preservative. Because it is under suspicion as a liver toxin, its use is not allowed in some countries. While there is no evidence of harm at the very low doses consumed in foods, animal studies show large doses can be lethal. Nevertheless, Pearson and Shaw's book *Life Extension* recommends huge doses of BHT as a herpes remedy. This has helped create a market for BHT pills. Some "health food" stores, most of which avoid foods with traces of BHT added to prevent rancidity, peddle megadoses of BHT in pill form. There is no evidence that BHT helps the herpes sufferer, but this "remedy" has landed some people in the hospital. Symptoms of BHT poisoning include severe abdominal cramping, nausea, vomiting, weakness, dizziness, confusion, and loss of consciousness.[21]

Biorhythms

The theory of biorhythms holds that there are three fixed cycles in the waxing and waning of our abilities and attributes.[22] The cycles are the physical, the emotional, and the intellectual. To make interpretations or predictions, the three cycles are plotted as curves on a graph. They all start at baseline level at birth, but from then on they are generally out of synch because the cycles have different lengths, twenty-three days, twenty-eight days, and thirty-three days, respectively. Performance during the half of each cycle above the baseline is allegedly better than performance on "down days." Moreover, a "critical day" is one in which a rhythm is changing from the up phase to the down phase or vice versa. Double and triple critical days are especially dreaded. These notions have given rise to a biorhythms industry that peddles books, calculators, games, and the like. Believers are said to use biorhythm charts to make personal and business decisions and to schedule travel, surgery, and other events.

There are, of course, many examples of biological rhythms: heartbeats, respiration, body temperature, sleep-wake cycles, ovulatory and menstrual cycles, and so on. But none of them is immutable. They all vary between individuals and for given individuals at different times. The concept of three fixed cycles that are the same for everyone at all times is preposterous. Moreover, scientific studies thoroughly refute it. Several studies of industrial accidents, aviation accidents, automobile accidents, worker productivity, and performance in a variety of sports show no correlation of performance with biorhythms.[23] It's just another superstition that is exploited for profit.

Blood Type → Personality Type

In Japan it is widely believed that personality is determined by the individual's blood type. People with type A blood are said to be industrious, punctual, good employees, patriotic, and patient. Those with type B blood are believed to be creative, inventive, passionate, individualistic, and anti-establishment. Those with type O blood are supposedly aggressive, realistic, optimistic, eloquent, and athletic. Hundreds of blood-type subfactors allegedly correlate with other personality traits. The concept is used in business, sports, romance, fashion, and other areas of life. Vending machines dispense daily readings for each type, much like astrology columns do in the U.S.

False doctrines are always inherently dangerous, but this blood-type theory may pose a social hazard as well as a physical one. Japanese proponents claim that in automobile factories, for example, engineers should be type A's, salesmen type O's, and idea men type B's. And the rare type AB's tend to have psychic powers, so they could be useful in special ways. The theory and the stereotypes have been popularized by Toshitaka Nomi of Tokyo and her late father Masahiko Nomi, a former medical professor at Tokyo University. They claim to have done decades of research and to have lots of data to support their contentions.

The concept has been brought to the United States in *You Are Your Blood Type* [Simon and Schuster, 1988], a book coauthored by Toshitaka Nomi and Californian Alexander Besher. I doubt that the book will inspire American employers to discriminate on the basis of blood types, but you never know.

Body Wraps and Contour Creams

Vegetable oils rubbed on the skin are not absorbed or incorporated into fatty tissue beneath the skin. Nor do people gain weight from oily suntan lotions and moisturizers. Yet millions of people buy the opposite idea—that rubbing various substances into the skin can get fat to come out. Fraudulent television and newspaper ads promote creams alleged to be effective for spot-reducing and body-wrap clinics that promise fantastic rates of weight loss. In the clinics, clients are covered with lotions containing vitamins and herbs, then wrapped up like mummies in plastic wrap. An hour or so later they are unwrapped, told they look better, and measured with a tape to "prove" the effectiveness of the treatment. (Of course, the tape is held more tightly after the treatment than before it.) The whole business, of course, is nonsense—as are sweat suits advertised for weight loss. The most this gimmickry can do is cause temporary weight loss due to evaporation of water from the body. The weight returns when the person rehydrates. Wrapping the entire body is not a good idea because it can cause overheating.

Carnitine

Carnitine is an amino acid that plays a role in fat metabolism. It is synthesized in the body from the amino acids lysine and methionine, so it is normally not necessary in the diet. In certain extremely rare congenital metabolic defects, however, as well as in some endocrine diseases and a few other conditions, carnitine deficiency can develop. In these cases carnitine supplements can be life-saving. Persons with heart disease may also benefit from supplements. However, anyone who needs carnitine supplements should be under the care of a physician and should use the prescription product Carnitor. The over-the-counter products sold in drugstores and "health food" stores may be subpotent and ineffective.

There is no evidence that carnitine supplements benefit anyone whose body makes normal amounts of it, which includes almost everyone. Nevertheless, it is not surprising that the "health food" industry has seized upon it as a miracle "vitamin" and now hucksters it as an aid to weight control, a preventer of heart disease, a booster of athletic performance, an energy enhancer, and an antiaging nutrient. None of these claims is supported by scientific evidence.

Carnivora

Carnivora is a patented extract of the insect-eating plant Venus's-flytrap. German physician Helmut Keller started using the extract on cancer patients in the 1980s and claimed some favorable results. German tabloids trumpeted the "miracle cancer cure," and demand for it skyrocketed in Europe. Desperate cancer patients pay $1,000 per week and more for the drug. German cancer specialists, however, say that Carnivora is worthless and that the whole affair is a delusion or a scam. Delusions and scams have a way of catching on with the public, so the Venus's-flytrap, with its limited population, may join the list of species endangered by health fraud and greed.

"Catalyst-Altered Water"

In 1980 the CBS show "60 Minutes" did a tongue-in-cheek story about some miracle water developed by John Willard, Professor Emeritus of the South Dakota School of Mines and Technology. Willard added a little castor oil, Epsom salt, sodium metasilicate, and calcium chloride to ordinary water and started marketing it as a miracle cure for everything that ails humans, animals, and plants. It was called Willard's Water and Catalyst Altered Water.

In 1982 the FDA prohibited Willard, his company, Catalyst Altered Water Industries, and all distributors from making unfounded claims about the product. More recently the product has been distributed by Fountain of Youth

International Trust, whose head is "Dr." Russ Michael. He calls himself "Dr." on the basis of a Doctor of Divinity from the Church of Humanity, which he founded. His literature claims that the product is an effective treatment for dozens of diseases and that it increases the lifespan of cells, increases the rate of protein production, and removes wrinkles. There is no evidence for the claims; it's all a preposterous scam.

Cell Salts

Also known as "tissue salts," these are infinitesimally small doses of common salts of magnesium, phosphorus, sodium, chloride, and potassium dissolved in a water-alcohol solution or mixed with lactose in tiny pills. They are not labeled as ordinary sodium chloride, magnesium phosphate, potassium sulfate, and the like. Rather, they are "natrum muriaticum," "magnesia phosphorica," "kali sulphuricum," et cetera, as though they are something special. After all, everyone knows sodium chloride is common table salt. Who would believe that a single grain could cure depression, headaches, constipation, anemia, hay fever, and the other symptoms it is advertised for? The so-called cell salts, promoted as cures for a wide variety of ailments, are available in much larger doses in a few bites of practically all common foods. The claims that these products are nutritionally significant, pharmacologically active, or in any way beneficial are complete nonsense. Their fancy names are terms used by alchemists several centuries ago.

Cell Therapy

Also known as live cell therapy, fresh cell therapy, and cellular therapy, the original "cell therapy" was invented by Swiss surgeon Dr. Paul Niehans, who died in 1971. Niehans created Clinique La Prairie in Montreux, Switzerland, a spa that specializes in injections of fetal lamb cells for the purpose of "rejuvenation." Cures of various diseases as well as greater fitness, libido, skin health, and general well-being, are said to result from the shots. The clinic has had dozens of celebrity clients, which has enhanced its mystique and increased its popularity—with the wealthy, that is, since the costs start at about $10,000. The clinic is so popular that reservations must be made months in advance.

Naturally, the tremendous financial success of Clinique La Prairie (CLP) has inspired imitators. CLP uses cells taken from fetal lambs whose mothers are slaughtered. It takes six animals for one series of treatments, three lambs and their mothers. But if lamb cells work, why not other fetuses and young animals? Why not cows, pigs, cats, and dogs? And who is to say what tissues are to be used and how they are to be prepared and administered? Various distasteful and grisly variations can be imagined, and some have begun to show up in fringe clinics and the mail-order marketplace. If competition drives down the price within range of the middle class, this form of quackery could become widespread and indeed goulish.

Although the large profits could provide adequate funds for research, neither CLP nor anyone else has done scientific studies, and there is no evidence the treatments do anything beneficial. They can, however, cause harm. Fever, fatigue, and pain at the injection site are common side effects. Viruses and other microbes may be transmitted from the animal to the patient, causing infection. Cell therapy can also cause severe allergic reactions and arthritis. These risks are very real. Any benefits, on the other hand, are surely illusory.

Christiaan Barnard, South Africa's pioneer heart transplant surgeon, who has served as director of research for CLP, has taken the treatment himself for arthritis and claims the injections exert an antiaging effect by promoting the repair of cellular damage. He has acknowledged that proof is lacking, but has promised it will come forth. In 1988 Barnard said, "within a year, we will have definite scientific evidence to prove forever that it's not a hoax."[24]

As we go to press, however, proof is still lacking that cell therapy is good for anything except making its promoters wealthy. In fact, in 1990, at least one scientific study showed that cell therapy had no effect on Down's syndrome children, for which it is often promoted. The study compared those treated with cell therapy to those not so treated. No improvement was found in IQ, motor skills, memory, language, social skills, or growth.[25] Such negative results are the likely outcome in all such studies. The treatment has been used for decades on thousands of people and has generated millions of dollars. Positive results, if they exist, should have been unequivocally demonstrated by now. Dr. Barnard's involvement with cell therapy is proof that even a highly-skilled and celebrated surgeon, a pioneer in his field, can succumb to fantasy and fuzzy thinking.

Chelation Therapy

The drug EDTA (ethylene diamine tetraacetic acid, or edetic acid) is a chelating agent, which, when injected intravenously, can attach itself to certain minerals and take them out of the body through excretion in the urine. EDTA is used to treat poisoning with lead, cadmium, and other toxic metals and to treat iron overdosage. In these uses there is always a danger of kidney damage that can lead to death. Although the FDA can regulate claims that manufacturers make about their products, it cannot stop licensed physicians from using approved drugs for unproven uses.

During the past few decades, some physicians have been using EDTA to treat coronary artery disease, angina, and other manifestations of atherosclerosis, as well as varicose veins, arthritis, multiple sclerosis, Alzheimer's disease, muscular dystrophy, cancer, and many other disorders. The theory regarding atherosclerosis is that the drug breaks up atheromas (fibrous calcium-cholesterol plaques in the arteries) and causes the material to be excreted in the urine. The rationale for chelation therapy in other diseases is less clear.

Each treatment takes several hours and is usually done in the practitioner's office. Some traveling chelation therapists do the treatments in hotel rooms. The usual course is twenty to fifty treatments, but some people are treated hundreds of times. The cost—typically $75 to $100 per treatment—is not covered by most insurance policies.

The problem with the theory is that if EDTA did remove calcium from the blood, hormones would cause the mineral to be released from the bones. There is no evidence that the mineral is removed from atheromas or that atherosclerosis can be cleared as the proponents claim. Calcium is a small part of an atheroma. Even if it could be removed, the fibrous tissue would remain and the artery would still be blocked. Although the therapy has been used on several hundred thousand patients, there is still no scientific evidence that it works. Moreover, the treatment can be dangerous.

Hazards of Chelation Therapy

The Food and Drug Administration has not approved the use of EDTA for atherosclerosis or other disease and considers such treatment hazardous. The American Heart Association, the American College of Physicians, and other professional groups also disapprove of the treatment. Potentially serious side effects include kidney damage and failure, bone marrow damage, irregular heart rhythm, hemolytic anemia, and severe phlebitis (inflammation of the vein EDTA enters). Other reported side effects include nausea, vomiting, muscle spasms, headaches, loss of appetite, malaise, and aching joints. Since the treatment removes body calcium, the mineral is leached from the bones (not from atheromas), which can promote osteoporosis. In one Louisiana clinic, thirteen deaths in two years were attributed to chelation therapy.[26]

Proponents state that the treatment is no longer dangerous because the dose has since been lowered. Regardless, the fact remains that people can be diverted from diet therapy, drug therapy, bypass surgery, or angioplasty, all of which have been proven beneficial to properly selected patients.

Chelation hucksters are aggressive promoters and claim to have high cure rates. They say the "medical establishment" wants to suppress their treatment because it's so effective it would put cardiologists out of business. This is absurd, since chelation is very lucrative and cardiologists could profit handsomely by using it.

Chelation therapists are often involved in other forms of quackery as well. For example, Ray Evers, M.D., who ran the Evers Health Center in Alabama, put out a fat, slick brochure hyping the wonderful "natural" therapies he used. They included hair analysis for trace minerals, applied kinesiology for allergy testing, chiropractic to "eliminate nerve interference," enemas and mineral baths "to remove toxins," and diagnosis with the Accupath 1000. These are all worthless methods. The latter is a "microcomputerized instrument used to analyze the electromagnetic energies of your body based on the principle of electroacupuncture diagnosis." We are told that it can detect disorders of every organ and tissue of the body in their earliest stages. It also was said to be "an excellent tool for the diagnosis and correction of allergies and toxicity due to environmental pollution." In reality, this device is nothing more than a pocket-picker, a "modern" version of the EAV device described in Chapter 4.

During the past two years, chelation proponents have been trumpeting the fact that the FDA has approved a protocol for testing whether chelation therapy is effective against intermittent claudication, a condition in which impaired circulation to the legs causes pain when the person walks. Although a clinical trial was started, its findings have not been publicly released, and it is not clear whether the study will ever be completed. Critics of chelation therapy believe that this experiment will find no benefit. Even if it does, that would not prove it is safe or effective for treating heart disease.

A variation of the chelation racket is "oral chelation." Never ones to miss a trick, the "health food" industry has promoted combinations of vitamins, minerals, enzymes, and other chemicals as chelating agents that will clean out and heal atherosclerotic arteries. Buyers are urged to take them for life. All such products are worthless, and some are dangerous because they contain potentially toxic amounts of vitamin A. Some have cost more than $100 for a month's supply. Although the FDA has ordered many manufacturers of "oral chelation" products to stop selling them, some are still being marketed.

Chinese Herbal Remedies

Hundreds of herbs used in Chinese medicine are gradually being tested for effectiveness and safety by the Chinese and others using modern scientific methods. Some show promise and may eventually be used or their components modified for use by scientific practitioners. Aside from ginseng and a few others, however, Chinese herbs are not widely available in the West outside of "Chinatowns" in large cities. Therefore, this discussion is limited to an important hazard associated with so-called Chinese herbal remedies in pill form.

These drugs are smuggled into the United States and sold in "health food" stores, specialty shops, by mail, and through other outlets. Typically, a few dozen pills are packaged in a cellophane bag or glass bottle with labeling or an illustration that suggests effectiveness against arthritis and similar conditions. The pills have been found to contain not only the powerful and hazardous drugs, but animal bones, horns and shells, toxic heavy metals, insect parts, and rodent droppings.

Since the late 1970s, Oriental arthritis remedies said to be "all-natural" herbal products have been illegally marketed in the United States under the names Chuifong Toukuwan, Black Pearls, and Miracle Herb. Government agencies have found that in addition to herbs, these products contain various potent drugs not listed on their labels. The drugs have included antianxiety agents (diazepam [Valium], chlordiazepoxide [Librium]), anti-inflammatory drugs (indomethacin, phenylbutazone, prednisone, dexamethasone), pain relievers (mefenamic acid, acetaminophen, aminopyrine), and the male sex hormone methyltestosterone. Aminopyrine was banned in the United States in 1938 because it can cause agranulocytosis, a life-threatening condition in which the body stops producing white blood cells. Prednisone and dexamethasone are steroids. Some batches of Chuifong Toukuwan have contained amounts of diazepam high enough to cause addiction. In 1975, four users of Chuifong Toukuwan were hospitalized with agranulocytosis and one died. The FDA has banned importation of the product and helped Texas authorities obtain criminal convictions against several marketers.

Chlorophyll

Chlorophyll is the green pigment that enables plants to trap energy from sunlight and use it in photosynthesis, the manufacture of carbohydrates from carbon dioxide and water. Chlorophyll is sometimes referred to as the "blood" of plants—but it is not. Although a small part of the molecule resembles a small part of hemoglobin, chlorophyll has absolutely no role in human metabolism. When consumed it is simply digested and used for energy; it doesn't get into the blood intact. These basic facts haven't kept quacks from promoting chlorophyll as a miracle treatment for ulcers, hypertension, colitis, arthritis, allergies, anemia, coughs, infections of all kinds, and dozens of other symptoms and disorders. Moreover, most so-called "chlorophyll" on the market isn't chlorophyll at all but a green soup of breakdown products produced by subjecting plants to acetone and other chemicals.

Clinical Ecology

Also called "environmental medicine," clinical ecology is a pseudoscience that deals with the diagnosis and treatment of so-called environmental or ecological disease. Related terms include universal allergy, universal reactivity or reactor, hypersensitivity syndrome, environmental illness, environmental hypersensitivity, twentieth-century disease, and cerebral allergy. I call it the everything-causes-everything disease.

The central contention of this dubious specialty is that a great many people are susceptible to and suffering from accumulated exposure to hundreds of contaminants in the air, water, and food. While most people can handle the small amounts of toxins that accost them every day, some allegedly suffer derangement of their immune systems, which leads to all kinds of mood and thought disorders, fatigue, abdominal symptoms, urinary symptoms, rashes, arthritis-like symptoms, heart palpitations, respiratory symptoms, and even psychotic episodes. So we are told.

The disorder cannot be diagnosed by standard allergy tests or other standard examinations. Instead, the practitioners use a dubious test called provocation and neutralization, in which suspected substances are given under the tongue or injected under the skin, and symptoms noted. Offending substances are then "neutralized" with lower doses of the same substances. Yes, people are actually given diluted doses of formaldehyde, toluene, and other petrochemicals to treat symptoms claimed to be caused by larger doses of the same chemicals. Some clinical ecologists diagnose illness and determine the offending substances by using crystals, pendulums, galvanometers, and the like.

In severe cases, patients may spend several weeks in an environmental control unit designed to remove them from exposure to airborne pollutants and synthetic substances that might cause adverse reactions. After fasting for several days, the patients are given "organically grown" foods and gradually exposed to environmental substances to see which ones cause symptoms to recur.

Once environmental illness is diagnosed, the treatments vary according to the symptoms, the patient's ability to pay for treatment, and the whims of the practitioner. Commonly prescribed strategies are mostly aimed at avoiding suspected offending chemicals. They include avoiding air pollution, smoke, volatile solvents, aerosols, perfumes, newspaper ink, and the like; eating only organically grown foods; drinking distilled water to avoid traces of contaminants; moving to a rural area; and living in a specially prepared trailer or other surroundings designed to be as free as possible of the allegedly offensive chemicals. Other remedies are purported to strengthen the immune system. They include taking an array of nutritional supplements and antifungal and alleged antifungal drugs, taking hormones and gamma globulin, inhaling pure oxygen, and drinking urine.

The concepts and practices of clinical ecology have been carefully studied and rejected by several scientific panels, including the American Academy of Allergy and Immunology, the California Medical Association Scientific Board Task Force on Clinical Ecology, and a committee on the subject established by the Minister of Health of Ontario, Canada. These groups all concluded that so-called environmental illness has not been proven to exist and that clinical ecology is not a valid medical discipline.[27,28] It does not deserve to be considered "experimental," because its proponents are not testing it with scientific methods. Studies have shown that people diagnosed with "environmental illness" suffer from no unifying pattern of symptoms, exhibit no pattern of physical signs or laboratory abnormalities, and don't respond predictably to any particular treatment. In other words, it is not a legitimate diagnosis.

These negative conclusions have not stopped practitioners from charging $400 to more than $12,000 per year for treatment. So far the patients themselves are bearing most of this burden. However, increasing numbers are demanding coverage by private and government insurance programs, including worker's compensation, and are suing employers. The epidemic of this imaginary disease could cost the public a great deal if allowed to get out of hand.

In addition to financial harm, clinical ecologists can cause two other types of harm. First, they can divert patients from proper evaluation and treatment of serious physical problems. Clinical ecologists tend to be zealots who, in their eagerness to diagnose yet another case of their favorite disease, may overlook the real cause of symptoms.[29] While the undiagnosed disease festers, the patient is sent off on an expensive wild-goose chase. Physical conditions that can get people labeled environmentally ill include: sinus infections, upper respiratory infections, mononucleosis, chronic middle ear infection, nasal and vocal polyps and tumors, thyroid dysfunction, diabetes, surreptitious drug abuse, and allergies (to specific substances, not the "universal" but nonexistent allergies of clinical ecology). Even malnutrition has been misdiagnosed as "environmental illness."

Second, clinical ecologists can harm patients by aggravating the emotional and psychosomatic disorders that may be at the root of the patient's problems. Millions of people suffer from anxiety syndromes, depression, somatization, and other emotional disorders that can cause severe physical symptoms. True, they may be temporarily relieved by news that their problem is physical. But it can hardly be healthy in the long run to convince people with psychogenic symptoms that there are terrible toxins in everything they eat, drink, breathe, and touch and that they must go off and live as a hermit far away from friends, family, and familiar surroundings.

Colonic Lavage

A colonic lavage or "colonic" is an enema in which very large amounts (typically five to twenty gallons) of water are infused into the large intestine for the purpose of washing out its contents. Colonics have long been a favorite practice with herbalists, naturopaths, chiropractors, and other fringe practitioners. The notion behind their use is that accumulated fecal wastes produce toxins that enter the blood and cause all kinds of disorders. Like bloodletting, colonic lavage is not used as a general treatment of disease by scientific practitioners. The hazards are significant, for the colon can become distended and therefore unresponsive to the normal stimulation provided by dietary bulk. The more enemas are used, the worse constipation gets.

In recent years, "colon therapy" clinics have opened in many U.S. cities. They are promoted with large, misleading newspaper and magazine ads and pamphlets distributed in "health food stores." Colonic lavage with the added gimmick of oxygenated water can, promoters claim, relieve colds, flu, fatigue, headaches, insomnia, loss of memory, depression, irritability, nausea, poor circulation, weak heart, obesity, sexual dysfunction, and even insanity and shock. The skin supposedly glows, and the person looks years younger. Some people are claimed to have lost twenty-five pounds just by getting their colon cleaned. All this is utter nonsense.

Most colon clinics are run by chiropractors, naturopaths, and/or laypersons, some of whom are associated with physicians who take x-ray films of referred clients. One typical newspaper ad shows photos of barium x-rays of diseased or distorted colons and says that such x-rays are definitely advisable for anyone who has ever suffered from headache, depression, irritability, weakness, fatigue, or low sex drive. This includes almost everyone. These examinations deliver at least fifty times as much radiation as a chest x-ray and are an unnecessary hazard to health.

Some ads say that the therapy removes tapeworms and other parasites, claimed to be present in 90 percent of people. But when I telephoned one clinic making this claim and asked whether they routinely check for parasites in the stool, they said no. Nor could they estimate how many people are relieved of parasites by their treatment. The parasite ploy is a scare tactic. Very few people in the United States have intestinal parasites, and those who do are not likely to be helped by enemas.

The treatment usually costs about $30 to $50, excluding x-rays. Most clients sign up for a series costing up to several hundred dollars.

Promoters claim that a series of treatments strengthens the intestinal muscles and improves their tone. This is false, of course; it is well known that repeated enemas can distend the colon and thereby cause chronic constipation. More important, the enema devices are not always properly designed or properly cleaned. Microbes from one person's intestines may contaminate a machine and be transmitted to other people's intestines. One outbreak of amebiasis in Colorado was traced to a chiropractor's enema machine. Ten of the victims required surgery because the infection had perforated the bowel. Seven of these died.[30] Others have died from ruptured appendix or other complications caused by enemas.

Some naturopaths and herbalists recommend coffee enemas. This is dangerous because the coffee leaches potassium and other elements from the body. The resulting electrolytic imbalance can be fatal.[31] The large dose of caffeine delivered this way can cause anxiety and promote diarrhea and dehydration.

In 1985 the California State Infectious Disease Branch of the Department of Health Services said, "Neither physicians nor chiropractors should be performing colonic irrigations. We are not aware of any scientifically proven health benefit of the procedure, yet we are well aware of the hazards." The report then cited cases of disease outbreaks and deaths associated with the procedure, including those cited above. If other state health departments took a similar stand against colonics, the dangerous and worthless practice might be curbed.

Colostrum

Colostrum is a fluid secreted by the female breast during the first few days of breast-feeding. It contains antibodies found in the mother's blood that apparently provide the newborn with a certain amount of immunity against some infections. Quackery promoters exploit every possible opportunity to peddle "immune-system enhancers" to the gullible, so this was a natural. Bovine colostrum in the form of pills, powders, and ointments has been promoted as a cure for cancer, arthritis, multiple sclerosis, and a variety of infections. There is no evidence to support the claims. They are, in fact, udder nonsense.

Cranial Osteopathy

Proponents of cranial osteopathy state that: (1) the brain beats rhythmically about ten to fourteen times per minute, (2) these movements are unrelated to the heart rate or breathing rate, (3) the brain's rhythmic movements cause the cranial bones to move a thousandth of an inch, (4) any restriction on the bones causes "binding" and interference with the pulsations, which leads to all kinds of disease and dysfunction, and (5) cranial adjustments free up the bones at their joints and allow the normal pulsations to resume and health to return. The high-tech tools of modern physiology have detected no such cranial pulsations, however, and anatomists insist that the skull bones are fused tightly by age two. But some dentists, osteopaths, and chiropractors claim they can feel the pulsations with their fingers and realign misaligned skull bones.

Neural Organization Technique (NOT) is a chiropractic variety of cranial osteopathy said to be an offshoot of applied kinesiology (described earlier in this chapter). NOT's originator, Carl A. Ferreri, D.C., of New York City, has trained hundreds of chiropractors in the use of his techniques.

NOT came to public attention in 1988 when chiropractors subjected children to it in a program sponsored by school officials in Del Norte County, California. For five months, dozens of children from age four to sixteen with epilepsy, Down's syndrome, cerebral palsy, dyslexia, and various other learning disorders were "treated" by having their skull compressed with viselike hand pressure. The children were also forced to endure painful thumb pressure against the roof of the mouth and finger pressure against their eyes.[32,33] Michael A. Corwin, D.C., who did most of the treatments, said that they "remove static from the nervous system."

According to news reports, the children struggled, cried, and screamed bloody murder to no avail as they were forcibly restrained. One reportedly experienced his first seizure when his eye sockets were "adjusted." Some of the children became violent, explosive, rebellious, uncontrollable, and lacking in self-motivation and drive.

The bruising, painful sessions, comprising 260 separate steps, were supposed to realign skull bones, which, chiropractors allege, are commonly out of position. These misalignments allegedly impede circulation of the cerebro-spinal fluid and thereby affect the brain and nervous system and cause all sorts of diseases and disorders. The chiropractors claim they can cure these problems, including learning disorders, cerebral palsy, schizophrenia, Down's syndrome, color blindness, bedwetting, and nightmares. There is no evidence to support these fantastic claims, but lack of evidence has never stopped chiropractors.

In 1987, the *Journal of Learning Disabilities* published a review of "controversial approaches" related to learning disabilities. The article warned that Ferrari's approach was not based on any known research but on anatomical concepts that are not held by the majority of anatomists. The article also noted that no research done others had replicated Ferrari's supposed cures and no follow-up research documented his claimed results.[34] This was a polite way of saying the whole thing is a lot of rubbish.

Neural Organization Technique is an example of the habit chiropractors have of dreaming up bizarre panaceas and promoting them with a religious zeal without even considering doing scientific studies first and without adequately considering potential harm to the patients. It also shows how easily the chiropractic leaders persuade the gullible and opportunistic in their profession to join in their latest fads and frauds and how easily they can persuade some of the most educated and responsible people in a community. It is distressing that some dentists have also fallen for the fad, and some naive dental societies have sponsored continuing education courses without carefully examining the course material.

Cryonics

Would you like a maximum lifespan and vigor into your eighties or nineties? That's nothing. Why not shoot for the stars and go for the whole schmier? Yes, immortality may be yours for only $100,000. With cryonics you can be frozen until a cure for what killed you and the ability to retore body function are developed. Then you will be defrosted and fixed up. Of course, all the cells in your body will be dead and will need to be regenerated. But we'll deal with that when we come to it—perhaps in 100 years. That's a personal promise. Now, if you want the economy accommodations (only $35,000), we'll just preserve your head and brain for later regeneration. These aren't the exact words of cryonics advocates, but should give you the flavor of their sales pitch.

National Council Against Health Fraud President William T. Jarvis, Ph.D., calls cryonics "quackery's last shot at you." In a recent interview he said:

> Cryonic technology has not been demonstrated to work in laboratory animals. Even if the rest of a person's body could be revived after hundreds of years, the brain could not. Brain cells deteriorate within minutes after death, and any still viable when the body is frozen would be burst by the freezing process. Cryonics might be a suitable subject for scientific research, but marketing an unproven method to the public is quackery.

Despite all this, promoters apparently do a brisk business. Sure, there's a scandal now and then about a head perhaps being removed before a person was quite dead, but liquid nitrogen vaults are being contracted for at a steady clip. People and their estates are paying to have their body or head maintained reasonably intact (can a severed head ever be reasonably intact?) until the Scientific Millennium arrives and the dead are made to live again. Not surprisingly, the center of cryonics is southern California, a significant consolation should the Great California Earthquake finally hit.

Crystal Healing

Superstitious people imagine that consciousness pervades inanimate objects, that magical powers emanate from them, and that the inanimate world cares about human beings. The more important objects, such as the sun, stars, oceans, and forests have gods associated with them. These beliefs are not confined to primitive or medieval cultures, but are widespread even in the most advanced societies. Astrology is the prime example. Crystal healing, a variant of radionics, is another.

Beliefs that various minerals, stones, gems, and jewels have magical powers date back to ancient times. These objects were supposed to confer wisdom and strength and to shield the owner from assorted dangers, including disease. In recent years these superstitions have been riding the crest of the New Age wave in the form of crystal healing. Quartz crystals are the most popular, but topaz, beryl, and others are also used. The powers attributed to them include healing just about any physical or mental condition, improving gas mileage when attached to your carburetor, making refrigerators run better, improving the taste of wine, and conferring psychic powers.

Proponents say that crystals are surrounded by an energy field (they don't say what kind of energy) and telepathically receive and store emotions and information. Used with meditation and breathing exercises, they supposedly can help you get in touch with your Higher Self, or with God. They are also said to emit negative ions that produce health benefits. Proponents state that the use of crystals in radios, transmitters, and watches provides a scientific basis for their claims. In electronic applications, however, energy is supplied by an external source. The crystals don't vibrate on their own or have any kind of energy field around them. Nor do they produce ions.

There is little agreement among promoters about what different crystals can do, how they should be used, or how to "cleanse" or "recharge" them. There is no evidence to support any of their claims, but that hasn't stopped the entrepreneurs from cashing in on the nonsense. "Health food" stores, metaphysical stores, jewelers, mail-order companies, crystal miners, as well as authors, publishers, and hucksters of books on crystal healing have enjoyed a boom since the early 1970s. Crystal quackery has become such a rage that beautiful formations in ancient caves are being ravaged for their quartz. This is analogous to the decimation of the black bear and black rhinos by poachers who sell the animals' gall bladders and horns to quacks for their alleged healing and aphrodisiac properties.

Cytotoxic Testing

Cytotoxic testing is a quack diagnostic technique that blitzed the country in the early 1980s with large ads in the *Wall Street Journal, The New York Times,* the *Los Angeles Times,* and many other publications. The test was touted as a scientific breakthrough that allowed laypersons to do simple blood tests to diagnose hundreds of food and chemical allergies said to be the cause of obesity, fatigue, confusion, asthma, depression, headaches, liver disease, hormonal imbalances, ulcers, baldness, and dozens of other diseases and conditions. Nutritional advice based on the tests would supposedly solve the problems. Ads were directed not only to people looking for a new approach to their health problems but also to potential investors in franchised operations.

For an investment of thirty to fifty thousand dollars, people who knew nothing about medicine could get to play doctor without having to get a permit, license, or malpractice insurance. Or so it appeared. With clients paying several hundred dollars for initial testing and more for supplements and follow-up testing, the profit potential would be high. Storefront clinics run by entrepreneurs rather than health professionals popped up in many parts of the country.

Cytotoxic testing, short for leukocytotoxic testing, involves exposing a person's white blood cells (leukocytes) to slides containing dried food extracts. If microscopic examination of the cells shows disintegration, collapse, or change of shape, the person is declared allergic to the substance and given long lists of foods to avoid and supplements to take, the latter sometimes peddled by the clinic.

According to experts on allergy and immunology, cytotoxic testing is worthless both theoretically and empirically. Allergic reactions affect not leukocytes but immunoglobulins in the far-less-numerous mast cells. These cells then release histamine, which causes the allergic symptoms. There is no evidence that an abnormal change in leukocytes indicates a change in mast cells. Moreover, the tests don't control for temperature, concentration, acidity, and other important factors that affect leukocytes. Above all, there is no evidence whatsoever that the technique is accurate.[35] Tests have shown that it diagnoses allergies where none really exist and can fail to detect those proven to exist by well-established techniques. It doesn't even give consistent results: blood tested one day or in one lab can test differently the next day or in another lab.

The standard food extracts used by clinics are subject to FDA regulation as drugs. They are used for diagnostic skin tests and allergy shots. Using the extracts for cytotoxic testing is an unapproved use. Enforcement actions by the FDA and several state agencies appears to have driven cytotoxic testing from the American marketplace.

One California cytotoxic testing company filed an antitrust lawsuit against the American Academy of Allergy and Immunology and several other groups and individuals for their efforts in exposing cytotoxic testing as worthless. The case was dismissed and the defendants awarded court costs in November 1989. This illustrates that responsible health professionals can prevail against entrepreneurs whose financial interests they harm when they blow the whistle on fraud.

Dental-Amalgam Phobia

Are millions of Americans being poisoned by the mercury in their silver-amalgam fillings? Some dentists, naturopaths, and chiropractors say yes. The American Dental Association and other expert sources say no.

It has been known for a long time that mercury poisoning can be very serious. Toxicity, of course, is a matter of dose. The tiny amounts of mercury normally found in our food, water, and air are harmless. If blood levels get too high, however, severe nerve damage can lead to tremors, difficulty walking or moving normally, and dementia. This is why industrial workers who use mercury take precautions to avoid contact with the metal. Dentists and their assistants who work with mercury must exercise care in handling the unhardened amalgam. Once amalgam has hardened, however, very little of the mercury can get out.

A few years ago it was found that even hardened amalgam can release infinitesimal amounts of mercury vapors during chewing. This led to the claim by a few dentists and other fringe practitioners that amalgam fillings can cause toxicity leading to headaches, depression, learning disabilities, arthritis, epilepsy, cancer, multiple sclerosis, and many other health problems.

Some of the mercury phobists, particularly those who believe in acupuncture, go further and say that all metals, including gold, should be removed from the teeth because they set up tiny electric currents that interfere with the flow of vital energy through "acupuncture meridians." They thereby cause illness, especially cancer, in distant organs on the same meridian as the teeth. The solution for this problem, say the phobists, is to drill out all the old fillings and replace them with plastic composites. Spectacular cures of stubborn diseases have been claimed, but the evidence is anecdotal and circumstantial rather than scientific. Removal and replacement of the fillings can be very expensive and can permanently weaken the teeth.

The anti-amalgam practitioners often use a mercury vapor analyzer or an "Amalgameter" that supposedly indicates whether dangerous levels of mercury are released by chewing. These devices are worthless for this purpose.[36] The correct way to tell whether someone has an overload of mercury is to test the person's blood and/or urine. Tests done on volunteers have shown that people with amalgam fillings don't have higher body mercury loads than those without the amalgam. Nor do most dentists who handle the material all the time. Even after several fillings are put in, repeated tests of urine and blood show no increase in mercury. This is because the mercury in fillings is securely bonded with copper, tin, and silver and is biologically inactive.

Body mercury levels can be increased by eating contaminated tuna and other deep-sea fish. But the average person would have to increase consumption tenfold to approach the danger zone.

Although a National Institutes of Health panel absolved amalgam fillings of mercury toxicity charges in August 1991, there is a trend away from amalgam for some fillings because more attractive composites are being developed. In some cases they are stronger and bond the tooth together better. They don't have amalgam's tendency to expand and cause little cracks to develop that can slowly split the teeth. They are also safer to handle and work with. This trend does not give legitimacy to the claims of the amalgam phobists and should not be used as justification for wholesale removal of amalgam. "Amalgam toxicity" is clearly a scare tactic used to promote unnecessary care and phony detoxifying diets, supplements, herbs, enemas, and other nostrums.

Diet Pills and Potions

Scores of products are promoted as weight-control aids. The most common are amino acid combinations, spirulina, bee pollen, herbs and herbal extracts, homeopathic products, "sugar blockers," fiber products, and the drugs phenyl-propanolamine and benzocaine. Only the last two are approved by the FDA, but the evidence for them is very flimsy.

Phenylpropanolamine (PPA) is a chemical cousin of amphetamine, a potentially addicting drug that was prescribed for weight loss for decades until its ineffectiveness and hazards were finally recognized. PPA is a decongestant used in products for colds, as well as an alleged appetite suppressant. It is the main ingredient in scores of nonprescription diet aids. Reported side effects include headache, nausea, anxiety, palpitations, nervousness, dizziness, and insomnia.[37] The most serious charge is that it causes or aggravates hypertension in some people, especially if caffeine is also consumed. PPA is contraindicated for people with heart disease, thyroid disorders, depression, diabetes, or hypertension. Since many people have these disorders without knowing it, the nonprescription status of PPA seems unjustified. Since there is little evidence of long-term effectiveness, its use in weight control is highly questionable.

Benzocaine is a local anesthetic. Added to candies and gum, it is alleged to decrease appetite by numbing the taste buds. It poses little hazard, but there is no evidence of long-term effectiveness in weight control.

Fiber products have been marketed throughout the 1980s and into the 1990s with large ads in newspapers and magazines across the country. Capsules and pills with names like Fat Magnet and Cal-Ban 3000 have been claimed to prevent digestion and absorption of carbohydrates or fat. They therefore allow you to eat all you want and still lose weight. These products consist of various plant fibers, especially cellulose and guar gum. None works as claimed. If they did, the unabsorbed nutrients would be digested by bacteria in the intestine, producing gas, bloating, diarrhea, cramps, and foul-smelling stools. In spite of their ineffectiveness, clever ad copy and ads disguised as articles in tabloid papers have made selling such products a multimillion-dollar business.

During 1990, Cal-Ban 3000 was driven from the marketplace by a series of enforcement actions by local, state, and federal agencies. The actions were triggered by reports of serious harm to users. The FDA collected reports of more than one hundred victims, fifty of whom needed medical intervention. The problems included esophageal obstruction, gastric obstruction, upper and lower intestinal obstruction, nausea, and vomiting. In 1992, prompted in part by the Cal-Ban situation, the FDA banned guar gum and 110 other ingredients from use in nonprescription weight-loss products. The ingredients include arginine, caffeine, kelp, lecithin, papaya enzymes, phenylalanine, tryptophan, and vitamin B_6.

So-called "sugar blockers" contain an extract of *Gymnema sylvestre,* a plant grown in India. They are claimed to cause weight loss by preventing sugar in the diet from being absorbed into the body. According to Purdue University's Varro E. Tyler, Ph.D., a leading authority on plant medicine, chewing the plant's leaves can prevent the taste sensation of sweetness. But there is no reliable evidence that the chemicals they contain can block the absorption of sugar into the body or produce weight loss.

The other products mentioned above (amino acids, spirulina, etc.) are discussed in separate entries. None has been proven to work as claimed. Weight control does not come in a bottle.

Diet Sodas

In television ads featuring slender, beautiful people, diet sodas sweetened with saccharin and aspartame are touted as aids in controlling weight. There is no evidence to support this contention. While diet sodas are essentially calorie-free, people typically substitute them for water rather than high-calorie snacks such as candies and potato chips. Most sodas, the "diet" ones included, contain at least two ingredients that tend to promote calcium excretion: caffeine and phosphoric acid. Heavy consumption might increase the risk of calcium deficiency, especially in women and children.

DMSO

Dimethyl sulfoxide, or DMSO, is a simple organic chemical with some remarkable properties that make it potentially useful in medical practice. It is a clear, colorless liquid that dissolves many substances and has been used for decades as an industrial solvent. DMSO can penetrate intact skin and carry other chemicals with it. Animal studies show it has anti-inflammatory, analgesic, vasodilatory, and other properties.

By the mid-1960s at least 100,000 persons had been treated by physicians with DMSO, which was reported to be effective for treating injuries and inflammation of muscles and connective tissues, arthritis, gout, viral and bacterial infections, skin parasites, burns, wound healing, scleroderma (a connective tissue disorder that first affects the skin, then internal organs), interstitial cystitis (a bladder disorder), and even mental and emotional problems. DMSO was also found to cause changes in the lenses of dogs, pigs, and rabbits, however, so all clinical studies were stopped. For about fifteen years, very few studies were done, but in 1980 the FDA revoked the restrictions on clinical testing because no evidence had been found of harm to the human eye, even after prolonged use.

The FDA and the National Academy of Sciences reviewed the thousands of scientific articles on DMSO and concluded that the evidence was adequate to approve the drug only for interstitial cystitis, but that further study was warranted because there were strong indications that DMSO might be effective for several other disorders and types of injury. Studies are being carried out, and the drug may eventually be approved for scleroderma, sprains, various types of arthritis, and possibly strokes.

DMSO is cheap and easy to make and get. A large market for it has been created by a blatant promotional story on CBS TV's "60 Minutes" and other media attention on its potential applications. Several states have even legalized the drug for human use under certain conditions, and some state medical societies have urged that it be approved for more uses. It is not surprising that entrepreneurs have capitalized on the situation by bottling DMSO and marketing it to the public.

DMSO is available by prescription as Rimso-50, a 50 percent solution for direct instillation into the urinary bladder for treating interstitial cystitis. A 90 percent gel is available for veterinary use in reducing swelling due to trauma. The one sold directly to the public is a 99 percent DMSO industrial degreaser that contains impurities. It is available in "health food stores," beauty parlors, novelty and gift shops, flea markets, and by mail. People rub it in and inject it without much concern about the contaminants or possible side effects.

Adverse Effects and Hazards

Common side effects of topical DMSO application include burning, itching, local and generalized dermatitis, and an unpleasant oysterlike odor of the breath, clothes, and furniture. Potential hazards are presented by the impurities, even if "guaranteed pure." Another problem is that some people are diverted from proper and effective treatment by quacks who make outrageous claims about curing cancer and other serious diseases with DMSO.

There are three types of DMSO preparation on the market. One, the diluted Rimso-50, is too weak to be useful in the strains, sprains, and arthritis for which most people use it. The other two do not fit the high standards of purity, effectiveness, and safety for human use. If the usual remedies for these disorders are not effective and you want to try DMSO, don't use an unproven, impure product. Instead, try to find a physician who is licensed to do clinical testing with pure preparations.

Although hundreds of drugs have been trumpeted as cure-alls in much the same way as DMSO, few of the promises have been fulfilled. DMSO is a remarkable substance that may find more of a place in the healing arts. Until its role is more clearly defined, however, caution is in order.

Electrical Muscle Stimulation

Electrical muscle stimulators (EMS) are devices that stimulate muscle contractions by electrical impulses. They are heavily promoted for body-shaping, figure-toning, cellulite removal, weight loss, and even wrinkle removal. Some health spas and slenderizing salons provide sessions with EMS devices for armchair joggers; they advertise that you can read or watch TV while sophisticated machines do all the work. The devices are often sold by mail order; ads in magazines claim they can provide the benefits of jogging for ten miles or doing thousands of sit-ups while you lie flat on your back.

EMS devices have legitimate uses in physical therapy, such as to relax muscle spasms, to prevent blood clots in leg muscles after surgery or a stroke, and to prevent muscle atrophy due to disuse. However, they are not effective for weight loss or body shaping, there are certain hazards in their use, and they are not supposed to be used by unlicensed practitioners. The FDA considers the use or promotion of muscle stimulators for purposes of weight loss or body toning to be fraudulent, even if a physician or other licensed practitioner is administering the device.[38]

EMS devices can cause electrical shocks and burns. They should not be used on pregnant women, persons with heart problems or pacemakers, or anyone with epilepsy or cancer. The electrodes should not be placed where a strong current could pass through the heart, brain, or spinal column. Many years ago, a muscle stimulator called the Relax-A-Cizor was banned after forty witnesses testified that they had been injured by the machine.

Fasting

Everyone "fasts" during sleep, and when people are sick, they tend to eat much less. This is natural, especially in the early and severe stages of illness, though intake may be large during recovery. Some writers advocate fasting regularly for one day to several weeks, whether sick or not. They cite numerous alleged benefits, such as "physiological rest" and "cleansing the system."

Many newly health-conscious people fast in order, they say, to flush out chemicals from junk food and drugs. The fast thus represents an "atonement" for past transgressions. If it makes them feel weak and sick, they believe it is because of the mobilization of poisons for disposal and is a sign that they need to fast. While it makes sense to greatly reduce food intake for a day or two after a bout of overindulgence, fasting on a regular basis makes no sense and can be hazardous, especially if prolonged, for the following reasons.

Fasting causes blood sugar levels to drop. This low supply of glucose leads to the breakdown of muscle and other protein tissue for energy and can cause weakness, fatigue, irritability, depression, decreased libido, and a sick feeling. The byproducts of protein breakdown, ammonia and urea, are normally handled easily by the liver and kidney. But these organs are severely hampered by inadequate nutrition. Far from "cleansing the system," fasting causes self-cannibalism and *decreases* the body's ability to destroy and excrete toxins.

Fasting leads to rapid loss of water, sodium, and potassium, which causes a decrease in blood volume, postural hypotension (low blood pressure upon standing up), and fainting. Severe potassium depletion can cause a distrurbance of heart rhythm that can be fatal. The body can't tell voluntary fasting from starvation, and deaths have occurred even during medically supervised fasts and near-fasts. The cause of death is usually kidney or heart failure. Those who survive prolonged fasts may suffer anemia, decreased resistance to infection, osteoporosis, and kidney and liver damage. Depression of digestive functions can continue for weeks or months, with even small amounts of food causing pain and discomfort. Besides being dangerous and destructive of lean, calorie-consuming tissue, fasting for weight loss almost never works. Even with large initial weight losses, the rate of return to the prefasting weight is well over 90 percent by most accounts. Obese people need good eating and exercise habits that last a lifetime, not short-term panaceas.

Feingold Diet

In the early 1970s Benjamin F. Feingold, M.D., a California allergist, started preaching that attention deficit disorder ("hyperactivity") in children is often caused by a reaction of the brain to certain items in the diet. He specified that artificial colors and flavors, as well as salicylate-like compounds naturally present in some foods, were the culprits. Later forms of this notion also blame white sugar. Dietary restrictions based on Feingold's ideas are commonly used by parents in attempts to improve the behavior of their children.

There has never been good theoretical support for the concept. Nor has there been experimental or clinical evidence in its favor. On the contrary, several controlled studies have shown that supposedly susceptible children do not behave badly when they ingest the substances in question.[39] The parents cannot accurately judge whether their kids were fed the "bad" foods or given the "bad" chemicals in a pill. After nearly twenty years, the theory lacks scientific support, yet it is widely believed and has achieved the status of a modern myth. Believing false doctrines is always harmful in the end, and the Feingold theory is no exception. Children should not be taught that their behavior is determined by the foods they eat rather than by their attitudes, feelings, and habits. And if they need psychological counseling or special teaching methods, time should not be wasted seeking a nonexistent dietary cure.

Firewalking

Since the early 1980s entrepreneurs have run an operation centered around the dubious art of firewalking, that is, walking barefoot on a bed of burning charcoal. For several hundred to several thousand dollars, you can be led through an experience that will make you a tiger in business and in bed. "Self-improvement" advocate Anthony Robbins has made a fortune with his firewalking business and inspired many imitators. His seminar supposedly lays the foundation for the profound experience by helping instill the state of mind and psychic energy required for success, including protection from harm from the fire. He promises to help his followers and clients achieve their wildest dreams by "tapping into rarely used parts of the brain." They chant "cool moss" as they cross the fire, convinced that failure to keep the positive image will lead to severe injury and perhaps death.

In promotional flyers, Robbins says he was a consultant to the U.S. Olympic Team and the U.S. Army, teaching "accelerated learning programs which have produced the most extraordinary results." While his primary business involves motivational seminars, books, tapes, and the like, he also teaches that the mind can control body processes to overcome disease and improve general health. His flyers and ads say he is "recognized as one of the world's leading experts on nutrition" and "Director of Nutrition at the Institute for Holistic Studies." However, he has no academic credentials in the fields of health, medicine, or nutrition. His book, *Unlimited Power* [Ballantine Books, 1986], refers to Harvey and Marilyn Diamond as his former partners and incorporates their theories wholesale (see Chapter 1). Robbins's writings about health and nutrition are sheer lunacy. In the book he denounces milk as "cow pus" and denies that germs cause disease. He also says that vultures look the way they do because they don't eat water-rich foods: "If you eat something that's dried and dead, guess what you're going to look like." Actually, the flesh of freshly dead animals, which is what vultures eat, is 60 percent water.

Life magazine described Robbins as "a freewheeling all-purpose savior" who travels around the country and performs $1000-an-hour "one stop" therapy promised to cure any psychological problem in a session. *Omni* observed, "It usually takes 5 to 15 minutes to effect cures of various neuroses, phobias, and other behavioral problems. . . . Stubborn problems like coma and autism may require from 15 to 45 minutes."

In 1985 Robbins brought his circus to Honolulu. His unusual and dramatic event naturally got substantial publicity from the local media. Even the University of Hawaii football team got involved. The desperate coach of the struggling team apparently bought into Robbins's nonsense about doing the impossible (winning a game in this case). For the discounted group price of some $2,000 to $5,000 (exact figures were hard to come by), the entire team was subjected to hours of mind-over-matter mumbo-jumbo followed by a cheap trick. The team went on to be named one of the nation's ten worst that year, but the university did not receive a refund from Robbins.

In response to this skullduggery, some friends and I held a firewalk and invited the public to join us for free. We received front-page newspaper coverage as well as coverage on local television news. In that event and others since, our coals have been at least as hot as Robbins's and our fire at least as long. We have been thanked for our demonstrations by grateful relatives for helping to dissuade loved ones from continuing to waste money on firewalking seminars and experiences. One mother said her daughter had already spent $35,000 following her firewalking guru to seminars and firewalks around the country. She paid geometrically increasing fees for what she had been led to believe were ever more important and advanced lessons.

In our events we have no seminar, positive thinking, or praying to invoke special powers or awaken dormant parts of our brains. In fact, following two minutes of safety instructions, our participants chant "hot coals" as they stride across the glowing bed. In over one hundred individual crossings, only one person was ever burned badly enough to raise a blister. Other groups of skeptics, most notably members of the Southern California Skeptics, have done similar demonstrations of firewalking. (Nevertheless, we all strongly urge against anyone trying to do it without advice and preferably direct supervision from an experienced person. Several safety and legal precautions are absolutely essential.)

Firewalking is a physical feat, not a mental one.[40] It is possible because charcoal, especially when coated with ashes, does not transfer heat rapidly to other objects. Its heat-transmission characteristics are similar to those of air. You can stick your hand into a very hot oven without burning yourself, but if you touch metal in the oven, you can be badly burned. The metal is no hotter than the air, but it transfers its heat much more quickly. I'd like to see Robbins and his disciples walk on hot metal at the same temperature as the coals. No "dormant areas" of their brains, chanting, or wishful thinking would save them from severe burns.

Glowing hot charcoals, of course, are not the same as hot air. The firewalkers walk (usually rapidly) on the charcoals—they don't stand around. If they did so they would be burned. Each foot is in contact with the heat for only about a second before being lifted. Moreover, the entire walk generally lasts less than seven seconds. Any longer exposure and the risk of burns is much greater.

Walking on hot coals without sustaining injury is not a miraculous feat. It is remarkable that it can be done, and it makes for exciting spectacles and fun social events that provide an adrenaline rush to the participants and the audience. But there is no magic and no psychic power involved, and there is certainly no evidence that buying into commercial firewalking seminars and experiences brings about the promised transformations in brain use, health, wealth, and happiness. On the contrary, the gullible may be severely burned in more ways than one.

Fish oils

Fish oils have been promoted by the "health food" industry as a safeguard against several ailments, especially heart disease. Studies have shown that eating a lot of fatty fish (with high levels of omega-3 fatty acids) may help lower cholesterol levels and prevent abnormal blood clotting. These have been cited to support the sales efforts. However, self-prescribed supplementation is not a good idea. The prevention and treatment of heart disease should be approached in a comprehensive manner, taking all risk factors into account, not just blood cholesterol level. If someone's cholesterol level is high, attention should be paid to both exercise and diet. A drug should not be considered unless dietary modification is unable to lower the cholesterol level sufficiently. If a drug is appropriate, the choice of the drug should depend on factors that are complicated enough to make professional help advisable.

Fish oil products have variable levels of oils, cholesterol, vitamins A and D, and other components. They also have lots of calories. In some cases, they raise cholesterol rather than lower it. It is much more sensible to get your omega-3 acids from fish itself. They are all good—even shellfish, which have much less cholesterol than previously believed and lots of omega-3 fatty acids.

People who don't like fish and want the benefits of unsaturated fatty acids can eat a variety of vegetables, especially beans. Don't believe the commercial hype about fish oil capsules. Like many "health food" products, they have not been proven safe or effective for use by the general public. In fact, fish oil supplements can lead to loose stools, belching, abdominal discomfort, and excessive thinning of the blood, with increased risk of stroke and hemorrhage.[41]

Fluoride Phobia

Fluoride is a basic entity, which, like its chemical cousin chloride, is widespread in nature. It is also a nutrient of great importance to teeth. Decades of animal research, epidemiological studies, and clinical research around the world prove this beyond a reasonable doubt. Nor is there any question that adjusting the level in drinking water to about one part fluoride to one million parts water is one of the most cost-effective public-health measures ever devised. That's why fluoridation has been endorsed by the American Public Health Association, the American Dental Association, the World Health Organization, the American Academy of Pediatrics, Consumers Union, and medical and dental associations in scores of countries. The average cost of fluoridating community water supplies is about fifty cents per person per year.

Unfortunately, while more than 135 million Americans now have access to naturally fluoridated water or water with supplemental fluoride, many others are denied the benefits. Amazingly, in many cases communities deprive themselves of the benefits by voting down fluoridation referenda or pressuring legislators voting on the issue. They elect tooth decay for one reason: a sophisticated campaign of lies has been waged for years by promoters of quackery who charge that fluoride is a deadly poison that causes cancer, birth defects, AIDS, Alzheimer's disease, and much more.

The aim of the campaign is to stir up distrust and paranoia. If quacks can convince people that the "medical establishment" would actually poison them by putting toxic chemicals in drinking water, it's much easier to persuade them that scientific health care doesn't work. It is no coincidence that most leaders of the antifluoridation movement make their living huckstering quack methods for serious diseases. While sincere but misled local antifluoridationists are frightened into doing the dirty work, the national leaders enjoy the profits generated by promoting paranoia.

Of course, organized quackery has always opposed important public-health measures, such as milk pasteurization and childhood immunization. But their antifluoride campaign has been their greatest "success" by far. The National Health Federation (NHF) has been most responsible for this success, and its members can be proud that they have made a tremendous contribution to the poor dental health of millions of Americans and even Europeans, many of whom have likewise opposed fluoridation on the basis of NHF disinformation.

Lies about fluoride have been thoroughly refuted in detail. Those who want to explore the matter further can consult literature from the American Dental Association and the U.S. Public Health Service. Many local and state health departments also have information available.[42]

Fluoride's most vigorous opponent has been John Yiamouyiannis, Ph.D., who led NHF's antifluoridation campaign from 1974 through 1980 and now works independently. A pamphlet he wrote, "Lifesavers Guide to Fluoridation," has been distributed in many communities where fluoridation was considered. The pamphlet cites 250 references to back up his many claims that fluoridation is ineffective and unsafe. Experts from the Ohio Department of Health who traced the references, however, found that almost half had no relevance to community water fluoridation and that many others actually support fluoridation but were selectively quoted and misrepresented.[43]

Fructose

Fructose is heavily promoted as a miracle food for energy and stamina and as an aid in weight control. It is half of the sucrose molecule (table sugar); glucose is the other half. Fructose is about 70% sweeter per calorie than other sugars, but this advantage must be weighed against its higher cost and tendency to lose its sweetening power with heating. Fructose does not promote tooth decay as much as sucrose does. It is claimed to be better for diabetics because of its relatively slow absorption. Even if true, this advantage is outweighed by evidence that fructose tends to increase blood lipids, at least in some people. There is no evidence that supplementary fructose helps any ailment, relieves fatigue, or provides any health benefit when substituted for sucrose.

Germanium

Germanium is a metallic element of the carbon family that has long been used in the electronics and aerospace industries. Because many trace elements turn out to be nutrients, toxins, or both, it is not surprising that interest in germanium's biological effects started decades ago. In the 1920s germanium dioxide was tested as a remedy for anemias and systemic infections, but was found ineffective. Later it was found to be toxic to the kidneys if taken for long. Germanium apparently has no role in normal nutrition or metabolism.[44]

Modern research on germanium has focused on an array of organic (carbon-containing) germanium compounds, some found in plants and some synthesized in laboratories. Two or three of these have exhibited some antitumor effects in certain mouse cancers, but so far most human trials have yielded negative results. Most cancer specialists don't consider it a promising subject for research.

Negative results in scientific studies, however, have never deterred zealots and quacks. Alhough there is no evidence to back the claims, various forms of organic germanium are now promoted as a prevention or cure for cancer, AIDS, osteoporosis, heart disease, allergies, liver disease, arthritis, chronic fatigue, sexual dysfunctions, brain and nerve disorders, and infections. We are assured that germanium can even confer immunity to infectious diseases like influenza and rubella, as well as regulate cholesterol levels, and prevent birth defects. PMS can be relieved by putting germanium tablets in panties, and headaches can be relieved by putting them on acupuncture points with bandaids. Germanium also has been described as an "electronutrient" that "optimizes life force," and acts as an "adaptogen" that "enhances the body's ability to deal with all stresses, challenges, and assaults."

It would be easier to list the few diseases the miracle drug isn't said to cure than the hundreds it allegedly does. Wholesale germanium products sell for about $2 per gram and retail for anywhere from $10 to $400 per gram, depending on the pills made, packaging used, and so on. An individual could spend up to $20 per day on recommended doses. The products are huckstered with all the sleaze experienced snake-oil peddlers can muster. For example, a supermarket tabloid runs a headline screaming that a new miracle drug cures everything. The article quotes some phony authority about some nonexistent studies and miraculous cures. And a nearby ad invites you to send a check for your first month's supply.

Kazuhiko Asai, Ph.D., a Japanese miner and metallurgist, found germanium in coal and developed an extraction process. He says his interest in the mineral was "the working of some supernormal inevitability," commanded by another will greater than his own. He synthesized his first germanium-containing organic compound in 1967, but later said it had been "divinely conferred."[44] The compound was germanium sesquioxide, a water-soluble organic germanium Asai called Ge-132. He claims he tested it on himself, and it cured his "severe polyrheumatism complicated by arthritis." He says he did animal tests and found that his miracle drug could cure all animals of all diseases. It works, he says, because all diseases are caused by lack of oxygen, and germanium carries the needed oxygen into the cells. Moreover, it was completely nontoxic at all dose levels. Convinced he had discovered the ultimate panacea, Asai founded the Organic Germanium Clinic near Tokyo, where virtually everything was treated with germanium.

At some point Asai must have seen that taking germanium isn't always followed by recovery, for he stipulated that three conditions are necessary for it to work: the patient must firmly believe it will work, must not be subjected to excessive mental stress, and must adhere to a balanced diet. If the drug doesn't work, one of these conditions must be the cause. Now, there's a miracle drug for the ages. The patient, though perhaps very ill and frightened, must not suffer mental stress and must have absolute faith in the remedy. *Real* drugs work in the absence of faith and despite the presence of stress. In fact, lack of dependence on faith, as proven by double-blind studies, defines an effective drug.

Promotional literature mentions Asai's "patients" and refers to him as simply "Dr." Asai, who "treats seriously ill people" with germanium. But Asai had no training in medicine or nutrition—just an obsession with germanium. In 1984 he died at age seventy-six. His miracle cure apparently afforded him no more than an average (for Japanese) life span. In fact, it may have resulted in a premature death, for he died of a bleeding ulcer that he treated with a germanium drug instead of getting modern therapy, which is usually very effective. You might say he got seduced by his own propaganda and done in by his own snake oil. How many other victims might there be?

In 1988 the FDA banned the importation of germanium products (except those intended for use in electronic equipment), because marketing claims had made them unproven drugs in the eyes of the law. Subsequently, the FDA took action against several American manufacturers, but germanium products are still widely available. I wonder whether the FDA has hit upon a strategy for reducing America's trade deficit and boosting its gross national product: No imported quackery will be allowed; if anyone is going to swindle and endanger Americans, it will be other Americans.

Gerovital

Procaine, a synthetic chemical related to cocaine, was first used in medical practice in 1905 and has played a vital role ever since. It is an excellent local anesthetic that is especially useful in dentistry. Most people who have had a tooth drilled or pulled have experienced its powerful numbing effect.

But some people think procaine (also called Novocain) is much more than a numbing agent. In the 1920s and 1930s Dr. Ferdinand Huneke of Germany experimented with procaine injections in hundreds of patients with various serious diseases and severe pain syndromes. He claimed remarkable results, but other physicians could not duplicate his successes, and many denounced him as a quack.

In the 1950s a Rumanian physician, Dr. Anna Aslan, started using procaine injections, mostly in older people with chronic diseases. She claimed spectacular success not only in the treatment of ulcers, arthritis, hypertension, and other specific ailments, but in retarding and reversing aging. She said that procaine, or GH3 as she called her procaine solutions, was a vitamin, in spite of the fact that it does not occur in nature and is purely synthetic. The scientific community was skeptical of Aslan's claims, but the world press quickly spread the word. For decades, thousands of people flocked every year to her spa-like clinic with hopes of rejuvenation and healing. The drug is also available in some other European countries and in one U.S. state, Nevada.

In the 1960s American supporters of Dr. Aslan formed a company to import procaine from Rumania and sell it under the brand name Gerovital. They applied to the FDA for permission to test the drug as an antidepressant in the elderly. The FDA agreed, but only if they would also test it on young people, since depression occurs in them too, and only if the name were changed, since "Gerovital" implies an antiaging effect, which had not been proven and which the company did not want to test. The application was eventually withdrawn, and scientific studies were not performed. Although the FDA has taken some enforcement actions against American promoters, the drug is still widely available.

Gerovital proponents claim that scientific studies have proven its value. But the nearly 300 reports of Dr. Aslan and others concerning the effects of Gerovital on their patients were reviewed and evaluated by the National Institute on Aging.[45] This review was highly critical of the methods used by the Gerovital proponents and concluded that the evidence for antiaging effects was unconvincing. The reviewers conceded that the drug may have a slight antidepressant effect but said that even this had not been proven.

"Glandulars"

Glandular remedies, or glandulars, are pills or capsules containing ground-up raw testes, ovaries, pancreas, adrenals, and other glands from animals. Nonglandular tissues are also used, including brain, liver, and kidney. The actual amount of tissue per pill or capsule is usually just a few milligrams, like a grain of salt. "Glandulars" are supposed to work wonders for the corresponding organs. Homeopaths, naturopaths, chiropractors, and "health food" store clerks recommend them for treating a wide assortment of conditions and symptoms, as well as for general prevention. There is, of course, no evidence for the claims. The concept is primitive and preposterous.

Grapefruit

There is a widespread myth that grapefruits contain something special that causes weight loss. Diets in which several grapefruits are eaten each day are supposed to magically melt fat away. Pills with extracts of grapefruit are marketed as modern miracles of weight control.

No plausible theory has ever explained why grapefruit should be so special. A "health food" store flyer for one product says, "This grapefruit extract contains fruit enzymes to promote digestion and ease your digestion's work. These enzymes help reduce fat by stimulating digestive metabolism."

This claim is absurd. There is no evidence that grapefruit or any grapefruit product helps digest food. And if they did enhance digestion, they would tend to increase body fat, not decrease it. Products that block digestion, if there were any, would tend to decrease body fat. People who write such ads and those who believe them are seriously confused about the workings of the human body.

Claims for grapefruit have not been limited to weight control. Several years ago the fruit and its juice were promoted in a nationwide ad campaign suggesting that they could boost athletic performance and remedy fatigue and hypertension. There is no evidence to support these claims. Grapefruit has substantial potassium and little sodium, but so do lots of other foods. They can all be part of a healthy diet, but none of them should be considered remedies for serious diseases or symptoms or as aids to athletic performance. The ads were sponsored by the Florida Department of Citrus, an agency of the state government. The ads were paid for by an excise tax on citrus fruits. Thus, consumers paid for propaganda designed to deceive them.

Hair Analysis

Hair analysis is a test in which a small sample of hair, usually from the nape of the neck, is sent to a laboratory for measurement of its mineral content. Proponents claim that the test can be used to detect "mineral imbalances" and is useful for determining what nutrients should be prescribed for a long list of diseases and conditions. These claims are false.

Hair consists primarily of protein. The small amounts of minerals present are of unknown significance and have never been proved to be related to body levels of minerals, vitamins, or other nutrients. The mineral content of hair can be affected by sex, race, age, the season of the year, and contact with shampoos, sprays, dyes, and other products. It does not provide reliable information about minerals or other substances in the blood or tissues.[46] In addition, most commercial laboratories that have done hair analyses have not done them accurately. The only real value of hair analysis is as a preliminary examination to detect toxic heavy metals such as lead, cadmium, arsenic, and mercury. The results are not definitive; they must be confirmed by blood and urine tests.

During the mid-1980s the Federal Trade Commission halted a mail-order scheme in which people were invited to submit hair samples for analysis, and the lab would return a computer printout telling them what vitamins and minerals they should take. The FDA had investigated the lab by submitting identical hair samples under different names. The reported mineral values were completely different from sample to sample.

The bogus nature of commercial hair-analysis operations was further demonstrated by Dr. Stephen Barrett, who sent fifty-two hair samples from two healthy teenagers under assumed names to thirteen commercial hair-analysis laboratories. The reported levels of minerals varied considerably between identical samples sent to the same lab and from lab to lab. The labs also disagreed about what was "normal" or "usual" for many of the minerals. Most reports contained computerized interpretations that were voluminous, bizarre, and potentially frightening to patients. Six labs recommended food supplements, but the types and amounts varied widely from report to report. One report diagnosed twenty-three "possible or probable conditions," including atherosclerosis and kidney failure, and recommended fifty-six supplement doses per day. Literature from most of the labs suggested falsely that their reports were useful against a wide variety of diseases and supposed nutrient imbalances. Dr. Barrett concluded that even if hair analysis were a valuable diagnostic tool—which it isn't—most of the labs were doing it inaccurately.[47]

Dr. Barrett's study, published in the *Journal of the American Medical Association,* generated enormous publicity and was followed by the closing of several labs. Although many chiropractors and fringe medical doctors still rely on hair analysis in their practice, it is no longer advertised openly to the public.

Herbs

Plants have been used for therapeutic purposes for thousands of years. No doubt the effects of many plants were discovered by accident when they were tried as food or when they contaminated drinking water. In other cases, the origin of an herb's use is morphological (based on shape), astrological, or otherwise superstitious. While usually ineffective for the purported uses, some plants have been found useful for other purposes. Folk healers around the world know that many plants have physiologic effects, but they have done little or nothing to elucidate the effects, benefits, and hazards of herbal products.

Scientific studies have shown that the physiological effects of herbs are due to chemical components such as alkaloids, glycosides, oils, gums, and resins. Useful alkaloids, for example, have included morphine, ergotamine, cocaine, physostigmine, atropine, vincristine, and reserpine. After herbs are proven to have therapeutic value, however, isolation of their effective chemical component usually leads to production of synthetic compounds that are purer, safer, and/or more effective. Thus, herbs as such are not used in scientific medical practice.

Despite this fact (or perhaps because of it), the sale of herbs is a large and rapidly growing segment of the "health food" and "alternative medicine" industries. Hundreds of herbs (as roots, stems, leaves, barks, flowers, seeds, and powders and extracts thereof) line the shelves of "health food" stores and herb shops and are also sold through the mail. They are prescribed by naturopaths, chiropractors, and other fringe practitioners. They are also hawked to friends, neighbors, and relatives by many thousands of people who market health-related products from person-to-person (see Chapter 4).

The reason for this boom is certainly not taste; with few exceptions, medicinal herbs taste awful. The appeal of the herbs is their alleged healing powers. Many people have been deceived into believing that herbs are natural healing gifts from God or Nature and that they can cure just about anything that ails them without the side effects of modern drugs. While some herbs are sources of important purified drugs used in precise doses, only a handful are useful for self-treatment in the whole form. The rest generally don't perform as advertised, and many are toxic. The herbal-drug industry has been able to thrive because the FDA has given little attention to regulating it.

Stores that sell medicinal herbs typically sell books and magazines that promote the herbs as panaceas. Most of the popular herbals (as the books are called) provide little or no information on the toxicity of what they recommend—they simply list ailments for which each herb has been used, even uses that have been proven invalid. Some authors add a disclaimer saying that they don't necessarily recommend specific herbs for specific conditions and are just providing "educational information." But enthusiastic recommendations within the books are likely to be given far more credence than any disclaimer.

Danger Lurking

Many herb enthusiasts imagine that nature is benign and cares about humans. They believe that very few plants are poisonous, that every disease has an herbal remedy somewhere, and practically every herb is a remedy for something. This can lead to a "shotgun" approach: if you take enough different herbs, you're bound to be cured by one of them. Combinations may also be taken "preventively" for many years on the advice of a practitioner. Unfortunately, a few herbs contain poisons that do slow but serious harm to various organs. The problem may not be recognizable until too late. Comfrey, for example, contains pyrrolizidine and other alkaloids that are carcinogenic[48] and can cause severe liver disease.[49] This disease is endemic in Jamaica, parts of India, and other places where the people gather wild herbs and regularly drink teas made from them.

Unscientific herbal texts list powerful purgatives and other "eliminators" as useful in a large number of diseases. For example, *Back to Eden* [Back to Eden Books, 1985], by Jethro Kloss, recommends a high enema and an herbal emetic for dog bites, snake bites, insect stings, liver disease, kidney stones, gallstones, colitis, cholera, epilepsy, flu, and many other ailments that cannot be helped by such treatment. Kloss's recommendation of the purgative buckthorn for appendicitis could be deadly.

All this eliminating is unnatural and hazardous. Sweat-producers have no use in modern medicine. Emetics are used only to rid the body of certain poisons that have been swallowed. Diuretics are useful only for a few specific conditions, and stimulant laxatives are rarely appropriate to prescribe. Purging and eliminating through various orifices is dangerous because it can cause dehydration and depletion of vital minerals. Purging is also unpleasant and exhausting.

Hydrogen Peroxide

The hydrogen peroxide (H_2O_2) commonly used to clean minor cuts and scrapes is a 3 percent solution. It is approved and marketed for external use only. No other hydrogen peroxide is approved for any medical use. Nevertheless, since the mid-1980s, industrial strength (35 percent) hydrogen peroxide, diluted with various substances, has been promoted as a remedy for AIDS, cancer, arthritis, chronic headaches, and dozens of other diseases. The peroxide is purchased in bulk from chemical plants and put in pint and quart containers for retailing as "food-grade peroxide," "biowater," or "H_2O_2." Promotional literature calls it "hyperoxygenation therapy" and presents testimonials claiming miraculous cures. Unfortunately, some products have been mistaken for plain water, with tragic results. In one case three children were poisoned; one died and two were hospitalized.[50]

The prime promoter of hydrogen peroxide has been Kurt Donsbach (see Chapter 2), who has advocated drinking it, bathing in it, douching with it, taking enemas with it, and even injecting it intravenously. In 1988 the U.S. Postal Service charged him with falsely representing that hydrogen peroxide is effective against cancer and arthritis. Without admitting liability, he signed a consent agreement pledging not to make such representations in mail-order sales. He continues to make such claims, however, through speeches and publications.

"Hypoglycemia"

Hypoglycemia is both a rare condition and a popular diagnosis used by naturopaths, megavitamin advocates, and other fringe practitioners. It was especially trendy in the 1960s and 1970s. While still overdiagnosed in "alternative medicine" circles, it has recently given ground to "candidiasis hypersensitivity" and "environmental illness."

Hypoglycemia is not a disease but an abnormally low level of blood glucose that can be caused by many different factors, including some diseases. Since the brain and nervous system depend on glucose for proper functioning, the symptoms can include weakness, fatigue, hunger, headache, sleepiness, forgetfulness, and irritability. Because low blood sugar tends to stimulate adrenaline secretion there may also be sweating, trembling, heart palpitations, and anxiety. Severe hypoglycemia can result in coma and death.

Causes of hypoglycemia include overdosage of insulin or diabetes pills, rare glandular disorders, liver disease, and a variety of drugs. Fasting and starving are obvious causes of low blood sugar—the stores of glycogen in liver and muscle are depleted in a few hours, and the conversion of body protein to glucose is not always efficient enough to prevent hypoglycemia. In each of these cases, it is necessary to treat the cause of the problem, not the end results or symptoms.

Reactive hypoglycemia is another form of the problem. In response to carbohydrates (and sometimes caffeine) the pancreatic islet cells overreact and secrete too much insulin. This causes the blood sugar to plunge, and the person feels weak, tired, and hungry. In the 1960s it became a fashionable disorder to diagnose and self-diagnose. Carlton Fredericks, the Hypoglycemia Foundation, and others have claimed that twenty to fifty million people unknowingly suffer from this problem, and that it causes depression, schizophrenia, chronic fatigue, drug addiction, criminal behavior, sexual impotence, and much more.

Most medical experts, including those with the American Diabetes Association, the Endocrine Society, and the American Medical Association, say that very few people suffer from reactive hypoglycemia and that the condition rarely contributes to nervous, mental, or behavioral problems. But this has not stopped the hypoglycemia faddists from exploiting the public with alleged remedies.

The fad test for the fad "disease" is the glucose tolerance test. The subject drinks a large dose of glucose in water on an empty stomach. Blood glucose, and sometimes insulin and other hormones, are then measured for the next two to six hours. If the blood glucose level drops very low and the typical symptoms appear, reactive hypoglycemia is said to be likely. Most experts consider the test unreliable, however, because it does not simulate real-life conditions.

The diagnosis of hypoglycemia should be reserved for patients who get symptoms two to four hours after eating, develop blood glucose levels below 45 mg per 100 ml whenever symptoms occur, and are immediately relieved of symptoms when blood sugar is raised. The most practical way to test for this is probably with a home testing device.

Some fringe practitioners are so obsessed with hypoglycemia they assume that all or almost all of their patients have it. They do a glucose tolerance test and misinterpret the results, diagnose the disorder by questionnaire, or simply assume hypoglycemia is present. Then they prescribe a low-carbohydrate diet and hefty doses of nutritional and pseudonutritional supplements that they peddle. They may also prescribe and peddle herbal drugs. Because of the widespread quackery associated with hypoglycemia, the diagnosis should not be accepted unless it is made by a medical doctor with skill and integrity, one who does not specialize in the diagnosis or prescribe or sell supplements, herbs, or other drugs as a remedy. Anyone with definite signs of hypoglycemia, as diagnosed by an internist or family practitioner, should be examined by an endocrinologist.

Ion Generators

Ions are positively or negatively charged atoms and molecules. They occur in chemical solutions, as byproducts of certain technologies, in living organisms, and in the atmosphere. In the 1950s some companies started marketing machines that generate ions in the air. They made fantastic claims that breathing the ions could cure all kinds of diseases, including cancer and heart disease. Some of these early ion generators produced hazardous levels of ozone. The FDA took action against the health claims, and interest in the devices waned.

In the 1970s, experiments with animals suggested that changing the ion level in the air could affect their behavior and ability to fight respiratory infections. The results of these preliminary studies were not definitive. Nevertheless, the market was soon flooded with negative ion generators that, the public was told, would make them more energetic and cheerful, and improve their health in a wide variety of ways. An industry had been born. Several hundred thousand units have been sold since then for use in homes, offices, and even hospitals.

Ion generators, however, have never been proven to fulfill the promises made for them. Ions may have effects on humans, but no one knows what levels have what effects. Some levels might be harmful. Moreover, there is no practical way of controlling the ion concentration, which varies with room size, ventilation, machine capacity, and other factors. Therefore, using an ion generator is like taking an unknown dose of a medicine that has unknown effects.

As they are generally used, the devices probably have no significant effects, positive or negative. A study done with two sets of office workers used some real ion generators and some fakes that looked just like the real ones. The occupational health experts could detect no difference in the health, energy, or comfort levels of the two sets of workers.[51]

Iridology

Iridology is a system of diagnosis based on examination of the irises of the eyes (the colored portions surrounding the pupils). According to the theory, the iris reflects the state of the organs and limbs in a precise way that can be read by trained iridologists. Iridology charts show the different parts of the body represented by the segments of the iris. Abnormal spots, lines, and colors develop when the corresponding organs are disturbed, we are told.

Examination of blown-up color photos of the iris is said to reveal drug deposits and diseases in organs, hereditary weaknesses, healing processes, and subconscious tensions. Even a person's life expectancy can be determined. In fact, it is so powerful a method that one pair of photos furnishes more accurate and detailed information than a series of blood tests, x-rays films, or biopsies and can be useful in very early diagnosis. So they say.

Naturally, such claims can be very appealing. Who wants to give flesh or blood for tests, be exposed to x-rays, or pay for such procedures? Iridologists (mostly chiropractors and naturopaths) find sympathetic listeners (and clients) when they claim medical science unfairly ignores their technique and keeps it out of the medical schools.

Medical science, of course, does not ignore the eyes for signs of illness and recognizes that jaundice, dilated pupils, bloodshot eyes, red spots, mineral deposits, and other changes can result from systemic disease. The iris is known to be affected in some cases of tuberculosis, diabetes, atherosclerosis, Crohn's disease, and other disorders. But these changes are not always seen with these disorders; nor are they confined to specific segments of the iris. Moreover, there is no anatomic or other evidence that certain parts of the iris are associated with certain organs.

Some years ago, a well-controlled study involving kidney disease was carried out by the researchers at the University of California and Veterans' Medical Center in San Diego.[52] Three practicing iridologists, including chiropractor Bernard Jensen, author of a popular text on the subject, participated. Twenty-four patients with severe kidney disease, twenty-four with moderate kidney disease, and ninety-five controls who had no kidney problems had photos taken of both eyes. The camera used belonged to one of the iridologists, and the slides were presented to them in their offices, at their leisure, and with the option of discarding any slides they thought unsatisfactory. They were asked to give an estimate of kidney function based on the photos.

The results were very interesting. None of the iridologists could predict the presence or absence of kidney disease with any accuracy. The best score had only a 2.5 percent predictive value. That is, of those in the general population identified as having kidney disease by this iridologist, only 2.5 percent really will. And others with serious kidney disease will be told their kidneys are fine. This contrasts sharply with scientific methods, which can correctly assess kidney function 95 percent of the time with one blood test (creatinine level) and, in the remaining cases, with one or two subsequent tests. In another study, Dutch iridologists were unable to determine which thirty-nine of seventy-eight patients had gallstones.[53]

Since even the master practitioners cannot come close to correctly assessing kidney function, why should we believe iridologists any more than palm readers? Serious psychological harm can be done when people are told they have a disease when they don't. Serious physical harm can result when a person is assured he does not have a disease when, in fact, he does.

Even iridologists apparently do not have as much confidence in their method as they used to. Instead of stating with certainty that this or that disease is present, they usually make vague diagnoses, such as "you have a weakness in your liver," or colon, adrenal glands, or other organs. They then prescribe expensive vitamins and other supplements, which they sell, to prevent the "weakness" from developing into disease.

Some iridologists also have the strange idea that only blue eyes are normal. They say that green and brown eyes are really blue eyes polluted with toxins and waste. If you were born with nonblue eyes, it is because your mother passed on her pollution and toxins to you. If you follow your iridologist's advice, your eyes will gradually turn blue. Sure.

Jason Winters Products

Jason Winters, a former Hollywood stuntman, has no education or credentials in health, medicine, or nutrition. Yet, he has convinced many people that he is an authority in these fields and has discovered miraculous healing herbs around the world. His products, we are told, cure cancer and heart disease, promote weight loss, enhance energy and libido, strengthen the immune system, and prolong life. He has written several books that promote both his products and a host of superstitious ideas about health. He claims, for example, that astrological signs determine health problems and that one's birth sign determines what herbs should be taken for life to enhance one's health.

Winters's products are marketed by Tri-Sun International, a company in Fargo, North Dakota. The main product is a tea made from three herbs, which sells for $30 to $80 a pound. Although its label makes no medicinal claims, Winters's speeches and books promote it for the prevention and treatment of cancer. His book, *Killing Cancer,* tells the story of his struggle with cancer of the throat. The book states that despite treatment with radiation, Winters was told by his physician that the cancer would kill him. So he went searching for a cure. First he went to Mexico and tried laetrile, which he says works for many people but failed in his case. Then he obtained herbs that were considered folk remedies for cancer: chaparral from the American southwest, red clover from England, and "herbaline" from China. He tried them separately with no apparent effects, but upon finishing his first cup of a combination tea, he claims, he could feel it working. Within one month the tumor was gone.

The tea does not cure anything, he says. It just "purifies the blood" so the body's immune system can do its job. He claims that more than a hundred thousand cancer victims are enjoying the same results he got using the tea, and many others are getting relief from arthritis, hypertension, and other problems. Like laetrile proponents and other cancer quacks, he claims that doctors and medical researchers are not interested in a real cure for cancer because that would endanger their livelihoods.

Many people find Jason Winters's story persuasive and drink his tea regularly. Tri-Sun's literature says that millions use it each day. I can assure you they don't drink it for its flavor; it tastes vile and can cause nausea and dizziness. They take it because they believe it is effective against cancer.

Winters's alleged experience proves nothing. He says he underwent such intensive cobalt radiation therapy that the right side of his face turned black and his hair fell out. Only after this did he start using herbs. I believe he was cured by the radiation therapy but gave all the credit to drinking tea.

The National Cancer Institute has tested large numbers of herbs with the hope of identifying substances effective against cancer. Chaparral has been tested and found too toxic. Winters is secretive about the "herbaline" or "special spice" listed on some of his product labels. It may be from the chrysanthemum flower, which is often used in the Orient, though not as a cancer cure. There is no evidence that it has any anticancer activity. His secretiveness would be understandable if the ingredient were a soft-drink flavoring. But it is supposed to be a vital ingredient in a spectacular cancer cure, and it is being kept secret— apparently for commercial purposes—by a man who accuses the medical profession of covering up or ignoring cancer cures for monetary purposes.

In scientific medicine, important developments are made available to scientists around the world for testing and, when proven, are offered to the public without secrets. If Jason Winters really has a cancer cure, he should prove it works and share it with researchers so they can verify his claims.

Winters claims his tea is nontoxic and completely safe at any level of intake. In fact, chaparral contains toxins that can cause nausea and vomiting, and it may have other adverse effects. Winters acknowledges that these symptoms can occur, but claims they represent stored toxins being flushed out of the body by the tea. This excuse is commonly used by herbalists when asked why their products make people sick.

Kirlian Photography

In the 1930s a Russian couple named Kirlian developed a cameraless photography in which an image on photographic paper is generated by the interaction of a high-voltage, high-frequency alternating electric field with the object being photographed. The resulting photographs show bright colors and halos surrounding the objects. This eerie quality has led to wild claims about psychic auras, energy bodies, healing energies, and the like. Since the 1960s fringe researchers and assorted con artists have promoted the photography as a marvelous diagnostic tool. They allege that Kirlian photos of fingers and hands contain colors and patterns that reveal diseases and even latent diseases, including incipient cancer and assorted organ weaknesses. Even nutritional deficiencies, drug abuse, confusion, and psychiatric illness are laid bare by the Kirlian photos. These "diseases" are then treated or prevented with vitamins, acupuncture, homeopathy, and whatever else the fringe therapist happens to sell.

Despite all the excitement, hype, and thousands of hours of research by psychologist Thelma Moss, at UCLA, and others, none of the fantastic claims has been verified. The interesting patterns and variations seen in the photos are not "bioplasma" or mystic auras but the results of such mundane factors as voltage, moisture, exposure time, and the amount of finger pressure applied to the apparatus.[54] Nevertheless, hucksters continue to promote Kirlian photography as a special and highly effective diagnostic technique. It is especially popular with oriental medical practitioners and is sometimes seen at "health fairs," where it is used to diagnose "malnutrition" and prescribe supplements. No use of Kirlian photography in diagnosing, treating, or preventing ill health of any type is legitimate.

Lecithin

Lecithin, a phospholipid extracted from soybeans, is sold in granule, liquid, and semisolid forms. It is alleged to lower blood cholesterol levels and to improve memory in normal and demented persons. There is some evidence for the first claim, but the effect is probably due to its polyunsaturated fat content, in which case it would be much cheaper to simply consume more vegetable oil than to take lecithin. Definitive studies on this question have not been done.

The other claim, that lecithin can improve memory, is based on the fact that it contains choline, a B-vitamin that is incorporated into a neurotransmitter, acetylcholine, which is involved in thought processes. Unfortunately, there is no evidence to support the claim of improved memory in either normal persons or those with memory deficits.

Live Cell Analysis

In live cell analysis, a drop of blood is magnified by dark-field microscopy and viewed on a television monitor. The red and white blood cells stand out vividly against a dark background. The effect is quite dramatic and impressive to the naive client, who is then told that various "abnormalities" mean various nutritional supplements must be taken, specifically the expensive "special" supplements the tester happens to sell.

Dark-field microscopy is a valid and useful tool for examining cells and tissues, but in the hands of the supplement peddlers it becomes just another tool for lying, cheating, and stealing. These operators, usually chiropractors or phony nutritionists, see abnormalities that don't exist and falsely claim certain features indicate nutritional deficiencies, all for the sole purpose of misleading the clients into buying pills they don't need.[55] Accepting nutritional or medical advice from them can be expensive and dangerous.

Live cell analysis was developed by James Privitera, M.D., a Californian who started two major companies in the field, Livcell Analysis and NutriScreen. He had previously been convicted of conspiracy to distribute laetrile as a cancer remedy and sentenced to six months in jail. He was a member of the board of governors of the National Health Federation, the quackery industry's main lobbying group, which initiated a letter-writing campaign on his behalf. After serving fifty-five days, Privitera was pardoned by Governor Jerry Brown, the very same Jerry Brown who recently campaigned for the Democratic presidential nomination. Brown's platform, incidentally, was relevant to this book. His national health insurance proposal includes coverage of chiropractors and acupuncturists.

Mineral Supplements

Excessive mineral ingestion can be dangerous. Iron, for example, can accumulate to high levels in the blood and organs and cause a wide range of toxic effects. The hazard is increased by supplementation with vitamin C, which increases iron absorption. Excessive iron may promote the growth of certain tumors.[56] Too much zinc can cause bone marrow depression, anemia, possibly elevated blood cholesterol, and other serious problems.[57] Too much calcium is risky for people with recurrent calcium oxalate kidney stones. Too much magnesium can cause diarrhea. Too much of any mineral can interfere with the absorption of other minerals. There is no doubt that mineral supplementation beyond RDA levels is risky and should be avoided unless prescribed by a reliable physician for a condition such as confirmed iron-deficiency anemia. Some women who menstruate heavily may need an RDA-level iron supplement. Women who habitually avoid dairy products may need supplementary calcium. Children raised in nonfluoridated communities should take a fluoride supplement. Aside from these situations, people who eat well rarely need any mineral supplementation.

"Organically Grown" Foods

Organically grown foods are said to be grown without chemical fertilizers or pesticides. Advocates claim they are more nutritious, taste better, and are safer because they lack pesticide residues. They say organic gardening and farming are also safer for the workers and do less harm to the environment. This hodgepodge of half-truths and nonsense has created an "organic foods" mythology and led to a bull market and premium prices for the products. Since many crops are very difficult to grow without some help from chemicals, and since the consumer can't really tell the difference, fraud is rampant.

The "organic" concept is a fraud. Plants absorb the same nutrients through their roots by the same processes whether the fertilizers come in a concentrated chemical form or a more dilute form such as manure. Their nutrient composition and flavor are determined mostly by their genes. There is no evidence that foods grown without chemicals are more nutritious or taste better.

But aren't organically grown foods safer? Not necessarily, because the level of pesticide residue is our food supply is insignificant. Most people are exposed to far more carcinogenic activity from "pesticides" naturally present in foods.[58] These chemicals have evolved to protect the plants from insects, fungi, and other pests. Then there are carcinogens created by cooking and otherwise processing foods. And there is fat itself, which seems to be at least a cocarcinogen under some circumstances. Moreover, there is the problem of fraud. Organic farmers often take over acreage with soil that has recently been treated with pesticides and has significant residues left. They raise crops and sell them as "organically grown" until the residues are used up, then move to other treated fields. In other cases produce raised with the aid of chemicals is simply misrepresented as organically grown.

There is no good reason for consumers to pay high prices for foods labeled "organically grown." Neither the human body nor laboratory tests can distinguish such products from those grown with the aid of concentrated chemicals.[59] But what about concerns for the environment and for agricultural workers? Isn't buying organic the socially responsible thing to do? The organic advocates have a slightly better case here. We don't want cheap produce at the cost of high disease rates among farm workers and damage to wildlife and water supplies. The concept of "organically grown" or "organic," however, is not appropriate to deal with these concerns. Chemical pesticides can be, and usually are, used in a safe manner that does not harm people or the earth. On the other hand, fertilizing with manure can result in higher oil and gas consumption (and consequent air pollution) necessary to move the heavy fertilizer around. Bacteria from the manure can pollute local streams, and its smell can disrupt the lives of local residents. The toxins of manure would also be recycled.

I agree that home gardeners should attempt to avoid the use of dangerous pesticides, almost to the point of just growing crops that don't need them. While occasional careful use is generally harmless, too many people don't read labels and may overexpose themselves and others to the toxic chemicals. Moreover, they don't always properly dispose of containers and unused products.

When it comes to shopping for food, however, there is no point in avoiding certain foods unless one is aware of specific abuses and harm to workers or the environment. Simply saying "they use chemicals" is not enough. A more rational approach is needed. The adoption of the "organic" concept by some states (and probably by the federal government in the near future) is another example of pseudoscience influencing legislation for the benefit of special interest groups promoting quackery or do-gooders with little insight.

Oxygen Inhalation

Oxygen has legitimate medical uses, such as in severe lung disease and during surgery. But there are also two major types of oxygen quackery. One is the use of hyperbaric oxygen chambers for unapproved therapies. The chambers, in which the patient sits or lies, are filled with high-pressure pure oxygen. Approved uses include decompression sickness ("the bends"), carbon monoxide poisoning, embolisms, and burns. Unapproved uses include cancer, arthritis, multiple sclerosis, acne, and many others. Moreover, the only approved chambers are made of stainless steel to exacting specifications. Entrepreneurs have peddled unapproved fiberglass chambers to hospitals, clinics, and fringe practitioners, with claims of amazing cures in a variety of diseases.

The other major form of oxygen quackery is the use of pure oxygen by athletes, especially professional, college, and high-school football players. The "playing time" of a football game—the time during which the players actually may be in motion—is about an hour. Since there are offensive and defensive teams, players generally are in the game for half this amount or less, much of which is spent in huddling, walking, or standing still. For most players, strenuous activity occurs in bursts of fifteen seconds or less, spread over a period of three hours. Yet they are so incapacitated with exhaustion that they need to inhale pure oxygen as they sit on the bench? Come on! These aren't elderly patients dying from emphysema; they are fit young men. They should be able to play two or three times as long as they do without any problem. Soccer players, marathoners, and many other athletes do much more than football players without the illusory aid of oxygen. It's nothing but a superstition and a placebo that causes money to be wasted and, in all likelihood, viruses and bacteria to be spread around by players sharing the apparatus. Coaches and school administrators should not be misled by the peddlers of oxygen-dispensing gadgets.

"Pangamic Acid"

"Pangamic" acid was one of the names given to various substances marketed years ago as "vitamin B_{15}." It was concocted and patented by Ernst T. Krebs, Jr., who also was the major developer of the quack cancer remedy laetrile. According to its purveyors, "vitamin B_{15}" could prevent and cure heart disease, cancer, asthma, arthritis, diabetes, eczema, neuritis, hangovers, emphysema, poisoning, headaches, mental retardation, insomnia, and premature aging. In reality, it prevented and cured nothing and was not a vitamin. "B_{15}" faded from the limelight after the FDA obtained injunctions against several companies marketing it. Krebs, too, faded from the limelight following brief imprisonment for promoting laetrile in violation of a court order.

Past-Life Therapy

Past-life therapy is based on the idea that psychological disorders arise from elements (traumas and personality traits) of one's alleged past lives intruding on the subconscious. Proponents say they use hypnosis, meditation, or guided imagery to "regress" the patient to early stages of life—first to early childhood and infancy, then to life in the womb, and then to earlier incarnations ("past lives"). As with Freudian psychoanalysis, exposing the destructive elements to consciousness is supposed to be therapeutic. The example of regressionist Dr. Bruce Goldberg, author of *Past Lives, Future Lives: Accounts of Regression and Progression Through Hypnosis* [New Castle, 1982], is discussed in the section on Oprah Winfrey in Chapter 6.

Contrary to popular belief, hypnosis is not akin to a truth serum; people can and do lie, fabricate, and confuse fantasy with reality while hypnotized.[60] The power of memory is not necessarily enhanced by the procedure but may, in fact, be weakened. So the words uttered by those entranced, far from being gospel, may be nothing more than fantasy. In fact, the misnamed phenomenon of hypnosis is characterized by focused concentration and heightened suggestibility, including susceptibility to illusion and delusion. The realities behind the alleged past lives are fantasy-prone personalities, hypnagogic and hypnopompic hallucinations (waking dreams), and cult therapists who lead their subjects to the wild beliefs. Health professionals who use past-life therapy not only abandon critical thinking and scientific method, but encourage their patients to substitute their dreams and delusions (and the delusions of the therapist) for reality. Goldberg's delusions are grander than most, for he can take you (through hypnosis) not only to your past lives, but to future lives as well.

Radionics

Radionics involves the use of instruments or inanimate objects to detect, magnify, store, or control alleged psychic and healing energies. Early shamans used sticks (the original magician's wand) to help communicate with spirits. Modern radionics practitioners use a wide variety of pendulums, crystals, black boxes, and electronic gadgets that may generate pulses of current or may have nonfunctional circuits. If you consult a radionics practitioner, here's what is likely to happen. First you will provide a drop of blood, lock of hair, nail clipping, or photograph, which will be placed in or on the radionics device. The practitioner then concentrates on you, holds a pendulum over the device, and asks a series of questions. Or the practitioner may hold a pendulum over an anatomical diagram and interpret its movements to decide what organs are diseased. The practitioner then focuses healing energy on your diseased parts or uses the machine to "treat" your drop of blood. You may also be advised to see a homeopath, aromatherapist, herbalist, or other fringe healer. Radionics is such a transparent fraud that few practitioners operate openly in the United States. Nevertheless, it is a tenacious type of quackery that takes many forms and never disappears completely. Currently popular forms include crystal healing and diagnosis by Kirlian photography.

Raw Milk

Raw (unpasteurized) milk illustrates how the quackery industry can take a dangerous product and market it as a "health food." It has long been a standard item in "health food" stores, though recent court decisions have severely restricted its distribution. The "health food" press claims that raw milk is nutritionally superior because pasteurization destroys valuable nutrients. Although about 10 percent of the heat-sensitive vitamins (vitamin C and thiamine) are destroyed in the pasteurizing process, milk is not a significant source of these nutrients to begin with.

Believers, who pay a premium price, sometimes pay with their life as well. Raw milk can harbor dangerous bacteria such as *Salmonella* and *Campylobacter*. Far from being a "health food," it can cause nausea, vomiting, diarrhea, abdominal cramps, stillbirths, and even death. Young children, elderly adults, and persons with a compromised immune system are the most susceptible to the illnesses and the most likely to suffer severe symptoms and death. Only pasteurization, heating the milk to 145°F for thirty minutes or 161°F for fifteen seconds, can ensure that harmful bacteria will not be present.

"Certified" But Still Dangerous

The "certified" label on a raw-milk carton does not mean that the milk has been tested and found safe by a government agency. The certification is done by a private group affiliated with the dairy that produces it. Moreover, no agency can guarantee that the milk does not contain dangerous salmonella bacteria; this is simply not possible with present technology. In fact, some experts believe most raw milk contains at least low levels of salmonella all the time.

Given this state of affairs, drinking raw milk, or eating cheese made from raw milk and not properly aged, is like playing Russian roulette. The unlucky ones get zapped by very nasty bugs. For example, a California mother who believed the "health food" propaganda gave raw milk to her infant daughter. Several weeks later the girl developed diarrhea, high fever, lethargy, and partial paralysis. It turned out that some raw milk had given her a *Salmonella dublin* infection that lodged in her brain and formed abscesses. Surgery and antibiotics saved her life.[61] Others have not been so lucky.

Poisoning and infection from milk have been problems ever since humans started drinking it. For hundreds of years, contaminated milk has caused outbreaks of typhoid fever, diphtheria, brucellosis, tuberculosis, listeriosis, and many types of salmonella infection.[62] A century ago Louis Pasteur discovered that milk could be made safe by heating it enough to kill the bacteria it contained. Since then most public-health agencies have discouraged raw milk consumption and more than half the state legislatures have banned the products.

The "Health Food" Industry Exposes Itself

Raw-milk dairies have fought for decades to save their profits from the meddling of public-health officials and concerned citizens. They have aggressively marketed their products as safer and more nutritious and especially good for infants, pregnant women, the sick, and the elderly. And they have sued people who told the truth and warned the public.[63] In 1984 the Alta-Dena Certified Dairy, of City of Industry, California, filed a $110 million lawsuit against John Bolton, M.D., and the American Academy of Pediatrics in an effort to intimidate and shut them up. In 1986 a Superior Court judge summarily dismissed the suit as meritless.[64]

For almost fifteen years the FDA studied, stalled, and refused to take action. Finally, in 1984, Public Citizen's Health Research Group, with support from the American Public Health Association and the American Academy of Pediatrics, filed suit to force them to ban interstate shipment of raw milk (except for the purpose of pasteurization). Three years later they won when a federal court judge ordered the FDA to promulgate the ban. The judge concluded: "It is undisputed that all types of raw milk are unsafe for human consumption and pose significant health risks. The appropriate remedy in this case is, therefore, an order compelling the agency to promulgate a regulation prohibiting interstate shipment."[65] She added that the FDA can also prohibit intrastate sale of raw milk. So far it has not done this.

In another case, Consumers Union and the American Public Health Association filed suit in California in 1985 to stop Alta-Dena (then doing business as Steuve's Natural) from advertising that their unpasteurized products are safe and nutritionally superior to pasteurized milk. For thirty-five years Alta-Dena had carried out a false and misleading ad campaign promoting its raw milk even to infants and invalids. Moreover, long after it was common knowledge that honey carries a risk of botulism to infants, Alta-Dena ads continued to suggest that its formula be made with honey, thereby adding to the risk of raw milk. And, in spite of conclusive evidence that raw milk is very hazardous to immune-deficient people, including those with HIV infection and those undergoing treatment for cancer, the dairy refused the advice of experts to put warning labels on the products. Many AIDS patients have been duped into thinking raw milk is more nutritious and have subjected themselves to severe risks by drinking it.

Warning: Killer Milk

In 1989 California Superior Court Judge John Sutter ruled against the dairy and ordered it to stop making false and misleading claims.[66] The decision also required that for the next ten years the dairy place the following notice on the label of every carton of raw milk:

> Warning: this milk may contain dangerous bacteria. Those facing the highest risk of disease or death include babies, pregnant women, the elderly, alcoholics, those with cancer, AIDS, or reduced immunity and those taking cortisone, antibiotics or antacids. Questions regarding the use of raw certified milk should be directed to your physician.

Moreover, the judge's ruling required that any advertising of raw milk claiming health or nutrition benefits must carry the following notice:

> Warning: The FDA has determined (1) that there is no satisfactory scientific proof that pasteurization significantly reduces the nutritional value of milk and (2) that the risks associated with consuming raw certified milk outweigh any of its alleged health benefits.

The judge also ordered the defendants to pay almost $2 million in civil penalties, restitution ($100,000 to be used by the State Attorney General to investigate false advertising), and plaintiffs' attorney fees.

The raw milk situation illustrates the "health food" industry in a nutshell. The industry will stop at nothing to protect its profits. It will fraudulently claim health advantages for it products. It will knowingly sell products that are either inherently dangerous or tainted with potentially lethal filth. It can endanger the health of its customers. It will battle public-health experts in the legislatures, using campaign donations as needed. And it may wage lawsuit terrorism with the hope of to suppressing and silencing its critics, honest health professionals whose sole motive is to provide the public with accurate information on important health issues.

Rebirthing

Birth trauma is much worse than anyone imagines, according to Leonard Orr, self-styled miracle healer and inventor of the "rebirthing" system of attaining health, happiness, and riches. It causes not only neuroses and psychoses, but also sleep (a symbolic return to the womb), disease, and death itself (the permanent return to the womb). If only we could do it over and be born without pain and fear, we could escape this and always be awake instead of wasting all that time sleeping.

Fortunately for humanity, in 1974 Orr discovered a method of inducing a rebirth experience, which is now available to all who can afford it. It can, Orr claims, cure cancer, diabetes, and other deadly diseases. Details on the moment of discovery are sketchy, but Orr says he was in his bathtub with a mask and snorkel on when he saw the light.

In the original version of rebirthing, after thorough indoctrination of the impending miracle, the rebirthee floats face down in a hot tub with a snorkel in his mouth. A "rebirther" standing at his side supports the rebirthee's hips and provides guidance, which consists almost entirely of urgings to hyperventilate. "Breathe deeper, keep breathing, faster, deeper," go the exhortations.

The subject often blacks out for a few seconds. When he comes to, the exhortations to hyperventilate continue. This goes on for fifteen to forty-five minutes. Then the rebirthee is pulled out of the water and lies down, sometimes unconscious, while the rebirther plays loving midwife-mother-father. Many subjects repeat the experience several times until they have the right experience or give up trying. The blacking out is said to be caused by "plugging into" the anesthetic used in the subject's birth and to confirm that return to the womb has actually been achieved. Strangely, no effort is made to determine whether an anesthetic was used in the birth of the subjects. According to several subjects I interviewed, however, the blacking out occurs regardless of method of birth or drug use at birth.

More recently, Orr has decided that hyperventilation and presence of the rebirther are the important factors, not the flotation in warm water. So the tubs have been largely dispensed with, and now the subject simply relaxes and hyperventilates with coaching by the rebirther. This has reduced the cost, since overhead for the hot tubs can be considerable. The fee is now about $25 to $100 per session (up to about an hour).

Is the fee for the coaching in hyperventilation? No, it covers the presence of the rebirther, who, at the moment of rebirth, telepathically absorbs the stirred-up psychic garbage and disposes of it, according to Orr. Without a trained bona fide, certified rebirther in the room, all the effort would be wasted.

The Hazards of Rebirthing

All this would be too absurd to even discuss were it not for the facts that Orr has advertised nationwide to get thousands to pay to be "reborn" and that prolonged hyperventilation, especially in a hot tub, can be dangerous. The blacking out has nothing to do with anesthetics but is caused by reduction of blood flow to the brain. Excessive heat causes the peripheral blood vessels to dilate. This leaves less blood for the brain and by itself can cause fainting.

Hyperventilation also decreases blood and oxygen supply to the brain. The arteries dilate in response to carbon dioxide in the blood and contract in its absence. This controls the brain blood supply. Hyperventilation throws off carbon dioxide, the blood levels drop, and the brain arteries contract. Loss of consciousness can result. (The oxygen level of the blood is not increased by hyperventilation because the oxygen is carried by hemoglobin, which is saturated by normal breathing. Carbon dioxide is carried mostly in solution and can be increased by holding the breath and decreased by hyperventilating.)

Regaining full consciousness and strength after a rebirthing session can take two or three hours. During this time, a mild to ferocious headache may develop. Orr, of course, attributes this to the mythical anesthetic. In reality, it is more likely due to the starvation of the brain for oxygen and the rebound rush of blood to the brain when the torture is finally ended. Such stress on the arteries and normal metabolism of the brain could be harmful, especially to those with high blood pressure or atherosclerotic cerebral arteries.

Royal Jelly

Royal jelly is a salivary secretion from worker bees that is fed to a bee selected to be the queen of a hive. Along with abundant honey, the enzymes or hormones in the secretions trigger changes that cause the queen to grow much larger, live much longer, and reproduce. There is no reason to believe that bee saliva of any type is beneficial to humans, but this hasn't stopped the charlatans from making fantastic claims about royal jelly.

One of the best-selling brands of bee saliva is *Regina Royal Jelly*. In full-page ads in various magazines, Madeline Balletta, founder and president of Bee-Alive, Inc., states that the product is used by the British Royal Family. The ads suggest that royal jelly is effective for preventing or treating chronic fatigue syndrome (which Ms. Balletta erroneously equates with Epstein-Barr virus infection), asthma, assorted childhood ailments, insomnia, and emotional disturbances. She also suggests that it can help athletes gain physical and mental stamina, boost the immune system, and slow the aging process. The ad quotes singer Pat Boone saying the product is "for everyone who is sick and tired of being sick and tired." During the 1970s, the Federal Trade Commission objected to ads in which Boone promoted an acne remedy with unsubstantiated claims. The case was settled by a consent agreement prohibiting the manufacturer and the advertising agency from making such claims in the future. Now, according to Ms. Balletta, he is a "leading advocate" of royal jelly.

Seawater

This unlikely snake oil must have one of the greatest profit margins ever. The promoters get seawater free and sell it for up to $10 per half pint. That may seem expensive, but if you don't live close to a clean ocean, it's not that easy to get drinkable seawater. But why would anyone want seawater badly enough to pay for it? Because, they are told and they believe, a teaspoon per day is a great nutritional supplement that supplies critical nutrients and thereby prevents and cures such "deficiency diseases" as cancer, heart disease, schizophrenia, baldness, and whatever else might ail them. Thousands of people have been swindled by the scam. FDA action has dampened business, but seawater as a miracle cure is likely to be around for a long time. In fact, the idea is not new. Hydrotherapy, popular in India and with naturopaths in turn-of-the-century America, often includes drinking seawater as part of "taking the waters."

Snake Blood

In Asia it is commonly believed that drinking fresh snake blood confers a host of health benefits. The elixir is said to cure an assortment of ailments and to rejuvenate and vitalize the mind and body, especially sexually. The more venomous, the more powerful the blood. There is no evidence that these claims are true, and no reason why they should be. They are superstitious in origin, deriving from primitive views of snakes as powerful, virulent, and possessed with magical powers.

In Thailand the snake-blood business has become so lucrative that the rat and mouse populations are soaring and devastating crops. By catching one good-sized snake and selling it to the local vendor, a peasant can earn the equivalent of a week's work in the fields. So more people are hunting down the farmers' allies while rodents tend to the crops. In some areas the situation is so bad that some farmers have given up and become snake-catchers. If you can't beat 'em, join 'em. As the snakes become scarce, their cash value increases, and the hunters bear down harder.

In rural Thailand some villages have stopped farming and become tourist towns for snake-blood drinkers and patrons of prostitution—often one and the same. Asian and Western tourists come by the planeload to sit in elegant (relative to the poverty of the villages) lounges and drink fresh snake blood, sometimes mixed with juice or liquor, from a wine glass—followed by their hoped-for sexual marathon. Some connoisseurs like the blood so fresh that, rather than drink it two minutes after it is squeezed from the butchered snake, they prefer to suck it directly from an incision near the snake's tail.

So far, drinking snake blood has not become the rage in America. With many Asian immigrants here and more arriving every day, however, it would not be surprising if the practice catches on in some communities. The situation illustrates how quackery can endanger wildlife and cause environmental and economic damage. There may be other dangers: eating any type of raw flesh carries some risk of contracting parasites and harmful germs. Studies on the potential risks of drinking raw snake blood are needed.

Snake Venom

For centuries, snakes have been symbols of healing—used in the official seal of medical groups—and their body parts and venoms have been used as medicines for various disorders. Yet these have not been effective drugs, and "snake oil" has become a synonym for quack remedy. In recent years, snake venoms have made a comeback as alleged remedies for arthritis, multiple sclerosis, and other chronic disorders. Venoms from water moccasins, cobras, kraits, and other snakes have been used, though no success has been documented.[67]

In sufficient doses, snake venoms can be lethal. Users have reported dizziness, headaches, visual disturbances, and other symptoms consistent with snake poisoning. Some have even died. Still, there always seems to be a market for the venoms. We hold snakes in awe, we revere and fear them, and this makes snake venom a powerful placebo, especially for disorders subject to spontaneous remissions. Most multiple sclerosis and arthritis patients, for example, experience somewhat dramatic improvement now and then. If they happen to be taking a drug they believe is powerful around the time they start to feel better, nothing on earth will convince them the drug was not responsible, or keep them from paying heavily for it.

Spirulina (Blue-Green Algae)

Blue-green algae are microscopic plants that can form mats ("pond scum") on the surfaces of ponds and lakes, creating a putrid smell and ruining the taste of the water. There are more than 1,500 species of blue-green algae, some that are useful as food and others that can cause gastroenteritis and hepatitis. One type of blue-green alga—called "spirulina—has been marketed as a "health food" for more than twenty years.

Spirulina got a big boost in 1981 when the *National Enquirer* published an article with a front-page headline touting it as an appetite suppressant. Although the FDA stated that spirulina could not be legally sold as an appetite suppressant, many "health food" entrepreneurs jumped on the bandwagon to market it. Proponents claim that spirulina is an excellent source of vitamin B_{12}, protein, vitamin A, minerals, and neuropeptides (amino acid chains that nourish the brain). It is also said to be a mental and physical stimulant and euphoriant and an effective treatment for migraine headaches, Alzheimer's disease, alcoholism, herpes, diabetes, warts, allergies, arthritis, drug addiction, jet lag, obesity, fatigue, depression, some cancers, mood swings, and much more. It wouldn't surprise me to hear that it enables one to walk on water.

The truth, of course, is less glamorous. The commonly recommended daily dose of spirulina contains less protein than half a slice of whole wheat bread and less vitamins and minerals than a large serving of broccoli.[68] Bread and broccoli (and many other common foods) taste much better, cost less, and are more nutritious than spirulina. Spirulin's alleged vitamin B_{12} content is more likely from fecal or insect contamination, or it is a chemical analogue of B_{12} that has no role in human nutrition.

The claims about the neuropeptides are nonsense; peptides are generally not absorbed intact, and if they were they would not penetrate the blood-brain barrier. The promoters' claims about brain nourishment and stimulant activity are untrue; only those who talk themselves into it will say they notice any change in physical strength, stamina, or mental acuity. The claims about algae products being useful against dozens of diseases are preposterous. Furthermore, their taste is vile.

Mountains of Lies and Money

All these fraudulent claims have been made so strenuously for so long that they have become "health food" folklore. Thousands of spirulina peddlers are multilevel distributors who continually accost their friends, neighbors, relatives, and coworkers with algae propaganda and try to sign them up as customers and fellow peddlers. They set up booths at health fairs, advertise in local papers and on bulletin boards, plant promotional articles in local shoppers, and proselytize at every opportunity.

Because the general climate for quackery is so favorable, spirulina peddlers are rarely called to account for their fraudulent activities. One major promoter of spirulina, Christopher Hills, founder of Microalgae International Sales Corp. of Boulder Creek, California, did make a $225,000 out-of-court settlement with California authorities who had charged him with false and misleading advertising.[69] The company had advertised that spirulina could provide all the nutrients essential for life and that a person could live off one drum of spirulina for seventeen years.

Hills and spirulina are still going strong, however. He founded and serves as board chairman of Light Force, Inc., a multilevel company that markets spirulina products with claims that they can suppress appetite, boost immunity, and increase energy. Company sales materials claim that spirulina is a "superfood" and "works to cleanse and detoxify the body." Its magazine, *The Enlightener,* has carried reports about users who lost weight or recovered from arthritis, cancer, multiple sclerosis and serious injuries while taking Light Force products.[70]

The Dangers of Spirulina

There are two obvious hazards to believing the algae propagandists: you might waste money better spent on tastier and more nutritious food, and you might forego proper health care in the belief that spirulina will cure what ails you. But there is another danger. Some strains of the algae contain toxins, notably saxitoxin, that can cause gastrointestinal symptoms such as nausea, gas, diarrhea, throat irritation, and fatigue.[68] In test animals injection of the toxic algae causes tumors, and larger doses can cause death within minutes. Batches of contaminated spirulina have been seized by the FDA. Since the toxins are not routinely tested for by all manufacturers, it would seem that using the algae is like playing Russian roulette. In addition, many of the products sold as spirulina contain large amounts of counterfeit filler, and some are completely devoid of spirulina.

The presence of various toxins in some batches of spirulina may explain the warnings given by some manufacturers and peddlers that use of the products may cause gastrointestinal distress, headache, fatigue, and a host of other symptoms. But they explain the symptoms away as effects of stored toxins being miraculously released and flushed from the body by the miracle food. This familiar lie is often heard from advocates of fasting, bizarre and inadequate diets, and various toxic herbs and poisons. Here again we have the "health food" industry at its finest, using lies heaped-upon lies to not only sell a foul-tasting scum that is only moderately nutritious and sometimes contaminated with filth and toxins, but to get a premium price for it by convincing people that the sickness it causes is really a healing.

The FDA has made some feeble attempts at controlling the industry and stopping the fraudulent claims, but it has had little effect. But then, what can we expect from a government agency whose will is weak and whose antiquackery budget is less than that of one major spirulina manufacturer? The entire spirulina industry is but a drop in the ocean of quackery, but its resources for battle dwarf those of the FDA.

Another alga promoted as a panacea is chlorella, which is marketed around the world by dozens of Japanese companies. While it is moderately nutritious, the cure-all claims made for it are completely unfounded.

Sports Drinks

About twenty-five years ago the Florida State Gators football team started drinking a sugar-water concoction with a dash of salt during and after games and practice. The drink was then commercialized, very successfully. Since then so-called sports drinks or performance drinks have been big sellers. Some twenty companies produce a half billion dollars worth each year. The product names and advertising imply that they confer a competitive edge by enhancing efficiency and stamina. There is no evidence to support the claims, however, and no good reason to think they are true. Nor are the products healthful in any special way. Of course, water replacement is essential during prolonged physical activity, but plain water is adequate for the vast majority of partici-pants, who usually exercise less than ninety minutes.

For intense exercise that lasts more than ninety minutes and calls for additional energy, dilute fruit juice, lemonade, or even Kool-Aid or soda should suffice. There is no reason to pay inflated prices for "performance drinks." For those who prefer these drinks, there is no harm in using them, and they do efficiently replenish body fluids after a marathon or near-marathon. But they provide no competitive edge over those drinking less costly fluids.

Subliminal Persuasion

The theory of subliminal persuasion holds that the subconscious mind can hear and understand sounds that are too dim or unclear (due to reverse dubbing or another masking technique) to register with the conscious mind. Furthermore, messages "heard" subliminally are more persuasive than those heard consciously. Supposedly, a subliminal message not to eat ice cream can counter the advertisements urging you to eat ice cream. It's a sort of homeopathic theory of psychological persuasion: the weaker the message, the more powerful its effect.

The concept has spawned an industry that promises its audiotapes, videotapes, books, and consultations can help you lose weight, kick the tobacco habit, sober up, think positively, remember better, make more money, stop your employees from stealing, make your kids behave, and realize that you were raped because in a past life you were a rapist. The tapes supposedly repeat the messages (inaudibly) hundreds of times per minute, many times faster than the human ear can process.

The subliminal concept has also spawned near-hysterical fears about mind control with masked messages inserted into rock music. Some parents have dragged musicians into court with multimillion dollar lawsuits alleging that hidden messages in their music have made children take their lives. Such plaintiffs have not yet won, but they seem to come closer each time. Their actions have cost the defendants millions of dollars in legal fees. If they ever win a case, recording companies and musicians may have to protect themselves by hiring attorneys to screen their music forward, backward, and at every possible speed, and to censor anything remotely risky.

The claims made for subliminal persuasion are fantastic and, as such, require extraordinary proof. But even meager evidence is lacking. Moreover, the theory of subliminal persuasion can be refuted *a priori*. If it were true, surely it would have been discovered thousands of years ago and used as a potent weapon. Imagine the possibilities! Pretenders to the throne and Rasputins would have waged subliminal whispering warfare against their enemies. War against other nations would have been waged by sending in whispering spies and saboteurs who would whip a population into a frenzy against its government. Of course, they would whisper so quietly that no one would notice them and have them arrested. If the technique works, why has no subliminal persuasion arms race developed? Why don't we have a Subliminal Voice of America that uses this super technology to get other nations to do our bidding? The answer is obvious: because it's all a lot of nonsense. The Spring 1992 issue of *Skeptical Inquirer* has excellent articles on the subject.

Superoxide Dismutase (SOD)

Superoxide dismutase (SOD) is an enzyme, naturally abundant in most cells, which breaks down highly reactive and harmful superoxide molecules. As a free radical scavenger, it is believed to reduce the rate of wear, tear, and aging in most of the tissues of the body and, thereby, may help prevent cataracts, arthritis, and other age-related disorders. It is not surprising that "health food" stores, drugstores, and mail-order distributors do a brisk business in SOD tablets. The product labels make no health claims, but promotional literature makes the pills sound like nothing less than the Fountain of Youth. Unfortunately, SOD, like all proteins, is destroyed in the digestive tract. So ingestion of even enormous doses will not increase tissue levels of the enzyme or decrease one's rate of aging or risk of developing degenerative disease. It's just another ripoff.

"Tanning Pills"

Suppose a pill could produce a beautiful tan all over your body without your spending a minute in the hot sun or a tanning booth. Products promised to do this have been entering the United States from Canada and Europe since the early 1980s. The main ingredient in these pills has been canthaxanthin, a red-orange pigment that also occurs in some plants as well as brine shrimp and other marine life. Flamingos and other water birds get their pink hue from eating these. So it is with humans, too. If you take "tanning" pills, which would be more accurately called dyeing pills, you will gradually take on an orange tint. The dye accumulates in the skin, fat, blood, and certain organs. The blood plasma becomes bright orange and the stools brick-red. Even the sweat contains the dye. The pills are generally taken in large doses for a couple of weeks, then in smaller maintenance doses when the desired color is achieved.[71]

Canthaxanthin is approved by the FDA as a dye for foods such as soups, fruit drinks, salad dressings, catsup, and margarine. But the doses in the "tanning" pills are much greater than the amounts ingested in an average diet. Despite warnings by the FDA, canthaxanthin has been illegally sold in tanning parlors and by mail as a tablet for skin tanning, under such names as Orobronze, Darker Tan, and BronzGlo. Ads for Darker Tan promised "a rich dark bronze glowing tan without risking skin cancer." A case has been reported of a twenty-year-old woman who took high doses and developed aplastic anemia, a serious condition in which the production of blood cells is impaired. Previous reports have linked canthaxanthin use to hepatitis, generalized itching, hives, and eye problems.[72]

Therapeutic Touch

Proponents of therapeutic touch claim that it is possible to use one's hands to "detect when a person is sick, pinpoint where the pain is, and stimulate the recuperative powers of the sick person." They also claim that their maneuvers produce changes in the body's "energy field" that can be demonstrated with Kirlian photography.

The leading proponent, Doris Krieger, Ph.D., R.N., says she became interested in this approach after participating in a study in which people who were touched by a healer reported that they felt better. "In the weeks to come," she wrote in her book *The Therapeutic Touch* [Prentice-Hall, 1979], "I was astounded by the number of medical reports or first person reports that told either of an amelioration of symptoms or actual disappearance of symptoms. ... Pancreatitis, brain tumor, emphysema, multiple endocrine disorders, rheumatism, arthritis, and congestive heart disease were but a few." Inspired by this, she did postdoctoral research, looked into yoga, Ayurvedic medicine, Tibetan medicine, and Chinese medicine, and developed elaborate theories about "energy transfer" that occurs during the laying on of hands or merely holding one's hands an inch or two above the subject's skin to smooth out imbalances and disturbances in the subject's "energy field." She went on to become a professor of nursing at New York University. Her book states that she has taught her techniques to thousands of nurses and explained the method on radio and television throughout the country, in workshops, and in many public articles. The one thing she has not done, as far as I can tell, is to carry out well-designed studies to test whether her methods work.

UFO Abduction Therapy

UFO abduction therapy is based on the premise that many people, perhaps thousands, have been abducted by aliens from other worlds and taken away for genetic and reproductive experimentation and sexual perversions, including rape. Bud Hopkins, the main proponent of this idea, is not a raving lunatic residing in a facility for dangerous paranoids, but a celebrated author of books on the subject[73,74] and a frequent guest on major talk shows. He can scratch just about anyone and discover another abductee. Do you remember a time at about three years old when just after being put to bed you floated up and out the window and went on a wonderful journey high above the earth? Later your parents laughed at your story and said it was a dream. And when you were eleven, did you not once sit in the woods or by the seashore, let your mind wander, and suddenly realize it was much later than you thought, as though you were missing time? Have you ever seen a light in the sky you couldn't identify? And do you not have at least one or two little scars you can't explain? Look carefully with a large magnifying glass over every inch of your body.

If you answer yes to two or more of these questions, there is no doubt that you have been abducted by aliens from another galaxy. The trauma of the abduction and the subsequent medical and sexual procedures (for genetic experiments) is likely the cause of all your emotional and psychosomatic problems. Therefore, the traumatic events must be fully explored in detail. The repressed memories will be dredged up with the aid of hypnosis, and the emotional demons will be exorcised. In this way, UFO abduction therapy encourages elaboration of fantasies upon fantasies, and belief in them.

Like past-life regression (discussed above), UFO abduction therapies rely heavily on hypnosis and the many myths about it. The alleged phenomena have been amply and eloquently exposed and debunked by Philip J. Klass. His book *UFO Abductions: A Dangerous Game* [Prometheus, 1988] concludes that the therapists promoting the concept are indulging in dangerous psychological quackery that exacerbates and creates confusion and emotional distress in their clients.

Vitamin Supplements

Vitamins are complex organic substances required in extremely small amounts for normal metabolism and normal health. They are easily obtained by eating a wide variety of foods. Deficiencies become a problem when: there is lack of food as in war, drought, overpopulation, and agricultural failure; a regional diet isn't varied enough, such as in southern states when pellagra was rampant because people ate little besides corn; or when eating habits are atrocious due to alcoholism, ignorance, or food faddism.

Vitamins (especially in pills, but also in powders, breakfast cereals, drinks, candy bars, and so on) are among the most lucrative and ubiquitous snake oils in America. They are advertised in every print and electronic medium and peddled in pharmacies, supermarkets, sporting goods stores, chiropractors' offices, and through the mail. Even our friends, neighbors, and relatives are peddling them. Large doses of vitamins are falsely claimed to be safe and effective remedies for both serious and minor ailments, to be immune enhancers and aphrodisiacs, and to enhance stamina and protect against stress.

Vitamania has become a religion. Self-proclaimed high priests of the vitamin cult (none of them nutrition scientists) have led millions of Americans on an expensive and dangerous wild-goose chase. There is no evidence that vitamin C supplements prevent colds or cure cancer, that niacin can cure schizophrenia, that vitamin E can cure heart disease, or that daily stress increases vitamin requirements. Yet vitamins have become sacraments that untold masses fervently believe will give them better health, eternal life, or something close to it. Like the polytheists who pray to all the gods to cover all the bases, most megamaniacs take large doses of all the vitamins, just to be sure.

Most of the high priests of the cult have their favorite gods and sacraments. Linus Pauling is the Prophet of Vitamin C. Abram Hoffer is the Prophet of Niacin. The Shute brothers were Prophets of Vitamin E. To those who think Pauling must be right because he's a famous Nobel Prize winner, keep in mind that he was wrong about the structure of DNA (he theorized a triple helix), a subject within his area of expertise. And Einstein was wrong about quantum mechanics ("God doesn't roll dice."). In science there are no infallible gurus or unimpeachable authorities, only facts.

In 1984, Pauling served as a witness for the defense in the California Boad of Medical Quality Assurance's proceedings against cancer quack Michael Gerber, M.D., who used scores of unproven remedies on one cancer patient. For some three hours Pauling defended the use of astronomical doses of vitamins C and A (100 times the RDA for both), coffee enemas, and chelation therapy. The defendant's use of laetrile, bee pollen, herbal teas, and other cancer snake oils apparently didn't bother Pauling either.

The public is exposed to a constant barrage of megavitamin propaganda and rarely told of the dangers of excessive vitamins. It is appropriate, therefore, to briefly summarize some of the hazards here.

In general, you can get all the vitamins you need by eating reasonably well. If you don't always eat as well as you should, it won't hurt to take a multivitamin-mineral supplement with doses of 25 to 100 percent of the RDAs of the nutrients. It shouldn't cost more than a nickel per day. Doses greater than this have no proven benefit and may cause harm. The most important hazards of large doses are the following.

• Vitamin A excess is toxic to the brain, liver, skin, muscles, and bone. Symptoms of toxicity include severe headaches, nausea, vomiting, diarrhea, jaundice, lethargy, weight loss, poor growth in children, insomnia, brittle nails, hair loss, constipation, irregular menses, emotional distress, bulging eyeballs, severely dry skin, and bone damage with extreme bone pain. If the excessive vitamin A is not withdrawn so the body can metabolize the excess, death can occur. Doses as low as 20,000 IU taken for several weeks can cause trouble. Alcoholics are especially vulnerable to vitamin A toxicity.

The huckstering of vitamin A by the "health food" industry for a wide range of ailments, especially as an alternative to chemotherapy for cancer, illustrates how it profiteers from deception that causes sickness and death. Again using the Big Lie technique, cancer quacks portray chemotherapy as worthless and poisonous, while presenting vitamin A as a natural and nontoxic remedy. In fact, chemotherapy has a good chance of working in many patients while vitamin A has none. Moreover, the transient sickness some patients experience from chemotherapy is usually minor compared to the pain and illness of vitamin A poisoning.

The wracking bone pain, splitting headaches, and constant nausea caused by vitamin A overdosage are so terrible that the cheap chemical would be the perfect tool for the torturers of the world if they weren't so fond of quicker, more hands-on methods. No one knows how commonly people are harmed by megavitamins, and the "health food" industry would like to keep it that way. In 1989 the National Nutritional Foods Association, showing its true colors, filed a petition to end the FDA's program of collecting toxicity reports associated with vitamins and minerals. The petition was denied, but there still haven't been adequate attempts to determine the incidence of poisoning from supplements.

• Niacin (vitamin B_3) excess can cause a very uncomfortable flushing of the skin, itching, nausea, diarrhea, stomach bleeding, headaches, heart arrhythmia, changes in blood sugar and uric acid, and severe liver toxicity. Slow-release niacin products are more toxic. Ironically in light of the megamaniacs' claim that niacin can cure schizophrenia, there is evidence it may actually activate a psychosis.[75] Niacin can be very valuable in helping people control abnormal blood cholesterol levels, but it should never be taken without close medical supervision.

• Pyridoxine (vitamin B_6) excess can cause severe nerve damage. Recovery following withdrawal of the vitamin can take many months.

• Vitamin C excess can cause diarrhea and a dependency state in which withdrawal of the large doses leads to symptoms of scurvy. Chewable vitamin C can cause dental erosion. Megadoses of vitamin C can cause severe illness and death in people with sickle cell anemia and those with a hereditary enzyme deficiency common in American blacks, Sephardic Jews, and some people of Mediterranean and Middle East origins. Excess vitamin C also screws up tests for urine sugar and colon cancer. It probably also increases kidney stone incidence in those susceptible to oxalate kidney stones, since it is converted to oxalic acid and increases the body load of oxalate. While scurvy certainly impairs immunity, excess vitamin C now appears to have a similar effect. Moreover, studies done with mice by a former associate of Pauling suggest that mega-C may stimulate some kinds of tumor growth.[76]

• Vitamin D excess can have devastating consequences, especially on the very young.[77] Infants given excessive doses, even as little as five times the RDA, have developed hardening of the arteries, severe mental retardation, distorted facial features, kidney damage, recurrent infections, loss of appetite, and failure to grow. Many so affected have died. Much of the damage is done by excessive calcium saturating the blood, flooding the organs and crystallizing in them. In adults excessive vitamin D can likewise cause calcium deposition in soft tissues and contribute to kidney stones and other problems.

• Vitamin E, like vitamins A and D, is fat-soluble and can accumulate to high levels in the body. This alone should give pause to the zealots who take massive doses. The picture is still fuzzy because adequate toxicity studies have not been done. However, it appears that excessive vitamin E can, at least in some people, cause decreased thyroxin levels, headaches, fatigue, nausea, blurred vision, dizziness, inflammation of the mouth, chapped lips, muscle weakness, low blood sugar, increased bleeding tendencies, inhibited wound healing, gastrointestinal disturbances, and elevated blood fats and cholesterol.[78]

• Combinations of megadoses of vitamins may have harmful effects that have not yet been discovered. A hint of a hidden epidemic is provided by the experience of a young chemist who took 1 gram of vitamin C and 100 micrograms of vitamin B_{12} every day.[79] After just one week of the regimen, he experienced nosebleed, spontaneous bleeding from the external ear, dry mouth, and decreased ejaculate volume. Repetitions of the experiment by him and others confirmed the effect.

The Megavitamin Fallacy

The fundamental flaw of the megavitamin theory, which reveals a misunderstanding of the biochemical role of vitamins, is the assumption that increasing vitamin concentrations somehow increase or improve the reactions the vitamins are involved in. Vitamins are enzyme cofactors that help catalyze cellular reactions necessary to life. Vitamin molecules, like enzymes, are reused millions of times before being excreted. If an excess is supplied, it is excreted or stored until needed; it cannot push the reactions faster or improve them in any way. It can, however, exert biochemical effects unrelated to the vitamin's normal role in metabolism. These effects are unnatural in that they don't occur with normal dietary levels of intake. They are pharmacologic effects; in high doses, vitamins are drugs. Their effects are rarely beneficial and frequently harmful. Moreover, the cost of a megavitamin program can easily reach hundreds or even thousands of dollars a year.

Wheat Germ Oil/Octacosanol

Wheat germ has long been promoted as a supernutritious food with special components not available in other foods. Wheat germ oil is said to be a concentrated source of the special nutrients that confer increased vigor and stamina. Octacosanol, said to be the main active ingredient, is marketed in capsules. In 1986, after being charged by the FTC with false advertising, A. H. Robins Company agreed to stop claiming that its Viobin Wheat Germ Oil could help consumers improve endurance, stamina, vigor, or other aspects of athletic fitness. While fraudulent advertising for octacosanol products has slowed to a trickle, the momentum from years of false advertising, as well as the continuing false claims in magazine articles in "health food" and bodybuilding magazines, perpetuate its mythology. The products continue to sell well.

Yeast Syndrome

The story of the so-called yeast syndrome illustrates the efficient opportunism of the "health food" industry. This alleged condition is also known as yeast hypersensitivity, yeast allergy, chronic yeast infection, chronic candidiasis, candidiasis hypersensitivity, etc. Substitute candida or candidiasis for yeast and add "systemic" and/or "syndrome." Mix and match for dozens of names. Whatever you call it (I prefer "yeast baloney"), it surely sets an unbeatable record for the nondisease with the most names.

A yeastlike fungus, *Candida albicans,* commonly referred to as "candida," is normally present in small amounts in the digestive tract from mouth to rectum, as well as in the vagina. It is kept in check by other microbes, primarily bacteria. If the normal digestive-tract or vaginal flora is disrupted by, say, prolonged treatment with certain antibiotics or corticosteroids, the candida organisms flourish. This overgrowth can results in white patches (thrush) in the mouth or a vaginal discharge.The infection usually clears up spontaneously when the drug is discontinued, but chronic cases may require the use of antifungal drugs.

Several years ago, Drs. C. Orian Truss and William G. Crook began saying that millions of Americans are suffering from a different kind of yeast disease, one not visible to the naked eye or even diagnosable by lab tests.[80,81] It didn't take long for health food industry manufacturers, retailers, and quacks to jump on the bandwagon with vitamins, herbs, diets, and other phony remedies for this invented disease.

Drs. Truss and Crook claim that certain diets and drugs cause hypersensitivity to yeast and its (unspecified) toxins, so that even normal levels in the body cause a multitude of symptoms and disorders—chronic fatigue, headaches, mood swings, anxiety, depression, weight gain, indigestion, and frequent infections, to name just a few. These people are not hypersensitive just to candida. All kinds of molds and fungi, as well as all the foods they supposedly thrive on and all things they are made into or contaminate, become agents of dysfunction and disease. Crook implies that even AIDS can result from yeast hypersensitivity.

The "yeast syndrome" is diagnosed by questionnaire rather than blood or tissue studies. Do you sometimes have any of the following symptoms? (The list is very long; yours are included whatever they may be.) Have you ever been exposed to birth control pills, corticosteroids, or antibiotics? No? Well, how about fluoride, preservatives, dental amalgam, pesticides, or a high-sugar diet? Aha, I thought so. Therefore, the yeast syndrome is probably the cause of all your mental and physical problems.

Conversion to this idea has a strong emotional appeal. It holds the potential for solving all our problems with drugs and diets. Physicians who don't want to prescribe Nystatin or a restrictive diet unnecessarily and try to convince self-diagnosed patients that they don't have a yeast problem often meet with religiouslike conviction and resistance.

Now that we know you have the dreaded yeast syndrome, you must adhere to this diet: no refined starches or sugar; no foods made with yeast such as leavened breads and pastries; no nutritional yeast or supplements made from them; no alcoholic beverages, vinegar, soy sauce, sour cream, buttermilk, or other products of yeast fermentation; no coffee or tea; no milk or cheese; no dried fruits, vegetables, or herbs; no smoked meats or fish; no fruits, especially melons and bottled or canned fruit juices; and no mushrooms or chocolate. Some foods must be cleaned with diluted bleach. Crook's meal plans tend to be high in fat and cholesterol.

And you must take important drugs, herbs, and supplements. The list varies, but usually includes the prescription drug Nystatin (or ketoconazole) plus "health food" store remedies that contain vitamins, minerals, oils, enzymes, sorbic acid, caprylic acid, *Lactobacillus acidophilus,* and herbs such as pau d'arco, echinacea, and aloe vera. Crook recommends one million units of Nystatin per day, even for infants and children. He instructs his patients to experiment to find the proper dose. Careful study has shown that the drug does not reduce systemic or psychological symptoms more than a placebo does in women presumed to have the syndrome.[82]

You must also avoid fluoride, artificial light, and electromagnetic fields, and you may require acupuncture and chiropractic treatments to strengthen your immune system. You may have to have all your fillings removed. You may even need "cell therapy," the injection of cells from young animals. Oh, and you may have to move to a less humid climate. If all this doesn't cure you and you still aren't bankrupt and cowering in neurotic fear of everything, we'll turn you over to our friends, the clinical ecologists. They'll finish the job.

As you can see, the remedy for candida syndrome is not as simple and straightforward as might first appear. Seduction by the candida theory can get you swept into a sea of quackery that may leave you sicker, poorer, and more confused than ever. The culprits in this lucrative business fall into four categories: irresponsible physicians who took their half-baked theories to the media instead of doing proper studies and taking their case to their colleagues for critical review; other irresponsible physicians who prematurely adopted the theories and applied them clinically; the opportunists of the "health food" industry who thrive on every new quack notion; and opportunistic fringe practitioners such as chiropractors, naturopaths, diploma-mill nutritionists, and herbalists who are fond of phony diagnoses and bogus treatments for them.

Not surprisingly, the books by the yeast doctors sell briskly at the "health food" stores that carry "natural yeast remedies." The sensationalist media have also played a major role, as is usual in such affairs. *Omni* and *Redbook* magazines ran misleading articles about the new "mystery illness." The *Redbook* article was accompanied by an ad for a phony yeast syndrome remedy. The "health food" press and the tabloids learned that little trick decades ago. The pill peddlers are happy because ads near supporting "articles" work; that is, they help sell supplements. But consumers are deceived and swindled.

Before you radically alter your diet, take all those pills, and spend all that money, consider what the experts have to say about the alleged disease. The American Academy of Allergy and Immunology strongly denounces the concept as speculative and the treatment as dangerous.[83] And the FDA has denounced "candidiasis hypersensitivity" and its trappings as one of the nation's top ten health frauds.[84] (The other nine on the agency's list were fraudulent arthritis products, spurious cancer clinics, bogus AIDS cures, instant weight-loss schemes, fraudulent sexual aids, false nutritional schemes, chelation therapy, and unproven use of muscle stimulators, and quack baldness remedies and other appearance modifiers.)

The Real Dangers of the "Yeast Syndrome"

As with all fad pseudodiseases and unproved therapies, the yeast syndrome dogma carries some serious risks. Taking antifungal drugs can produce resistant strains (that may really make you sick some day), liver toxicity, chronic fatigue (!), anxiety, depression, and other side effects. Taking the recommended megavitamins and herbal remedies could make you sick. Unnecessarily forbidding dozens of nutritious and tasty foods may decrease the quality of your diet as well as your eating pleasure. Moreover, you might accept a mistaken diagnosis while the real problem is left to fester.

Finally, if you happen to have a real yeast infection and you rely on "health food" store advice and remedies or if you consult a chiropractor or naturopath, you could develop a life-threatening case because only prescription drugs can help. All other remedies are bogus. Enforcement actions by the FDA and FTC have stopped several manufacturers from making unsubstantiated claims for their "anti-yeast" products, but some are still being marketed.

References

1. V.E. Tyler: Pau D'Arco. *Nutrition Forum* 2:8, 1985.
2. J. Lowell: The Gerson Clinic. *Nutrition Forum* 3:9–12, 1986.
3. J. Dwyer: The macrobiotic diet: no cancer cure. *Nutrition Forum* 7:9–11, 1990.
4. American Cancer Society: Questionable methods of cancer management: hydrogen peroxide and other "hyperoxygenation" therapies. *Ca: A Cancer Journal for Clinicians* (in press).
5. S. Green: 'Antineoplastons: an unproved cancer therapy. *Journal of the American Medical Association* 267:2924–2928, 1992.
6. V. Herbert: Laetrile: the cult of cyanide. *American Journal of Nutrition* 32:1121–1158, 1975.
7. C.G. Moertel et al.: A clinical trial of amygdalin (laetrile) in the treatment of human cancer. *New England Journal of Medicine* 306:201–206, 1982.
8. J. Lowell: Mexican cancer clinics. In *Dubious Cancer Treatment* (S. Barrett and B.R. Cassileth, eds). Tampa, American Cancer Society, Florida Division, 1990.
9. Cancer "cure" challenged. *Consumer Reports Health Letter* 2:21–22, 1990.
10. American Cancer Society: Questionable methods of cancer management: immunoaugmentative therapy (IAT). *Ca: A Cancer Journal for Clinicians* 41:357–363, 1991.
11. American Cancer Society: Unproven methods of cancer management: Greek cancer cure. *Ca: A Cancer Journal for Clinicians* 40:368–371, 1990.
12. B.R. Cassileth et al.: Survival and quality of life among patients receiving unproven as compared with conventional cancer therapy. *New England Journal of Medicine* 324:1180–1985, 1991.
13. E.R. Friedlander: Mental imagery. In *Dubious Cancer Treatment* (S. Barrett

and B.R. Cassileth, eds.). Tampa, American Cancer Society, Florida Division, 1990.

14. M.L. Kamb et al.: Eosinophilia-myalgia syndrome in L-tryptophan-exposed patients. *Journal of the American Medical Association* 267:77–82, 1992.

15. M.A. Patmas: Eosinophilia-myalgia syndrome not associated with L-tryptophan. *New Jersey Medicine* 89:285–286, 1992.

16. G. von Nostitz et al.: *Magic Muscle Pills!! Health and Fitness Quackery in Nutrition Supplements*. New York City Department of Consumer Affairs, May 1992. Available for $5 from Communications Division, New York City Dept. of Consumer Affairs, 42 Broadway, New York, NY 10004.

17. Clinical ecologist guilty in child's near-death. *NCAHF Newsletter*, May/June 1989.

18. J.J. Kenney et al.: Applied kinesiology unreliable for assessing nutrient status. *Journal of the American Dietetic Association* 88:698–704, 1988.

19. *Nutrition Perspectives*, Nov. 1988.

20. T. Larkin: Bee pollen as a health food. *FDA Consumer* 18(3):21–22, 1984

21. D.M. Shilian: Toxicity of BHT. *New England Journal of Medicine* 314:648, 1986.

22. B. Gittleson: *Biorhythm: A Personal Science*. New York, Warner Books, 1988.

23. T.M. Hines: Biorhythm theory: a critical review. *Skeptical Inquirer* 3(4):26–36, 1979.

24. D. Greenburg: "O bury me not. . ." *Playboy*, July 1988.

25. D.C. Van Dyke et al.: Cell therapy in children with Down syndrome: a retrospective study. *Pediatrics* 85:79–84, 1990.

26. Chelation therapy: sound or risky atherosclerosis treatment? *Medical World News*, April 23, 1984.

27. J.A. Anderson et al.: Position statement on clinical ecology. *Journal of Allergy and Clinical Immunology* 78:269–270, 1986.

28. W.C. Wiederholt et al.: Clinical ecology—a critical appraisal. *Western Journal of Medicine* 144:239–245, 1986.

29. E.J. Bardano and A. Montanero: "Chemically sensitive" patients: avoiding the pitfalls. *Journal of Respiratory Diseases* 10:32–45, 1989.

30. Amebiasis associated with colonic irrigation. *Morbidity and Mortality Weekly Report* 30:101, 1981.

31. J.W. Eisele and D.T. Reay: Deaths from coffee enemas. *Journal of the American Medical Association* 244:1608–1609, 1980.

32. Unorthodox "cure" for kids spawns lawsuits, outrage. *San Francisco Examiner*, March 6, 1988.

33. P. Cooke: The Crescent City cure. *Hippocrates* 2(6):60-70, 1988.
34. L.B. Silver: "Magic cures": a review of the current controversial approaches for treating learning disabilities. *Journal of Learning Disabilities* 20:498–512, 1987.
35. R.E. Reisman: American Academy of Allergy: Position statements—controversial techniques. *Journal of Allergy and Clinical Immunology* 67:333–338, 1981.
36. The mercury scare. *Consumer Reports* 51:150–152, 1986.
37. Jitters over diet pill and coffee combo. *Medical Tribune,* Aug. 11, 1988.
38. R.W. Miller: EMS: fraudulent flab remover. *FDA Consumer* 17(4):29–32, 1983.
39. Red jello and the Feingold diet. *Nutrition Perspectives,* April 1989.
40. D.J. Leikind and W.J. McCarthy: An investigation of firewalking. *Skeptical Inquirer* 10(1): 23–34, 1985.
41. G. Schectman et al.: Can the hypotriglyceridemic effect of fish oil concentrate be sustained? *Annals of Internal Medicine* 110:346–352, 1989.
42. For the serious debator, I recommend: *Reply to Board of Supervisors on Questions about Fluoridation.* San Francisco Health Department, 1985.
43. C. Wulf et al.: *Abuse of the Scientific Literature in an Antifluoridation Pamphlet, ed.2.* Columbus, American Oral Health Institute, 1988.
44. J.A. Lowell: Organic germanium: another health food store junk food. *Nutrition Forum* 5:53–57, 1988.
45. A. Ostfeld: The systemic use of procaine in the treatment of the elderly: a review. *Journal of the American Geriatrics Society* 25:1, 1977.
45. K.M. Hambidge: Hair analysis: worthless for vitamins, limited for minerals. *American Journal of Clinical Nutrition* 36:943–949, 1982.
47. S. Barrett: Commerical hair analysis: science or scam? *Journal of the American Medical Association* 254:1041–1045, 1985.
48. I. Hirono et al.: Carcinogenic acitivity of *Symphytum officinale. Journal of the National Cancer Institute* 61:865–869, 1978.
49. Liver injury, drugs, and popular poisons. *British Medical Journal* 1:574, 1979.
50. Death caused by hydrogen peroxide. *Nutrition Forum* 6:23, 1989.
51. M.J. Finnegan et al.: Effects of negative ion generators in a sick building. *British Medical Journal* 294:1195–1196, 1987.
52. A. Simon et al.: An evaluation of iridology. *Journal of the American Medical Association* 242:1385–1387, 1979.
53. P. Knipschild: Looking for gallbladder disease in the patient's iris. *British Medical Journal* 297:1578–1581, 1988.
54. A.J. Watkins and W.S. Bickel: A study of the Kirlian effect. *Skeptical*

Inquirer 10(3):244–257, 1986.
55. J. Lowell: Live cell analysis: high-tech hokum. *Nutrition Forum* 3:81–85, Nov. 1986.
56. Effects of iron on tumor growth. *American Family Physician* 40:317, 1989.
57. E.R. Broun et al.: Excessive zinc ingestion. *Journal of the American Medical Association* 264:1441–1443, 1990.
58. B.N. Ames: Dietary carcinogens and anticarcinogens. *Science* 221:1256–1264, 1983.
59. R. Newsome: Organically grown foods: a scientific status summary by the Institute of Food Technologists' expert panel on food safety and nutrition. *Food Technology* 44(12):123–130, 1990.
60. E.R. Hilgard: Hypnosis gives rise to fantasy and is not a truth serum. *Skeptical Inquirer* 5(3):26, 1981.
61. Raw milk: elixir of life or deadly potion? *NCAHF Newsletter,* Jan./Feb. 1984.
62. M.E. Potter et al.: Unpasteurized milk: the hazards of a health fetish. *Journal of the American Medical Association* 252:2050–2054, 1984.
63. Raw milk involved in legal battles. *Nutrition Forum* 2:64, 1985.
64. Suit against raw milk dismissed. *Nutrition Forum* 3:23, 1986.
65. Court orders raw milk ban. *Nutrition Forum* 4:12, 1987
66. Raw milk creamed in California court. *Nutrition Forum* 6:21, 1989.
67. A. Hecht: Snake venom or medicine? No proof yet. *FDA Consumer* 15(7):18–21, 1981.
68. M. Paros: Can Super Blue-Green help save the world? *Nutrition Forum* 5:17–19, 1988
69. Spirulina promoter pays $225,000 fine. *NCAHF Newsletter,* March/April 1982.
70. S. Barrett: The multilevel mirage. *Priorities,* Summer 1991, 38–40.
71. L. Fenner: The tanning pill, a questionable inside dye job. *FDA Consumer* 16:23–25,1982.
72. R. Bluhm et al:. Aplastic anemia associated with canthaxanthin ingested for 'tanning purposes.' *Journal of the American Medical Association* 264:1141–1142, 1990.
73. B. Hopkins: *Missing Time.* Berkeley Books, 1983.
74. B. Hopkins: *Intruders.* New York, Random House, 1987.
75. J. Fried: *Vitamin Politics.* Buffalo, Prometheus Books, 1984, 44–45, 130.
76. Lowell: Some notes on Linus Pauling. *Nutrition Forum* 2:33–36, 1985.
77. M.S. Selig: Vitamin D and cardiovascular, renal and brain damage in infancy and childhood. *Annals of the New York Academy of Science* 147:537, 1969.

78. A.C. Tsai et al.: Study on effect of vitamin E supplementation in man. *American Journal of Clinical Nutrition* 31:831–837, 1978.
79. G.N. Schrauzer: Ascorbic acid abuse. *International Journal of Vitamin and Nutrition Research* 43:201, 1973.
80. C.O. Truss: *The Missing Diagnosis.* Birmingham, The Missing Diagnosis, Inc., 1983.
81. W.G. Crook: *The Yeast Connection: A Medical Breakthrough.* Jackson, Tenn., Professional Books, 1983, 1984, 1986.
82. W.E. Dismukes et al.: A randomized double-blind trial of nystatin therapy for the candidiasis hypersensitivity syndrome. *New England Journal of Medicine* 323:1717–1723, 1990.
83. J.A. Anderson et al.: Position statement on candidiasis hypersensitivity. *Journal of Allergy Clinical Immunology* 78: 271–273, 1986.
84. Top 10 health frauds. *FDA Consumer* 23(8):29-31, 1989.

6

How Tabloid Journalism Promotes Quackery

We've all seen the headlines:

Girl Raised by Goats—Eats Tin Cans!
Unfaithful Husband's Head Explodes (Doc Blames Guilt)!
I Gave Birth to an Extraterrestrial!
Miracle Herb Wards off Cancer!
Faith Healer Zaps Arthritis!
Seven-Up Lowers Cholesterol!

I'm not sure how many people believe such stories and how many buy tabloid newspapers for laughs. But surely most educated people would deny that they rely on them for news, health information, or serious commentary. The tabloids—*National Enquirer, Globe, National Examiner, Sun,* and *Weekly World News*—often publish atrocious health misinformation in ads and articles. *The essence of the tabloids is that they sensationalize and deceive with exaggeration, imbalance, and omission.*

As bad as they are, however, tabloid newspapers are much less influential and therefore less dangerous than the talk shows that reach huge audiences. Several years ago I became so concerned about the situation that I began to monitor the major shows closely. When I couldn't tune in, I had a friend or relative keep tabs. Whenever the subject concerned health, fitness, diet, medical treatment, mystical claptrap, or the like, one of us watched and took notes. In many cases, I was able to obtain transcripts as well. My opinions, as expressed in this chapter, reflect a minimum of two years of monitoring each

231

show discussed. This chapter emphasizes television talk shows but includes other forums with nationwide impact.

Phil Donahue

Among talk-show hosts, Phil Donahue is the champion promoter of medical and nutrition quackery. He seems to have a special fondness for authors of quackery-promoting books and has turned his show into a soapbox for many of them. Despite complaints to Donahue and the Federal Communications Commission from responsible health professionals, he continues to promote quackery while rarely airing responsible dissent. His shows dealing with nutrition and health are seldom more than hour-long plugs for the guests' books, supplements, or other commercial enterprises.

Donahue and/or his producers don't seem to care what type of health information they promote as long as it is offbeat. On one of his shows, Harvey and Marilyn Diamond, authors of *Fit for Life,* said that our diet should be 90% carbohydrate, mostly sugar, and only 4 to 5 percent protein and that we shouldn't take supplements. But on another show, his guests Linus Pauling and Jack LaLanne blasted sugar and said that that everyone should take huge amounts of supplementary nutrients. (LaLanne said he took 100 pills a day.) Both views can't be right and, in fact, they are both terribly wrong. Yet Donahue treated all four like brave discoverers of great truths.

AIDS Cures, Miracle Diets. You Name it, Phil's Got it.

On another "Donahue" show, Robert Cathcart, M.D., was represented as having successfully treated AIDS patients with massive doses of intravenous vitamin C. Other guests have been permitted to claim success in treating multiple sclerosis, arthritis, and other serious diseases with vitamins. In none of these cases were responsible experts invited to provide dissenting views. On one show that included Gary Null, who promotes laetrile and other cancer snake oils, a member of the audience bragged that she had injected cancer patients with laetrile in her home. Donahue didn't bat an eyelash. Perhaps he thought that treating friends with quack cancer remedies was a neighborly thing to do. No one bothered to inform Donahue's huge audience that laetrile has been proven worthless against cancer and is toxic because it contains cyanide. Or that experts have likened the laetrile movement to the activities of Jim Jones's People's Temple, which ended in 1978 with a mass murder-suicide in the jungle of Guyana. Both movements involved the same poison.

When Donahue hosted the Diamonds, he let them get away with one looney statement after another without expressing the slightest doubt. Their brilliant insights included:

Only fruit should be eaten in the morning.
Carrot juice prevents cellulite and wrinkles.
People don't get protein from eating protein foods.
Dairy products rob calcium from our bones.
Eating protein and starch together causes weight gain and disease.
Children benefit from their diet.
It doesn't matter what or how much you eat, just what time and in what combinations. (This statement, of course, contradicted many of the other things they said.)

Through an hour of this nonsense, Donahue expressed no skepticism. To the contrary, he defended the Diamonds from a skeptical caller with the comment, "There's a part of you that has got to believe they've got something here . . . . Now if you want all kinds of credentials about nutrition, I mean, they are all arguing about this out there," implying that the Diamonds' mail-order training left them as qualified as professional nutritionists with a real master's or doctoral degree and/or recognition as a registered dietitian. Donahue didn't mention that the Diamonds' guru, high-school dropout T.C. Fry, "Dean" of the so-called "college" from which they obtained their "credentials," teaches that viruses don't exist and that AIDS and polio are phony diseases concocted by a government-drug industry conspiracy designed to foist unnecessary drugs and vaccines on the public. (See Chapter 1 for more information about the Diamonds.)

Donahue's promotion of Stuart Berger, M.D., has probably made Berger a millionaire. According to *People Magazine*, during the three days after Donahue plugged *Dr. Berger's Immune Power Diet*, 50,000 copies of the book were sold. For Berger's *What Your Doctor Didn't Learn in Medical School*, Donahue conducted his show like a class, taking the audience through the book systematically and conducting little pop quizzes to make sure everyone was paying attention and absorbing Berger's baloney about problems with yeast infections and chronic fatigue and the mean-old-doctors who don't give sufficient recognition to these diagnoses.

During 1990, "Inside Edition" exposed Berger as a rogue who diagnosed "yeast problems" and "chronic fatigue syndrome" in practically everyone who consulted him and then prescribed expensive but worthless supplement regimens. Did Donahue finally host critics of Berger to undo some of the damage? Is the Pope a Hindu?

Hey, Phil, How About a Little Glasnost!

On his shows with Soviet spokesman Vladimir Posner, Donahue, radiating smugness and superiority, was critical of censorship in the Soviet Union and strongly supportive of Glasnost, the movement toward openness. Yet Donahue censors skeptics and responsible health professionals and, with rare exceptions, allows only quacks to have their say on his show. Is censorship by Communist bureaucrats any worse than censorship by multimillionaire capitalist talk-show hosts?

If Donahue loves glasnost so much, why doesn't he allow it on his own show? The answer is simple: money. Sensational claims attract bigger audiences, which mean more advertising revenues. Skeptics are excluded for purely commercial reasons. For Donahue to invite skeptics to critique the quacks would be like the *National Enquirer* asking magician James Randi to write an article exposing psychic fraud.

Donahue Is Worse than the Tabloids

Donahue does far more damage than other tabloids (print or electronic) because he has greater credibility. On an otherwise excellent "Nightline" show called "Tabloid Television," ABC's Ted Koppel, interviewing Donahue, called his show an oasis of rationality in a desert of unreason. He ignored Donahue's promotion of quackery and made him seem responsible compared to Geraldo and other sensationalists. In fact, Donahue does far more damage than all the other tabloid TV stars combined by hosting and promoting more quacks than the others and lending them credibility.

Vaccinations have prevented millions of Americans from becoming seriously ill during their childhood. But Donahue's guests have encouraged parents to play viral roulette with their children's health. On one show, he made no objection when actress Lisa Bonet said that childhood vaccinations cause cancer, leukemia, multiple sclerosis, and sudden infant death. On other shows, he provided an audience for the fearmongering of Robert Mendelsohn, M.D. (discussed below and in Chapter 2).

"Nightline" itself has not been immune to the New Age bug. In June 1991, Barbara Walters, substituting for Ted Koppel, focused on the growing problem of the publishing industry's profiteering from sensationalism and trash. But the target was not the dangerous diet-hoax books or New Age-hoax books that foster childish magical thinking. No, Walters was concerned about unauthorized celebrity biographies. Her main guest was none other than Shirley MacLaine, the High Priestess of the New Age, who, like Carlos Castaneda (author of books on "Don Juan," an alleged sorcerer) and many other writers, has demonstrated that silly ghost stories can make millions if they are presented as factual. Walters presented MacLaine as the principled one who had not stooped to writing sensational memoirs about her lovers. Instead she writes on metaphysics and spirituality, and she's so sincere. There was no mention of the millions MacLaine makes from her books, seminars, and promotion of the psychic surgery fraud, which can kill people by diverting them from proper therapy. Nor was there any discussion of the amoral, irrational, and anti-intellectual nature of MacLaine's philosophy. Moreover, on a June 1987 "Nightline" show on UFOs, hosted by Ted Koppel, airtime for proponents exceeded airtime for skeptics by four to one.

While Donahue is more likely to promote medical and nutrition quackery than New Age psychic nonsense and astrology, he also has a fondness for the latter. He did an entire show with Nancy Reagan's astrologer Joan Quigley as the only guest. At one point she said, "Look, Phil, the reason I wrote this book was because I wanted to explain what astrology was capable of doing at the highest level of government . . . . It's not a joke, it's a serious science." Donahue replied, "I believe you." For once, I believe him.

Incredibly, Donahue has won *nine* Emmy Awards. This is akin to the *National Enquirer* winning Pulitzer Prizes. Apparently, the Academy of Television Arts and Sciences, which awards the Emmys, does not consider endangering the public as a mark against the nominees.

Geraldo Rivera

Geraldo was once a crack investigative journalist with ABC's "20/20." I recall a brilliant exposé he did of the floating slums of the Philippines, large fishing barges that served as homes for hundreds of young boys who, for a square yard of living space and a few crumbs to eat, do dangerous diving chores for twelve hours a day. I was optimistic that his new talk show would be equally gutsy and honest. I could not have been more wrong.

During the first weeks of his show, Geraldo hosted a parade of psychics, UFO abductees, witches, and other kooks and cultists. These New Age heroes of tabloid television informed us about the wonders of love potions, past lives, and rape by extraterrestrials, all without a trace of disbelief from the host. On one show, psychics told audience members that they have undiagnosed kidney disease, gynecological problems, stomach disorders, and vitamin deficiencies. Others were told they are having, have had, or will have car trouble or an accident. One young man was told he was surrounded by animals. He replied that he had a parakeet. On the basis of these brilliant performances, Geraldo pronounced the psychics 80 percent accurate.

At one point, I must admit, he made a token gesture to sanity. When the psychic diagnosis and prescribing threatened to become the show's focus, Geraldo said that people should see their doctors for health problems. (It's O.K. to get bogus psychological, marital, financial and employment advice from so-called psychics. But if you are sick, see a doctor.) "I hate to be a skeptic," he said. "I hate to ruin the fun." Geraldo used to care about the truth; as a journalist he was a professional skeptic. Now all he seems to care about is ratings and "fun."

Ghosts, Witches, and Satan

On a show about haunted houses and exorcism, Geraldo had four "victims," two "exorcists" (one Catholic, one Protestant), and a clinical psychologist, Dr. Mark Stern, President of the American Humanistic Psychological Association. Geraldo introduced Stern as the "resident skeptic for the day." For an instant I thought that the show might cast at least a shadow of doubt on the hocus-pocus, even though the skeptic was outnumbered six to one on the panel. (Actually, seven to one including Geraldo.) But Stern immediately denied being a skeptic and said that it doesn't matter whether there is actual possession or not, that what's important is what people believe.

Since there is nothing humanistic about disregarding truth and encouraging delusional thinking, perhaps Stern's group should change its name to the American New Age Psychological Association. The one constant in New Age thinking is total disbelief in the concept of objective reality. As Shirley MacLaine and other leaders of the movement have said repeatedly, we all make and have our own realities, truths, and morals.

On the same show, one of the victims called herself a "witch" and claimed to have levitated, caused car accidents with her mind, and harmed her enemies by sticking pins into voodoo dolls. Geraldo expressed no skepticism. The "witch" also said she had been repeatedly raped and otherwise abused as a child. It didn't occur to Geraldo that this may have made the woman nutty for life and, therefore, an unreliable reporter. And when two other guests told about ghosts rampaging through their house, Geraldo displayed a polygraph report as evidence that they were telling the truth. He failed to mention that polygraphs are not accepted in courts of law because they are unreliable, a fact previously demonstrated in an excellent exposé by his ex-colleagues on "20/20."

Geraldo has hosted several shows that presented Satanic worship as an enormous problem spreading across the country like a plague. Critics have said he distorted the facts and greatly exaggerated the problem's extent—but much of this criticism missed the real mark. Whether or not he has exaggerated, he and other talk-show hosts who promote irrational and magical thinking surely contribute to whatever problem exists. Once someone accepts crystal healing, psychic healing, and "white magic," there is little reason not to believe in "black magic." If someone else's thoughts can heal you magically, then surely they can also kill you. Geraldo helps perpetuate superstitions and delusions while simultaneously decrying the inevitable results of such beliefs: cultism and bizarre and dangerous behavior.

Pssst! Want to Buy Some Aphrodisiac. . .?

In an article I wrote for a Honolulu newspaper, I predicted that when Geraldo ran out of psychic hucksters and the like he would start hosting diet peddlers and other quacks. Sure enough, shortly thereafter he did a show boosting a phony herbal aphrodisiac. The format was purely promotional without the slightest hint of skepticism from Geraldo or anyone else on the stage or in the audience. The address for ordering the junk was given several times. It amounted to an hour-long commercial.

Since there are many phony aphrodisiacs on the market, I wondered why Geraldo chose to promote this one. Did the manufacturers pay for the promotion? I wrote, but never received a reply. Why did Geraldo serve as a program-length commercial for the phony aphrodisiac? Why do Phil Donahue, Larry King, Sonya Friedman, Oprah Winfrey, and other media stars repeatedly do much the same with a wide assortment of quackery?

. . . Or Miracle Diets and Cancer Cures?

Another "Geraldo" show, called "New Age Weight-Loss Techniques," promoted general health and weight loss through the use of crystals, laser acupuncture, psychic channeling, and other rubbish. One of his panelists, comedienne Renee Taylor, promoted a "food du jour" diet. On day one you eat just fruit, the next day just bagels, then chicken, then pasta, then vegetables, then just grains. On the seventh day you eat just cake and ice cream. This surely is one of the kookiest diets ever dreamed up, but the comedienne did not appear to be joking. Other panelists told about getting diet tips and recipes psychically from the long-dead Adelle Davis and James Beard. Geraldo ate it all up.

Perhaps the most irresponsible of Geraldo's shows was one he did with Robert Atkins, M.D., premier promoter of "alternative medicine." A man who told his story from the audience said that he had had a malignant melanoma (an often lethal skin cancer) removed by a surgeon. He said that after a pathologist had studied the excised tissue, the surgeon recommended removing a nearby lymph node because it might contain cancerous cells that could spread to vital organs. Nervous about surgery, he consulted Atkins, who referred him to an unnamed "German physician." Instead of having the node removed, he underwent unspecified "alternative" therapy. A skeptical physician from the audience tried to explain why such a decision was unwise. But Geraldo cut him off, saying "I don't want to get into a debate about alternative medicine."

Geraldo did have a brief vacation to earth with his show "Now It Can Be Told." In October 1991 he did an excellent piece on nutrient supplements for bodybuilders during which Dr. Victor Herbert was interviewed and called the products a "scam" and a "lie." Geraldo agreed with him. Not long afterward, however, he hosted a segment featuring two women promoters of these pills and potions.

Michael Jackson

Popular KABC Radio (Los Angeles) talk-show host Michael Jackson is bright, witty, articulate, and charming. He is well informed about most of the important national and international issues of the day, and he's an excellent interviewer. Because of these assets, he has a great deal of credibility. Unfortunately, in covering health, medical, and nutrition issues, Jackson has been grossly unfair, intellectually dishonest, and a hazard to the public. His show was syndicated nationally for several years to an audience of millions. He still has a large audience in Southern California.

Jackson has regularly hosted promoters of laetrile, homeopathy, megavitamins, and other quack nostrums, while rarely providing rebuttal opportunities to dissenting experts. He has been quick to host authors of one quack diet book after another, yet has rarely hosted anyone with real credentials in nutrition. He has also helped promote fear of such public health measures as immunizations and water fluoridation by hosting cranks who oppose these measures, but not experts who support them. He likes to brag that he strives to present a balanced view of controversial issues. Apparently he doesn't consider expensive or dangerous quackery to be controversial.

Jackson's favorite "nutrition" guru seems to be Earl Mindell (see Chapter 2). In introducing him on one occasion, Jackson said, "He's been here so many times he hardly needs an introduction." Yes, and on each show Jackson has given Mindell carte blanche to promote his supplement scams.

For years, Jackson's "resident physician" was Dr. Robert Mendelsohn (see Chapter 2), the whiney-voiced crackpot who made a career of telling Americans that their doctors are out to rob and kill them. Mendelsohn urged everyone to avoid medical doctors and go instead to chiropractors, naturopaths, and "health food" store clerks for health care and advice. He also preached incessantly against vaccinations. Given the endless hours Jackson afforded Mendelsohn to propagandize, it seems likely that the show (then nationally syndicated) inspired thousands of parents to deny their children immunizations. I wonder how many children have died or suffered permanent brain damage from whooping cough, measles, or other preventable diseases as a result of Mendelsohn's dangerous advice.

While providing an outlet for Mendelsohn's ravings about the alleged evils of Modern Medicine, Jackson never asked him about the activities of the National Health Federation (NHF) or the American Quack Association (AQA). Mendelsohn spent a year as NHF's president and gave talks at AQA meetings. NHF's main purpose is to promote the right to peddle snake oils without interference from the government. AQA's apparent purpose was to ridicule quackery's critics.

Another of Jackson's favorite guests has been journalist Peter Barry Chowka, who has made a career of promoting "alternative" cancer treatments. On one show he claimed Steve McQueen's life was prolonged by treatments he received in Mexico. In fact, McQueen was ripped off and his life probably shortened by his Mexican experience. Chowka encourages cancer patients to give up conventional treatment and go to Mexican clinics whose methods are considered worthless by the scientific medical community. But Jackson never made a skeptical noise.

Jackson's charm is so great that even after hearing him promote dangerous quackery on many occasions, I still had hope that he would recognize the truth if it were shown to him. He seemed too intelligent, honest, caring, and fair to continue promoting quackery once he understood the damage it does. My optimism was heightened when the publisher of my first book, *The Best Medicine,* arranged for me to be on his show. The book is a preventive medicine handbook with passages exposing much of the very same quackery that Jackson promotes. The book had won high praise from the *Library Journal, Kirkus Reviews,* the National Council Against Health Fraud, *Nutrition Forum,* and other responsible critics. Jackson had been sent a copy before I was invited to be his guest. Thinking he was secure enough to accept criticism of his show, I wrote the following poem, which I planned to read on the air. I figured he would accept the criticism with his usual good humor, then discuss the problem in a serious way.

Ode to Michael Jackson:

Come now fellow peddlers / of oils of the snake
Our savior has arrived / now a fortune we can make
An opening to the world / a market of millions
If we use him right / we can make billions
His name is Michael Jackson / a wonder to behold
He is bright, sharp and witty / but his mind we can mold
He holds forth daily / with people of great power
But several times a week / he holds a snake oilers' hour
The world is listening / there is money to earn
The truth about us / he has yet to learn
So come quickly now / you diploma-mill docs
Michael is with us / we've got him in a box
He may ask tough questions / of the political rat
But to those in our field / he's just a pussy cat
No embarrassing questions / will he throw in our face
Or dissenting experts / to put us in our place
Mega-this and mega-that / whatever you have to sell
The dangers and the costs / Michael won't make you tell
We're all thyroid deficient / we're all hypoglycemic
When it comes to hogwash / Michael is bulimic
He gives us many hours / no critics expose our crimes
He makes the *National Enquirer* / look like *The New York Times*
So God bless Michael Jackson / give thanks for his creation
He owes his soul / to the National Health Federation

Unfortunately, I never got a chance to read the poem because my appearance was canceled. While I was sitting in KABC's lounge chatting with New York Mayor Ed Koch and Jackson was interviewing Barbara Bush, news of the tragic explosion of the *Challenger* space shuttle hit the station. All scheduled guests were then canceled so the station could focus on the *Challenger* disaster.

Before I left the studio, the producer rescheduled me for the next morning, so I stayed in Los Angeles another night. The next morning, the producer phoned to say that I was postponed again, but, if I couldn't wait another day, I could return to Hawaii and do the show by telephone on the following day. I agreed to that option and went home. The next morning, the producer called me about twenty minutes before my scheduled appearance and said they had decided not to have me on after all. Ever. I asked why, and he said he couldn't discuss it. I asked whether this was his decision, and he said only that Michael

Jackson "agreed with the decision."

During subsequent weeks, the show had several segments without any guests, just Jackson talking to callers about miscellaneous subjects. There were also segments with quackery-promoting guests. My repeated written inquiries and offers to do the show any time by telephone, and to serve as a critical expert to comment on the claims of some of his guests, were ignored. My complaint to the Federal Communications Commission evoked a form letter and brochure indicating that the great guardian of our airwaves does not attempt to compel talk-show producers to abide by anyone else's concept of balance.

Was my appearance canceled because Jackson read the book and realized that it was not another quack diet book? Having traveled from Hawaii to Los Angeles to do the show, I had expected a little courtesy, at the least. What I got was a door slammed in my face.

Larry King

Now let's consider a rock-solid talk-show host with impeccable credentials and indisputable intelligence. That would be Larry King, the eloquent, articulate intellectual who is equally at ease with world leaders, presidential candidates, rock stars, and astronauts. But on programs when he hosted Whitley Strieber, who writes tall tales of being abducted and sodomized by ETs, King was more cheerleader than journalist.

Strieber has also been interviewed by Rona Barrett, who substitutes for King. On one show I watched, she gave a few minutes to UFO expert and skeptic Philip J. Klass, who is senior editor for *Aviation Week & Space Technology* and author of books that debunk and expose UFO frauds. Wonderful, I thought. After endless hours of free and unchallenged promotion of Strieber's books on dozens of talk shows, an expert skeptic would finally get a chance to address Strieber's fantastic claims.

Klass briefly pointed out that there has never been a shred of physical evidence that UFOs or ETs have visited our earth, in spite of thousands of alleged cases. But when asked how he would explain Strieber's extremely vivid and realistic experiences, he was not permitted to answer. One feasible explanation is that Strieber is a fantasy-prone person. Another possibility, according to a psychiatrist whom Strieber consulted and quoted in his own book, *Communion* [William Morrow, 1987], is that he has an abnormality of the temporal lobe of the brain—perhaps temporal lobe epilepsy—which sometimes results in vivid hallucinations. But as Klass started to make a point along these lines, Barrett cut him off.

Larry King was putty in the hands of Harvey and Marilyn Diamond. Before their last appearance on his show, I sent King some literature from the "college" that awarded their bogus credentials. The material states that its graduates can cure cancer, schizophrenia, "so-called AIDS," herpes, and many other serious diseases with nutritional methods. King didn't ask the Diamonds about any of this. Instead, like Phil Donahue, he gave them hundreds of thousands of dollars worth of free publicity and promotion.

In December 1989, King hosted Bernie Siegel, M.D., author of *Love, Medicine & Miracles* [Harper & Row, 1986] and *Peace, Love & Healing* [Harper & Row, 1989]. Siegel is a surgeon who espouses meditation, support-group meetings, and other psychological approaches for the treatment of cancer patients. He claims that "happy people generally don't get sick" and that "one's attitude toward oneself is the single most important factor in healing or staying well." He also states that "a vigorous immune system can overcome cancer if it is not interfered with, and emotional growth toward greater self-acceptance and fulfillment helps keep the immune system strong." But he has done no research to test these notions. On the "King" show, Siegel said that people have gotten over AIDS with positive thinking. King missed the boat by failing to ask who the people were and why they hadn't come forward to announce this wonderful message of hope.

Perhaps King's darkest moment was with Barrie Konicov, who makes and markets audiotapes that supposedly help people who have been sexually abused as children or raped. He claims that his tapes regress victims to a past life as a sex offender to show that they were responsible for what happened to them—that victimization was in their "karma." Although Konicov calls himself a hypnotherapist, he has no credentials in psychology. He said he had taken four weekend courses in hypnosis.

On the same show, Anne Seymour of the National Victim Center did her best to convince King and his viewers that Konicov's revictimizing the victim could have disastrous consequences. Victims of sex abuse, especially rape and incest, often suffer tremendous guilt for years, even decades. An essential part of recovering from the trauma is to stop self-blame. But throughout the show, King defended Konicov with comments like, "What's wrong with using the tapes if they help?" He didn't show the slightest skepticism toward the blame-the-victim approach. Instead he put *Seymour* on the defensive.

Most of the callers, both men and women, expressed dismay and disgust. One called Konicov a charlatan and scolded King for having him on. King replied that he has no say on who appears on the show, that he just talks with whomever the producer sends in. Should we really believe that this prominent radio and television star has no power whatsoever to suggest or veto guests? And that he is obligated to help advocate the position of every flimflamming creep who comes into his studio? It's hard to believe he would sign a contract that gives a producer so much power over his reputation.

When told Konicov would be on, King could have said, "Look, if I'm going to do a show on helping rape victims, it will be with responsible professionals who have a proven track record. If we get into Konicov and his magical tapes it will be to expose him as a quack. Ask Anne Seymour to find a rape or incest victim who has been harmed by Konicov's tapes." (Seymour said she knew such victims.) But no; he gave kookery the spotlight and put the rational guest on the defensive.

Oprah

Well, you might say, maybe I have a point about Donahue and the others. Maybe they are naive and unfair on health issues. But you gotta love Oprah. She's so earthy, practical, and real. Okay, I'll grant you, Oprah is likable and bright. But even this intelligent woman is prone to extreme gullibility and foolishness. For example, she hosted Dr. Bruce Goldberg, a dentist who dabbles in psychology and claims to have done some 24,000 hypnotic "past-life regressions." He did a couple more for the audience. In these silly demonstrations he led his subjects, eyes closed, to imagine scenes and situations from "past lives." The "memories" they dutifully produced struck me as nothing more than fragments of old movies and novels, but Oprah appeared impressed.

Goldberg told the audience that more than a thousand of his subjects remember and speak foreign languages when regressed to past lives. He claimed that five-year-olds have spoken Latin and ancient African and Germanic dialects. He said his regressions are successful against major illnesses. If true, these claims would revolutionize not only psychology, but philosophy and even medicine. Goldberg might even qualify for a Nobel Prize. But surely a serious scholar would tape-record these amazing episodes. Could we hear some of these tapes? Have expert linguists verified that the subjects really were speaking archaic languages? Does he use the techniques in his dental practice? Has he submitted his amazing finding to scientific journals? Does he collect health insurance and Medicaid payments for these treatments? Does he advocate that we all submit to hypnotic regression and have entries in our medical records about our past lives?

Oprah didn't ask.

Oprah also has done shows with Shirley MacLaine, self-styled UFO abductees, psychics, faith healers, crystal healers, and the like. She rarely has so much as a token skeptic on to rebut the nonsense. Moreover, she rarely expresses any skepticism, and she seems to believe it all. True Belief is what it all boils down to. Blind faith in the whole grab bag of New Age nuttery. Scientific skeptics like myself are not the only ones who object to the biased presentations. Religious friends of mine also find them deeply offensive.

One Tabloid Attacks Another

At least one tabloid has accused Oprah of sensationalism, callousness, and indifference to the possible harm her show can do to her audience. The *National Enquirer* blamed her for the death of at least two viewers and quoted medical experts to back it up. The show in question focused on a sexual practice that can result in strangulation. According to the *National Enquirer,* Oprah and her producer ignored a warning by psychiatrist Park Dietz. In a letter published in the May 1989 issue of *Journal of Forensic Sciences,* Dietz described the circumstances:

> I could think of no worse format for the exploration of [the practice] than the show in question. I informed the member of the production staff who called me that, if the show she described were aired, it would foreseeably result in one or more deaths. She seemed so insensitive to the prospect of her show killing human beings that I informed her directly that if the show were aired, I expected one day to serve as an expert witness in a lawsuit against the show and other responsible parties for their reckless and negligent conduct . . . . The show aired, replete with statements by the host that it was not suitable for children, as if that would cause a child to turn it off rather than to become more fully attentive. Not long thereafter, I learned of the death . . . of a teenaged boy . . . after viewing the show. The case report . . . brings the death toll to two from this show, and still counting.

San Francisco Medical Examiner Boyd Stephens, M.D., also was quoted by the *National Enquirer.* He called the program "irresponsible . . . like teaching people how to make explosives out of household chemicals." He said that Oprah aired the episode "to make the show more sensational." And he added, "I wouldn't watch the Oprah show if you tied me to a chair in front of the television. The Oprah show should be banned!" Curiously, the page before the *Enquirer*'s article on Oprah contained a large ad for Cal-Ban 3000, a bogus diet product that later was accused of killing one person and causing many others to become seriously ill (see Chapter 5).

On one occasion, Oprah actually had a quackery-related program on which no quack appeared. All but one of the guests had been victims of quackery or were the survivors of victims. One family, for example, described how their diabetic daughter had died after a quack had persuaded them to stop her insulin. The other guest was John Renner, M.D., a prominent "quackbuster" who came prepared to discuss how to avoid being victimized. He was interviewed only briefly. The program capitalized on the misfortunes of its guests but failed to convey practical information to the audience.

Sonya Friedman

Now let's consider another of talk television's best and brightest, Dr. Sonya Friedman, a psychologist who is attractive, witty, and compassionate. With a master's degree in education, a Ph.D. in psychology from Wayne State University, and many years of experience as a radio and television psychologist, she seemed to be the perfect choice to hostess a CNN talk show, now called "Sonya Live." I was optimistic when the show started. I thought she was rational, competent, and responsible. You can judge for yourself.

Crystal Healing, Astrology, and Ancestral Spirits

Sonya has repeatedly hosted self-styled "psychics" and "healers." On at least two occasions she hosted crystal healers for half-hour segments. On each occasion she sat wide-eyed at the wonder of it all, never once expressing a skeptical thought, even at one young woman's claim that amethyst crystals are very helpful for people with AIDS. When a caller expressed skepticism, she replied, "We're talking about intuitive knowledge, not scientific knowledge" and hung up.

In 1988 ex-White House chief of staff Ron Regan reported that Nancy Reagan had used advice from an astrologer in making President Reagan's schedule and for other purposes. On the very next day, Sonya hosted a professional astrologer in order to "tell you why it's OK to believe in astrology." She kept her promise. The show was an hour of astrological gobbledygook without a single mention that scientific studies have repeatedly shown astrology to be nonsense. "Sonya Live" and other Cable News Network shows frequently host astrologers to help the viewers run their lives. They also present Jeane Dixon as someone with paranormal powers, even though there is no evidence that her guesses about future events are any better than yours or mine.

For her first show of 1990, Sonya hosted a panel of astrologers and asked them, in all seriousness, what was in store for the world politically and economically. She asked about the stock market, Panama, Europe, ozone, and more. One of her illustrious guests said that since Saturn was in Capricorn, ethical considerations would remain very important for at least another year and that we should expect more ethical scandals. Another said, "Everyone who follows astrology knows it works." Sonya could have countered, "How come astrologers failed to predict the massacre at Tiananmen Square, the fall of Communism in Eastern Europe, and the San Francisco earthquake?" But, of course, she did not. Nor did she compare the previous year's predictions by her guests with reality.

Why do Sonya and CNN, "the world's most important network," encourage Americans to believe in an ancient and thoroughly discredited superstition as we approach the twenty-first century? Several excellent books have utterly trashed astrological theory and practice. I have sent Sonya information about these books and suggested that she have the authors on to explain their findings, but she has ignored me. Why doesn't this woman, who has a Ph.D. in a field that is supposedly scientific in its outlook and methods, want to look at what scientists say about astrology? Why does she shield her audience from knowledgable skeptics?

On one show Sonya helped promote the Harmonic Convergence of August 1987, a celebration that was supposed to usher in a New Age of spiritual healing, love, and peace throughout the world. When a caller expressed skepticism, Sonya seemed bewildered. She couldn't understand why the caller was so negative about the event, and she seemed to pity him. The art historian who started the Harmonic Convergence claimed that it derived from astronomical and astrological facts, as well as ancient Mayan religion. Maya historians, archaeologists and astronomers have scoffed, but Sonya presented it as undisputed fact.

I once wrote an article critical of "Sonya Live" for a Honolulu paper and sent her a copy. Her producer, Scott Leon, vehemently protested. "Our goals here," he wrote, "are to present viewpoints as objectively as possible. We leave it up to our viewers to make up their own minds. Apparently you do not think they are intelligent enough to do that . . . typical of the scientific community."

Hogwash, Mr. Leon! It is you and like-minded producers and hosts who don't respect the viewers' intelligence. Don't you think they can handle an intelligent discussion of astrology, crystal healing, UFO abduction, or past-life regressions from a skeptical, show-me viewpoint? Why do you give them nothing but promotional pap while refusing skeptics an opportunity to rebut? Even geniuses can't find their way to the truth if exposed to nothing but lies.

Of course, my little article had no effect on Sonya's show. A few months later she hosted Michael Talbot, who claims to be a channeler (medium) for the spirits of dead folks. She encouraged her audience to call in to get in touch with their deceased loved ones. He went on and on about uncovering one's hundreds of past lives with the help of psychics. Then he cautioned viewers to be very careful about choosing a psychic, because "there are lots of kooks out there." Sonya never asked him how one can tell the difference between a past life and a figment of one's imagination or between a genuine psychic and a kook. Why didn't she ask him how we can be sure he isn't a kook? Her last words to him on this, the first of many times he would be her guest, were, "Thanks for joining us—you've certainly given us a lot of information." At the time I thought, there's no limit now; next it will be fairies, ghosts, and unicorns.

Even Unicorns and UFO Abductees

Lo and behold! A month later Sonya hosted a man who wrote a book about his adventures in wild Africa and his discovery of a unicorn. He showed the book's photos of a magnificent white horse with a long flowing mane and a single straight horn protruding about a foot from its forehead. Strangely, in one of the photos the beautiful beast was wearing a wreath or lei of flowers around its neck. Sonya did not ask how this came about. Nor did she ask the opinion of any biologist, photographic expert, or skeptic familiar with the history of such hoaxes. Nor did she ask why he didn't have a videotape or movie of the animal, which would have been much harder to fake.

I would wager Sonya any amount of money that the photos are fakes and the book is a hoax. I would also wager that if the hoax is fully exposed, we will not hear about it from her and she will not apologize for her gullibility. Her last words to her guest were, "Congratulations for finding the unicorn." This is somewhat akin to saying to a delusional paranoid, "Congratulations for realizing that you're Napoleon." I wonder what kind of advice and guidance she gave clients when she was a practicing psychologist. My letters asking about the author and publisher of the book have gone unanswered.

On another show Sonya introduced science-fiction author Whitley Strieber, who claims to have been repeatedly abducted and raped by extraterrestrials, as a "UFO expert." This makes as much sense as calling a person who has nightmares about monsters a zoologist.

On another show, when Sonya introduced her guest, alleged psychic Mary T. Browne, she said, "She doesn't use hocus-pocus, but she sure does work magic." Sonya asked Browne how a skeptic can know a psychic is real. Browne said the psychic must demonstrate access to some secret or private knowledge. Here was the perfect opportunity for Sonya to ask for such a demonstration, but she didn't! She apparently considers Browne's powers beyond question. It didn't even occur to her that the audience might have some doubts and would appreciate some evidence. She invited calls, saying, "This is your chance of a lifetime." Not to test the "psychic," of course, but to use her miraculous powers. Browne went on to say, "I do a lot of work with cancer and AIDS patients." This invitation to desperate people didn't appear to bother Sonya in the least.

On another show, Sonya introduced Andrew Weil, M.D.—who has written books promoting strange health notions—as one of America's finest physicians and a teacher of "natural healing." (The term was not defined by either host or guest.) She fawned over him and expressed exasperation that "traditional medicine" ignored his ideas. She apparently meant scientific medicine, which is nontraditional, iconoclastic, and ideally based on the latest and best evidence available. Actually, the term "traditional medicine" means folk medicine, which is based mainly on superstition, dogma, and mere tradition (we've always done it this way, so we always will). Doctor-bashers frequently misuse the term as Sonya did.

As usual, Sonya was not the least bit skeptical of even Weil's most preposterous claims, such as if you eat raw garlic with the right attitude (which he did not describe or define), it will not make your breath smelly. She may be even further out than Weil. She asked about Bach Flower Remedies, a line of flower scents that are claimed to restore health by correcting negative emotional states that underlie all disease. Weil said that they were most likely just placebos, meaning that any benefit would affect symptoms only and be due to belief in the products rather than their inherent worth. Sonya said she didn't see anything wrong with that. She apparently opposes the most fundamental consumer protection principle in the health marketplace, that drugs be proven *effective* for their intended use. Would she prefer to bring back the days of patent medicines and bathtub-manufactured remedies?

On another show, Sonya hosted pop-psychologist Paul C. Roud, author of *Making Miracles* [Warner Books, 1990]. Like Bernie Siegel—who wrote the foreword to his book—Roud bases his theories on anecdotal evidence rather than controlled studies. When Sonya asked him what one must do to make a "miraculous recovery" from a serious disease, he replied, "It's a very individual matter. I help people intuit what they must do to get well." Then a woman who had survived breast cancer said that she believes people aren't responsible for getting cancer, but once they get it they are responsible for curing themselves. This is the kind of twisted thinking fostered by the "alternative medicine" movement. The truth, of course, is quite the opposite. The risk of getting cancer can be greatly decreased by not smoking, avoiding the sun, preventing certain sexually transmitted diseases, and eating a well-balanced diet. But if cancer strikes, the chance of cure without scientific medical care is virtually zero. Sonya made no challenge to the magical thinking of her guests.

Sonya's one-page biography distributed by CNN's public relations department says, "The common denominator of everything with which Sonya is associated is the credibility, professionalism, care and thought which exemplify her work." Yet, there is apparently nothing too kooky for Sonya to espouse without the slightest hesitation. I realize that she was trained in psychology and is not a journalist, but I have always assumed that psychologists have a modicum of common sense and are trained to tell the difference between fantasy, delusion, deceit, and reality. Sonya seems incapable of mustering a skeptical thought, yet she has received numerous awards including Outstanding Achievement of the Year Award from American Women in Radio and Television, and Best Talk Show from the same group. The media have helped make her one of America's most influential educators and psychologists. This illustrates the appalling state of talk television today.

Program-Length Commercials

Back in the 1960s, half-hour television commercials promoted chinchilla farming. Buy a breeding-pair and pretty soon you'll have thousands to sell for making fur coats, audiences were told. In 1973 the Federal Communications Commission stated that program-length commercials (PLCs) violated its guidelines and limited the time a broadcaster could devote to ads. But in 1984, guided by President Reagan's deregulation philosophy, the FCC reversed itself and abolished limits on the length of commercials. The result has been an explosion of PLCs masquerading as talk shows, documentaries, investigative reports, and even public service announcements.

The products most commonly promoted on PLCs have been get-rich-quick schemes and a wide assortment of snake oils including weight-loss systems, baldness cures, aphrodisiacs, and bee pollen. "The Michael Reagan Show" promoted the Eurotrym Diet Patch, a piece of adhesive to stick on "the appetite control center's acupuncture point" on the wrist. The "homeopathic" preparation on the tape supposedly acts on the alleged "acupuncture point" to reduce appetite. Set up to look like a regular talk show with a studio audience and "expert" panelists (doctors with questionable intelligence and less ethics), the show even had "commercial breaks" to provide the toll-free number for ordering a month's supply for some $55. This scam was finally shut down by the Federal Trade Commission.

Another PLC produced by the company that made "The Michael Reagan Show" promoted a product called Oncor, a purported "sexual-enhancing" or "male potency" formula. People in the audience (who I suspect were paid actors) praised its wonders for both impotent men and those who simply want to increase their libidos. They said they experienced increased libido, firmer erections, and greater pleasure. Even some women said they used it and were very happy with the results. Like Reagan's diet patch, Oncor was said to be an approved homeopathic product. The cover of the official *Homeopathic Pharmacopeia* was shown, and the active ingredient was identified as the herb *Venus sativa*. Dr. Dudley Chapman, touted as a frequent guest on the CBS "Morning Show" and ABC's "Good Morning America," strongly endorsed the product—which also sold for $55 a month.

During the past year the FTC sent a resounding message to the infomercial industry by cracking down on several health-related scams. The blizzard of PLCs for phony health-related products has abated for now, but there is no guarantee it won't resume.

Sally Jesse Raphael

Sally Jesse Raphael appears to take pride in bringing "unusual and interesting guests" to her audience. She is somewhat more likely than the other major hosts to ask penetrating questions and have critics on shows that promote "alternative" methods. But practitioners and "true believers" invariably outnumber the critics.

For a show on psychic surgery her producer put four believers and one skeptic on the panel. Andrea Cagan, author of an incredibly gullible and foolish book promoting the scam, was captioned a "psychic surgery expert" rather than a "psychic surgery believer." Sally let her have her say, then let skeptic Richard Busch, the real expert on psychic surgery, demonstrate the hoax and explain why people fall for it.

But alas, even Sally cannot be relied upon to present controversial health issues in a responsible way. Her February 1988 show on Dr. Stanislaw Burzynski's unproven cancer treatment was an atrocity. She began the show by introducing four "miracles" who, she said, were "cancer-free." The patients then gave testimony that Dr. Burzynski had cured them when conventional methods had failed. Although a rebuttal expert was invited to comment briefly, she could not evaluate these claims because she could not investigate the cases before the show. Four years later, "Inside Edition" reported that two of the four patients had died and a third was having a recurrence of her cancer. (The fourth patient had bladder cancer treated by conventional means before he saw Dr. Burzynski. Bladder cancer has a good prognosis.) The widow of one of the deceased TV guests stated that her husband and five others from the same city had sought treatment after learning about Burzynski from a television broadcast—and that none had been helped, and all were dead. When a doctor who had worked with Burzynski was asked how many patients walk out of Burzynski's clinic without evidence of cancer, he replied, "The only patients who walked out without cancer came in with no evidence of cancer—and he treats a lot of those."

A 1988 program on "Alien Encounters" included three guests who said they had been abducted by aliens, one "alien abduction investigator" who said he believed hundreds of abductions had taken place, and Dr. Paul Kurtz, chairman of the Committee for the Scientific Investigation of Claims of the Paranormal (CSICOP). Dr. Kurtz, a philosophy professor who has devoted his professional career to understanding how people's beliefs lead them astray, made some telling points, but a four-against-one setup is hardly an ideal forum for arriving at the truth. Sally's parting advice to her listeners was: "I think we've heard three very interesting stories. Now, most people don't believe, I guess it's up to you. You listen and make your own decision."

For a 1989 program titled "Exorcisms: Fact or Fiction?" the guests were stacked the same way: one "exorcist," four of his satisfied clients, a medical doctor who knew and endorsed the exorcist, and a lone critic. Once again, this is not a format for ferreting out the truth. On a recent program featuring "clinical ecologist" Doris Rapp, M.D., no expert critic was permitted to challenge her unproven notions about the nature of allergies.

In April 1992, while editing this book, Dr. Stephen Barrett was asked by a staff member of the "Sally Jesse Raphael Show" whether he knew enough to appear with a man who claimed that he could enlarge women's breasts with hypnosis. Dr. Barrett was told that the hypnotist was scheduled to appear in about a week with two of his satisfied clients. Dr. Barrett replied that the only way to evaluate the claim was to take before-and-after measurements. The caller replied that they were attempting to do this, but with the show scheduled so soon it might be difficult. Delay until the evidence was in was impractical, the caller explained, "because if we don't have him right away, other talk shows will and we'll have to wait in line."

Are There Any Good Guys?

The one bright spot among the tabloids is "Inside Edition," a half-hour show syndicated to many cities throughout the U.S. Its editors and producers appear to have a special dislike for health frauds. During the past three years they have broadcast at least a dozen programs on this subject. Their producers typically pretend to be "patients" and capture what takes place with a hidden camera. Chapter 1 describes how they did this with Stuart Berger, M.D. Other exposés have attacked Cal-Ban (see Chapter 5), "clinical ecology," diploma mills, multilevel companies, and bogus diagnostic tests.

But even the best cannot resist the temptation to "tabloidize" some subjects. "Inside Edition" has a weakness for UFO stories and has presented some of the most biased ones I have seen. By presenting UFO cultists as "UFO experts" and not presenting rebuttal by responsible skeptics, the show has done a disservice to its viewers. A show featuring the likes of consumer advocate Ralph Nader and investigative journalist Jack Anderson has no business promoting the UFO madness that is so trendy these days.

John Stossel of ABC also deserves special praise for his excellent and merciless exposés of astrology, dowsing (water divining), and cosmetic quackery. For one "20/20" episode he investigated electrical facial toning, a multimillion dollar business. He had three women in their fifties and sixties undergo the $1700 series of twenty treatments (for which ABC paid) on just one side of their faces, then compared the treated and untreated sides. There was no difference whatsoever. He pointed out that women who undergo the procedure are told they have to come back for maintenance treatments for life. Stossel and "20/20" showed rare journalistic courage when they took on pet foods. They told the nation that the cheaper varieties are just as nutritious and tasty (to the animals) as the expensive ones, which are often deceptively promoted as better for the pets' health. This is remarkable in view of the fact that pet food manufacturers are among ABC's biggest advertisers.

Rationalists also appreciate the work of comedian and talk-show host Johnny Carson, who recently retired. During his long career, he frequently lampooned and exposed occultists. His "Carnak the Great" routine was a good satire of psychics and fortune tellers. And instead of hosting phony channelers and the like, Carson preferred James Randi, the brilliant magician who has made a second career of exposing psychic fraud. Unfortunately, however, Carson did make the horrendous mistake of hosting Dr. Lendon Smith several times and helped launch Smith's career as an M.D., that is, Media Doctor.

A few other television personalities should be commended. First, the "residents docs" of all three network broadcast morning shows are outstanding. Dr. Art Ulene, formerly of NBC, Dr. Timothy Johnson of ABC, and Dr. Bob Arnot of CBS have provided consistently excellent coverage of health and medical news and issues. Unfortunately, they rarely discuss fringe medicine and the two- and three-minute spots these responsible physicians get have little impact compared to the half-hour and hour-long promotions of quackery on the major shows. Dr. Dean Edell, whose television and radio shows are syndicated, is also excellent. He addresses controversial issues frequently and pulls no punches when it comes to quackery. Dr. Gabe Mirkin is another outstanding performer. He has been CBS-Radio's fitness commentator and has hosted a radio and television call-in shows for many years.

Unfortunately, there is no guarantee these islands of sanity will endure. As we prepare to go to press, we see less of Dr. Johnson on ABC's "Good Morning America" and more of Dr. Nancy Snyderman, who seems blithely unaware that there is such a thing as health fraud. In April 1992, she presented a five-part series on "alternative medicine." The uncritical series, heavily hyped by ABC, amounted to little more than a promotion for herbal medicine, acupuncture, naturopathy, chiropractic, and other fringe practices.

The fundamental problem here is that television producers, reporters, and talk-show hosts too often treat health issues as just more fodder for their entertainment mill rather than serious subjects deserving their best journalistic efforts and highest professional standards. They almost never do in-depth investigations before their shows with charlatans, or even read their books, and they are not competent to challenge assertions made by the quacks. Their token attempts at skepticism are less than inadequate because their ignorance makes the quacks appear reasonable. The shows almost invariably end up as positive promotions for questionable methods.

If the media must give inordinate attention and publicity to fringe healing methods, they should at least give equal coverage to responsible experts who consider the methods quackery.

7

How to Fight Back

The previous chapters illustrate how health fraud is running wild in all sectors of our society. The business of peddling worthless health products and services is so widespread that, in some respects, it has become institutionalized and legitimized—even chic and prestigious. The makers, peddlers, and promoters of quack nostrums provide employment, vote, and pay taxes. So many people have been fooled or have their fingers in the pie that few people have the will to raise their voice in protest.

Our society has little tolerance for gasoline pumps rigged to overcharge or for toys and tools that injure. We throw counterfeiters of currency, jewels, and stocks into jail. Yet we tolerate innumerable kinds of health fraud and glorify and enrich the promoters and hucksters of modern-day snake oils. A "health food" retailer who rigged his produce scale so he could overcharge a penny or two per pound might be heavily fined, perhaps even jailed, if caught. But if he sells a worthless or poisonous cancer or arthritis remedy for $50 for a week's supply, prosecution is unlikely even if the authorities detect the fraud.

Despite all this, the change in public attitudes toward smoking gives me hope that quackery can be curbed. Thirty years ago, cigarette smoking was considered natural and an inalienable right. Most adults smoked throughout their waking hours. Manufacturers, wholesalers, retailers, advertisers, and government tax coffers all profited from cigarette sales. Movies and television glamorized smoking. Few people questioned it. Nevertheless, since the 1964 Surgeon General's report on the dangers of smoking and the ensuing public education campaigns, the number of smokers and the social acceptance of smoking have steadily eroded. Most people now understand that smoking is a foolish and dangerous habit. Smoke-free zones in public areas and the work-

255

place are increasing in number and size.

Society's gullible and tolerant attitude toward medical and nutrition quackery must likewise be changed. Health is more precious than any stocks or jewels. Money spent on snake oils is just as wasted as that lost to pickpockets and burglars. Reformers should work to raise the level of awareness of the problem and make it a consumer-protection issue. Far from innocuous, health fraud is the worst kind of consumer fraud. It should be seen as such and treated as such.

As with smoking, the primary tools for curbing quackery are legal action, legislative action, and education. Almost anyone can do something about this problem. This chapter tells how.

What Consumers Can Do

Consumers should understand that health products are not like the defendant in a criminal trial who is presumed innocent until proven guilty. Health methods should be presumed worthless and possibly dangerous unless proper studies have shown them to be safe and effective. This is a fundamental tenet of scientific medicine as well as consumer-protection law. Without it, systematic progress in health care would be impossible, and consumers would be at the mercy of snake-oil peddlers.

Our society has strayed from this principle. The media tend to regard products as newsworthy until proven worthless, and the laws against marketing unproven remedies are only weakly enforced. Thus, for the most part, consumers must ferret out the truth for themselves.

Remember and assert your rights under the fundamental principle of consumer protection in the health-care field, a principle that is self-evident and just and has the potential to slow the quackery juggernaut considerably should it be widely accepted: *Unproved treatment and preventive measures, be they nutritional, herbal, pharmaceutical, manipulative, or any other mode, are—at best—experimental.* No patient or client should be subjected to an experimental method without full informed consent regarding potential risks and benefits. Moreover, no one should be required to pay for an experimental treatment. There are, of course, gray areas—remedies that appear to make sense and have attained some preliminary clinical success, but for which further studies are needed. This status can be explained to the patient, and payment can be negotiated with insurance companies and other parties.

Learn what you can from reliable sources such as those listed at the end of this chapter. Utilize a personal physician (a medical doctor, not a chiropractor, naturopath, acupuncturist, herbalist, or other fringe practitioner) who knows you and can rationally evaluate any symptoms you develop, answer your questions, and provide basic health care such as physical examinations and other appropriate screening tests. Everyone should also have a carefully chosen personal dentist.

Be extremely skeptical of information sources that contradict your reliable sources and personal physician. The odds are overwhelming that such information is false, misleading, and potentially dangerous, especially if it comes from a "health food" store, a popular diet book, a women's magazine, or a radio or television talk show. Remember that thousands of enthusiasts and scammers are willing to separate you from your money by making dubious health claims for some product or service, and many are masterful at getting favorable publicity from the naive, irresponsible, and sometimes corrupt mass media.

Keep in mind that the quackery industry's propaganda mills run overtime, and their handiwork is sophisticated enough to fool people from all walks of life. During their school years, millions of Americans absorb a great deal of information without learning the art of critical thinking. Such people are naive and easily misled by slick snake-oil propaganda that uses biochemical terms and pseudoscientific jargon. Many make perfect mugging victims by repeatedly coming back for more.

If you are harmed by a dubious health-related product (including a book) or by following the advice of a suspected quack, you may be able to recover damages from the retailer, fringe practitioner, or even from an author, publisher, or talk-show producer. The National Council Against Health Fraud's Task Force on Victim Redress may be able to help. It offers a free medicolegal analysis, referrals to attorneys and expert witnesses, and information on many types of quackery. These services are available to individuals, insurance companies, attorneys, and law-enforcement agencies. Its address is P.O. Box 1747, Allentown, PA 18105.

Of course, even if you haven't been victimized, joining the National Council Against Health Fraud is a good idea. Its 1,200-member network is the backbone of organized antiquackery activity in the United States. Members receive a bimonthly newsletter and discounts on various publications. The Council's address is P.O. Box 1276, Loma Linda, CA 92354.

Be Skeptical of Health Advertising

Many media outlets are willing to publish ads for health products and services that they know are fraudulent. These include worthless weight-loss products, dangerous diet books, body wraps, fake muscle-building pills, herbal aphrodisiacs, superenergy vitamin supplements, high colonics, astrological services, cult recruiting propaganda, naturopathic clinics, and the like.

The Council of Better Business Bureaus and the FDA are eager to help newspapers, magazines, and radio and television stations identify misleading advertising claims for health and beauty products. In 1984 these agencies sent a joint mailing urging nearly 20,000 media outlets to carefully review health claims before accepting ads. Although some recipients may have had their consciousness raised, many media outlets will publish any health-related ad that someone is willing to pay for.

Be Skeptical of Tabloid Television

Broadcasters profit from advertising revenue, and talk shows increase their ratings by sensationalizing and pandering. Many programs promote health frauds, while very few expose them.

Book Publishers to Beware of

Health pornography is an enormous business. Hundreds of millions of dollars are made by miracle-mongering, pandering, and peddling snake oils and paranoia. Some of the worst offenders are mentioned below. Their track records are so bad that anything they publish relating to health, nutrition, or medicine should be viewed with suspicion.

• Avery Publishing Group markets its own books plus those of several other publishers. Its *Prescription for Nutritional Healing,* by James and Phyllis Balch, recommends supplements and/or herbs for AIDS, cancer, diabetes, heart disease, multiple sclerosis, and more than a hundred other health problems. (The "health food" industry loves this book because it makes claims that manufacturers and retailers cannot legally make for their products.) Avery's catalog lists books promoting iridology, polarity therapy, macrobiotics, cancer quackery, homeopathy, chelation therapy, and a score of other dubious practices.

• Bantam Books, a German publisher, has feasted on Americans' love of hogwash. Its large stable of quackery-promoting titles includes *The Anti-Craving Weight Loss Diet,* by Elliot Abravanel, *The Yeast Connection,* by William Crook, *Quantum Healing,* by Deepak Chopra, *Dr. Atkins' Nutrition Breakthrough,* and *The Last Chance Diet,* by Robert Linn.

• Keats Publishing, with more than three hundred titles in print, is the primary publisher of books and booklets promoting "alternative methods," particularly methods involving nutrition.

• MacMillan Publishing Co. has made millions on *The Beverly Hills Diet* by Judy Mazel.

• McGraw-Hill has sold almost three million copies of *Nutrition Almanac,* by Lavon J. Dunne and John D. Kirschmann, who apparently have no credentials in the health field. The cover proclaims, "The Bestselling Guide to Better Eating for Better Health. . . . Millions of health-conscious individuals and nutrition professionals have turned with confidence to this book again and again for simple and sensible information about nutrition." Among the many fallacies in the book are these: pangamic acid is a vitamin (B_{15}) a deficiency of which causes nervous disorders; the herb skullcap is "one of the best nerve tonics ever discovered" and is useful in all disorders of the nervous system including epilepsy, rabies, tetanus, and assorted poisonings; and comfrey is a good source of various nutrients and an effective treatment for a variety of serious diseases. McGraw-Hill has also published several misleading books by Lendon Smith. Although the company is a respected publisher of medical textbooks, its books for the general public are not held to scientific standards.

• New American Library has published many unreliable books on nutrition, including several by Adelle Davis, Stuart Berger, M.D., and Robert Haas.

• Rodale Press has published many books promoting unproven nutritional methods and has marketed many more such books through its Prevention Book Club.

• Simon and Schuster has published many books that promote worthless and dangerous healing methods and superstitions. Its titles include *Maximum Immunity* by Michael Weiner; *Awakening the Healer Within* (on the wonders of psychic surgery) by Andrea Cagan, a crystal healer; *Numerology Has Your Number* by Ellin Dodge; *Tarot Made Easy* by Nancy Caren; *You Are Your Blood Type* by Nomi and Besher; *Supernutrition* by Richard A. Passwater; *The Encyclopedia of Alternative Health Care* by Kristin Olsen; *Celestial Bodies: An Astrological Path to Total Health* by Kathleen Johnson; *The Amino Revolution,* by "nutrition expert" Robert Erdman; *How to Beat Arthritis with Immune Power Boosters,* by "world renowned medical authority" Carson Wade; *Numerology Has Your Number,* by Ellin Dodge, and others by Carlton Fredericks, Lendon Smith, and Stuart Berger.

• Warner Books has hit the jackpot with *Fit for Life* by Harvey and Marilyn Diamond, *Life Extension* by Durk Pearson and Sandy Shaw, *The Medical Heretic* by Robert Mendelsohn, *Biorhythm: A Personal Science* by Bernard Gittelson, *Earl Mindell's Vitamin Bible,* and a series of books promoting Edgar Casey's ideas, edited by Hugh L. Cayce.

Periodicals: A Mixed Bag

The types of periodicals that cannot be relied on to provide accurate information on health and medicine include the following:

• "Health food" and fitness-industry propaganda outlets such as *Longevity, Let's Live, Total Health,* and *Muscle & Fitness* have one purpose: to sell the public on scores of worthless supplements and so-called natural remedies. *Vegetarian Times* is a promoter of unproven remedies and unnecessary supplements. It recently paid $11,000 to several "quackbusters" in return for a promise not to file suit over an article making false and defamatory claims about them. Cult-oriented magazines such as *New Age Journal* and *East West Natural Health* (which primarily promotes macrobiotics) are also unreliable. Beware of magazines that run ads for questionable products such as those discussed in Chapter Five. *Prevention,* long a major source of health misinformation, has greatly improved in recent years, but it still carries misleading ads for supplement products and encourages inappropriate use of supplements.

• Sensationalist tabloids that feature celebrity gossip and bizarre tales about UFO abductions, psychic powers, and the like cannot be relied on to report health news accurately. Some of them seem to be in cahoots with quack industries in defrauding the public with worthless weight-loss gimmicks, baldness remedies, arthritis cures, and the like. For example, a headline will scream about a wonder drug for arthritis or obesity, and the article will quote a "scientist" or two. On the same page, or a nearby page, an ad for the product will appear.

• Women's magazines vary considerably in the quality of their information about health. The primary purpose of some of them appears to be to promote the products of their advertisers. Every few years the American Council on Science and Health rates the quality of nutrition information in popular magazines. Their 1988 survey rated *Vogue,* the *Saturday Evening Post,* and *Good Housekeeping* among the best, and *Cosmopolitan* and *Ladies Home Journal* among the worst. The new advertisement-free *Ms.* also looks reliable.

• Metropolitan dailies, with few exceptions, cannot be relied on to consistently provide accurate information on health-related topics. The Honolulu *Star-Bulletin* illustrates this point. Its "Advertising Standards," published in each edition, says, "Advertising that is deceptive or misleading is never knowingly accepted." Yet the paper has run many ads for patently phony weight-loss products and ads that fraudulently state or imply that chiropractic treatment is effective for such ailments as allergies and ulcers. One ad for a quack cancer clinic promised "proven effective cancer treatment... remarkable results in all types of cancer using ... homeopathic treatment." My complaints about the ads have not stopped their publication.

Obviously, the *Star-Bulletin* editors have chosen to ignore the FDA/ Better Business Bureau offer to help ferret out false ads. Like most other editors of dailies, they have also ignored repeated requests to publish a small disclaimer with their astrology column to the effect that the column is for entertainment only and that astrology has no scientific merit. Apparently, they feel little obligation to print the truth or to protect the welfare of their readers. The paper's "science and environment" reporter is fond of things paranormal and mystical. In January 1991, she greeted the new year with gobbledygook about tarot cards, psychics, astrologers, and enlightened masters. The religion editor has run articles promoting the "workshops" of psychic healers, including a well-known psychic-surgery scam artist. All this is typical of hundreds of mediocre dailies around the country. A few larger papers, most notably the *Los Angeles Times,* do considerably better.

What AIDS and Cancer Patients Can Do

The sewer of exploitation that quacks wallow in seems to have no bottom. There is no depth to which this species will not sink. For several decades their swindling of cancer patients with laetrile and the like set the standard for their ilk. Now the advent of AIDS has opened new avenues of opportunity for them. They not only sap AIDS patients of financial resources and sap them of their health with toxic nostrums, they convince their victims to agitate against those who expose their scams.

The behavior of AIDS activists in attempting to disrupt the 1990 National Health Fraud Conference in Kansas City is a sad illustration of how victims can be manipulated into doing quackery's dirty work. Some participants distributed flyers stating, "The goal of this conference is to directly challenge any type of treatment that does not currently meet AMA guidelines or FDA approval! . . . It is not to eliminate any real health fraud that is out there! It represents the efforts of the AMA and the big drug companies to suppress their competition, and the insurance industry to reduce their coverage!" Other participants marched outside the conference hotel shouting slogans like, "AMA. FDA. Racist, sexist, anti-gay!" and demanding the right to pursue acupuncture, homeopathy, and other "alternatives" without government interference. Apparently, snake-oil peddlers and their sophisticated propaganda have confused many HIV-positive people about who their friends are.

AIDS and cancer patients should understand that there are sharks out there anxious to exploit them, as well as sincere but misguided zealots who have been duped by the quacks. There has been a great deal of progress in the treatment of AIDS and most types of cancer. Not one iota of this progress has come from "alternative medicine," "complementary medicine," "wholistic healing," "oriental medicine," or any of the rest.

What Arthritis Patients Can Do

Warning: if you have rheumatoid arthritis or osteoarthritis, beware! You are a prime target for quackery. Arthritis patients are the ideal prey because the disease is not curable and the debilitating and frustrating symptoms often wax and wane unpredictably. People who take a phony nostrum before a period of remission may become convinced that it works and continue to use it. By the time they realize it doesn't work they may have wasted hundreds or even thousands of dollars. Many patients go from one arthritis snake oil to another for years.

Proper therapy for rheumatoid arthritis and osteoarthritis is essential to minimize pain, inflammation, and joint damage and to keep joints functioning. It involves proper exercise, rest, and certain medications. Some drugs have proven value in these diseases, but they should be carefully prescribed, usually one at a time, by a physician who follows the patient closely. Beware of everything else.

Especially beware of promises of a cure, "secret formulas," testimonials, dietary remedies, and nutritional supplements. And stay away from vaccines, hormones, snake and bee venoms, herbs, drugs such as Gerovital and Liefcort (a dangerous hormone cocktail), cocaine, copper bracelets, holy water, homeopathy, Chinese herbs and pills, chiropractic, acupuncture, reflexology, "metabolic therapy," folk remedies, yucca extracts, mussel extracts, mud packs, manure poultices, DMSO, ointments, magnets, colored lights, assorted radiation, and all kinds of gadgets and devices. Don't buy books that promise amazing results. And stay away from clinics in Mexico and other neighboring countries where quacks prey on Americans.

If you have any questions about a purported arthritis remedy, contact the nearest chapter of the Arthritis Foundation and talk with your doctor. If your doctor's advice conflicts with that of the Arthritis Foundation, consult another medical doctor, preferably a rheumatologist.

What Physicians Can Do

Although the vast majority of physicians are not involved in unscientific practices, most physicians seem willing to tolerate those who are.

Fad diagnoses, unnecessary and incompetent surgery (especially cosmetic surgery), irrational and excessive drug prescribing, and inept communication create fertile soil for medical quacks to till.

Physicians, individually and as a profession, can help combat quackery by addressing each of these points. They can learn about the various forms of quackery, educate their patients about them, and consider them in the diagnosis of symptoms as well as in overall health care of patients. Cult medicine can lead to malnutrition, vitamin poisoning, herb poisoning, chronic cyanide poisoning, injuries from inappropriate manipulations, and delay in seeking proper help.

Some physicians are so naive about quackery that they wink at "alternative" and "complementary" therapies that may be harming their patients. Sometimes this tolerance reaches absurd dimensions. In Honolulu large "health fairs" are sponsored by Kaiser Permanente, the Hawaii Medical Services Association (HMSA), and other mainstream health-care groups. The governor and mayor issue supporting proclamations and declare Health Week for the week of the fair. The fun family event is held in a city-owned exhibition hall and is covered with enthusiasm by all the local media. Unfortunately, among the health-related products and services offered are invariably a plethora of snake oils.

For example, Kaiser's 1989 Health and Fitness Expo, held in conjunction with the prestigious Great Aloha Run marathon, included exhibits for a phony dental mercury tester, homeopathic remedies, healing crystals, miracle hair nutrients, and assorted megavitamin and amino acid supplements fraudulently promoted as weight-loss miracles, muscle builders, and energizers. Chiropractors in force gave free spinal examinations and set up appointments for further examination (not free) and treatment of alleged subluxations, which, according to chiropractic flyers, could cause all kinds of serious diseases. Most outrageous of all was a naturopath who claimed that his electronic gadget could measure a person's electromagnetic field and thereby determine blood mineral levels. These would be used to determine the proper therapy for a wide range of symptoms and disorders. For the half day I was there, the line at this exhibit was far longer than any other, including those for cholesterol and blood pressure checks!

Similar health fairs in this same city facility and in cities across the country promote all the above quackery as well as such nostrums as psychic surgery, urine-drinking for cancer, colostrum for everything, and herbal snake oils of every kind. It is reprehensible that responsible physicians so willingly associate with blatant health-fraud promotions. By so doing, they give the snake oils credibility and help mislead the public. Organizers of these events must keep the quackery out, even if it means some booths go unrented. Responsible health professionals should complain to government officials who endorse quackery-promoting fairs and allow them to be held in public facilities. We wouldn't allow con artists to huckster fake diamonds from a city exhibition hall; why should quacks be permitted to sell fake cancer and arthritis cures with the blessings of the mayor?

A doctor who winks at a patient's going off to a fringe practitioner for "complementary" therapy risks an unpleasant confrontation with the quack later. One doctor told me that a hypertensive patient of his went to a naturopath who prescribed an assortment of herbs and megavitamins. The physician challenged him to "see if you can find in your dusty tomes the interactions of your herbal drugs with the ACE inhibitor I prescribe, which is working very well without your meddling. And be warned that you will be liable for any harm to the patient." The naturopath then tried to convince the patient to stop taking the prescribed drug. In such cases a formal warning letter may be in order. Such letters can be effective tools in combating quackery in all its forms, especially if they are written by physicians and other experts. A warning letter should state the facts clearly and warn of the dangers posed by the recipient's actions. It should make clear that if harm results from said actions, a copy of the letter will be made available to the injured parties and their attorneys. This removes ignorance as a possible defense in subsequent litigation, and it might be enough to cause the recipient to stop the dangerous activities. The letter should be dated and sent by certified mail.

The formal warning letter can be a powerful antiquackery weapon. In California it is illegal for the media, print or electronic, to knowingly print false or deceptive claims in advertising. Suppose a physician knows that patients are put at risk by a worthless product advertised in a local paper or on television. Instead of writing to the FDA and waiting months for nothing to happen, the doctor could try sending warning letters to the promoters of the product and to the media that run the ads. Since this is a criminal matter, a copy of each letter should be sent to the Attorney General. Such warning letters might even make it possible for victims of the scams to recover damages from the media as well as the promoter, provided the advertisement was a major factor in the decision to purchase and try the product.

It is also essential that physicians clean their own house. Too many incompetent and crooked doctors are in business and doing a lot of harm. Efforts to weed them out must be stepped up to protect the public and to hold the line on malpractice insurance rates. The risks of libel and antitrust suits tend to discourage whistle-blowing and even participation in peer review. Peer review carries no serious risk, however, when done correctly, with due process, in good faith, and aimed at improving health care rather than harming a competitor.

Neither is it risky to write to a licensing board to complain about a doctor's misconduct and *ask for an investigation.* On the other hand, ignoring or condoning a colleague's misconduct could get anyone remotely associated with that individual dragged into court.

Physicians should also support and participate in studies to determine the appropriateness, effectiveness, and safety of many of their cherished tests, procedures, and remedies. While coronary artery bypass, carotid endarterectomy, pacemaker implantation, hysterectomy, and the like are life-saving in some situations, they are expensive quackery in others. Only scientific research can provide proper guidelines. Good physicians will keep up with the research and adjust their practices as warranted.

Physicians must learn the right lessons from the *Wilk* v. *AMA* decision and not overreact and clam up on the subject of chiropractic and other health fraud. Responsible health professionals have a right and a responsibility to tell their patients and the public the truth about chiropractic's dogma and the rampant quackery among its practitioners. Of course, as long as mainstream medicine tolerates the practice of homeopathy by M.D.'s, its complaints about unscientific medicine will ring rather hollow. Nevertheless, individual doctors should speak up. In fact, doctors not associated with large group practices, health maintenance organizations, or the AMA may be seen as more concerned about their patients and the public welfare rather than turf battles and may be taken more seriously by legislators.

What Nutritionists Can Do

Nutrition quackery, in the form of dangerous diets, worthless supplements, and bogus nutritional "cures," is the most widespread category of health fraud. Most of the quackery discussed in this book involves nutritional products. Diploma-mill and self-proclaimed nutritionists have become a national plague. Their ability to confuse and mislead the public is an enormous problem that real nutritionists should not ignore.

Registered dietitians and other legitimate nutritionists can fight back by learning about quack nutrition and taking the time to explain the fallacies and dangers to their clients and the public. They should talk to reporters and go on radio and television talk shows to refute the claims of the phonies. They should write letters to the editors of newspapers and magazines that do shoddy stories on nutrition-related subjects and glowing reviews of dingbat diet books. They can help school and community librarians make rational choices for their nutrition sections. Quacks have an inherent advantage in the media: they get publicity because their far-fetched claims are judged "newsworthy."

What Pharmacists Can Do

Pharmacists are trained in pharmacology, an exacting science whose findings and principles they are ethically bound to apply in their work of preparing and dispensing drugs and giving advice. As professionals, their job ought to go beyond filling prescriptions, being alert to prescribing errors and drug interactions, and advising customers about nonprescription remedies. But pharmacists are also business people who may have to watch the bottom line. When they see the "health food" stores selling tons of megavitamins, amino acids, and other unnecessary concoctions, they can be understandably envious. So they sell them too.

Large drug companies have advertised deceptively to both the public and to health professionals. E. R. Squibb & Sons, for example, advertised for a few years that Theragran (their high-dose multivitamin) was selected by the U. S. Olympic Team. They neglected to say that they bought the right to make the claim for $500,000. It was a meaningless and deceptive advertising ploy. (Of course, it would help if the Olympic Committee refrained from endorsing health-related products unless the endorsements are based on scientific tests rather than payola.) Supplements are the biggest money-makers for "health food" stores and among the biggest for drugstores. The biggest supplier of both is Hoffmann-La Roche, which supplies the raw materials for most of the vitamins that are manufactured. Roche, too, has engaged in misleading advertising.

Of course, unnecessary supplements aren't the only questionable products sold in drugstores. Of the thousands of remedies for dozens of symptoms and ailments, most people can benefit from just a handful through a lifetime. Whole categories of nonprescription products are either worthless or vastly overrated. This includes products for weight control, constipation (except bulk remedies), nausea (though some motion sickness products work), vomiting, over-indulgence, insomnia, and hemorrhoids (except petrolatum and zinc oxide).

Most of the cold cocktails, the multidrug pills touted to relieve up to a dozen symptoms simultaneously, are unnecessary, irrational, and overpriced. Colds usually come in stages, with one or two symptoms at a time. If one must use drugs, it makes sense to use just a throat spray or lozenge for the first day or two when sore throat is usually the dominant symptom. Nothing should be taken for a runny nose. A nasal spray can be used later for a day or two if stuffiness occurs. Severe muscle aches, fever, and headache may indicate influenza, so call a physician. Aspirin or acetaminophen may relieve these symptoms, but they may increase nasal stuffiness and even slow recovery.

Ibuprofen may be a better choice.

Pharmacists generally have a good reputation with the public; they are seen as professionals who can be trusted. Physicians encourage this trust and so does the FDA, which in the 1980s joined in a campaign with the Pharmaceutical Advertising Agency that encouraged the public to "ask your pharmacist" about questionable claims for health products. Unfortunately, if you do this, the recommended product may be something you don't need. In March 1986, *Consumer Reports* revealed that many pharmacists give poor advice and fail to advise consumers to consult a physician rather than buy a nonprescription remedy. When thirty pharmacists were asked whether a vitamin would relieve symptoms of nervousness or fatigue, most suggested buying a product and few recommended seeing a doctor.

Pharmacists say they are in a difficult position because they stand to lose money by telling people the truth about products commonly sold in drugstores. Many rationalize that if they don't sell all the junk to their customers, someone else will. But they should consider another angle. If they are consistently honest and always advise what is best for the customer, even if it means less immediate profit, they may gain long-term loyalty and ultimately more profit. They may also sleep better at night.

Pharmacists should take a stand against all kinds of quackery, including unnecessary supplements and bogus nutritional remedies. Their organizations and publications should help educate the public, as well as discourage pharmacists from profiteering from quackery.

What Nurses Can Do

Nurses frequently have opportunities to educate patients on health-related matters and usually do a good job. However, the profession is not exempt from the tidal wave of quackery afflicting all sectors of society. Far too many nurses have fallen for New Age and "alternative" therapies and are passing kooky ideas on to their patients. Some of the quackery gets official blessings. For example, nurses in California can get continuing education credits for classes in crystal healing, acupressure, and visits to quack cancer clinics in Tijuana.

This nonsense obviously should be stopped. Nurses should help patients and clients develop rational attitudes toward prevention, self-care, and professional care. Beyond this, nurses are in a good position to combat quackery by providing some of the elements that physicians sometimes don't provide. They can listen, sympathize, encourage, make comfortable, soothe, massage, hold, and just be there for patients. A quack will do all these things plus indulge in a lot of herbal, nutritional, homeopathic, or mystical mumbo-jumbo and charge ten times as much while likely endangering the patient's health.

Nurses who believe certain therapies are underutilized should encourage their use in a responsible and conservative manner. For example, nurses who want to introduce therapeutic touch (see Chapter 5) into their wards should stick to the simple facts and avoid talk about "balancing the body's energies" and other mystical and unscientific jargon. A foot massage can be a pleasant, relaxing experience that can relieve various symptoms. Period. There is no need to resort to acupressure dogma and other silly theories dreamed up centuries ago by people who had no idea how the human body works.

By providing the human touch that sick (and well but worried) people crave, nurses can decrease the impulse to consult a phony "wholistic healer" or "natural, organic doctor." Thus, they can essentially co-opt the elements of "alternative medicine" that really do work while helping society discard the rest into the dustbin of history.

What Dentists Can Do

Dentistry deserves credit for advances in the treatment and prevention of tooth and gum disease. The oral health of the American people has never been better. Unfortunately, some dentists perform dubious procedures. Some of these are even being taught in continuing education courses that naive and careless authorities have accredited. The following types of quackery are the most popular with misguided dentists.

• Amalgam phobia, the fear of mercury poisoning from dental fillings. The dentist who made a living for twenty years putting amalgam into carious teeth and now thinks he has nothing to do, or hasn't the skills to do other procedures, can spend the next twenty years removing the fillings and putting in plastic ones. There is no good reason for it, but it generates income.

• TMJ treatments. This is a very murky area with dozens of unproven diagnostic techniques and remedies for the apparent dysfunction of the temporomandibular joints that connect the jaw to the skull. Experts believe the condition usually resolves by itself and the symptoms disappear in the vast majority of cases, though some patience may be required. In other cases, simple remedies suffice, such as not chewing too much gum or otherwise overworking the jaw. In only a very small minority of cases is treatment necessary. Yet some dentists diagnose TMJ syndrome every day and recommend expensive treatments. Some are even teamed up with shyster lawyers and crooked clients to defraud insurance companies of compensation for accidents. Practically any kind of accident could conceivably cause TMJ dysfunction, and it can be difficult to prove it didn't in any given case.

• Bogus nutrition. Some dentists promote fad diets and unnecessary supplements, including megavitamins.

• Cranial osteopathy, or cranial adjustments. Dentists who believe in this unsubstantiated theory believe their dental treatments can affect the health of the whole body by causing "binding" of the skull bones and preventing their alleged pulsations. It's all nonsense.

• Applied kinesiology (or dental kinesiology). Some dentists believe that each tooth is related by purported acupuncture meridians to muscles, glands, and other organs. These misguided dentists claim that disease in a tooth, or even an allegedly abnormal electrical activity in a healthy tooth, can cause disease in the corresponding organ.

• Acupuncture and acupressure. Some dentists take courses in acupuncture and dabble in electroacupuncture.

• "Holistic dentistry." The word "holistic" (or "wholistic") no longer means a rational approach that considers all factors affecting a patient's life. Instead it has become a buzzword for marketing a whole gamut of unscientific treatments. Patients should watch out for the "holistic dentist." While the American Dental Association evaluates dental devices, materials, and instruments for safety and effectiveness, it does not evaluate procedures. Perhaps it should start doing so. At the very least it could take a stand when utter nonsense and egregious fraud gain a beachhead in the profession. Like the American Cancer Society does for cancer quackery, the ADA could compile and publicize a list of dubious treatments and procedures used by dentists. The public could be informed that the vast majority of dentists disapprove of the treatments. And it certainly should not allow continuing education credits to be granted for courses that teach the quackery.

It would also help if the dental schools put more emphasis on the scientific basis of clinical dentistry. Expert critics say that too often students are taught clinical procedures from older dentists in an authoritarian manner with lots of memorization rather than understanding. They don't take courses about the scientific method, and they don't do research. Later most of them set up solo practices where their work is not judged by colleagues. The isolation and lack of peer review make them more susceptible to fallacies and illusions. Rigorous training in how clinical science proceeds could help remedy this.

What Chiropractors Can Do

Most chiropractors still distance themselves from other health professionals by clinging to cult dogma and using unethical techniques to peddle a vast array of unproved methods and medicines. If they ever want peace with rational professionals, if they want respect and referrals, they must change their ways. There can be no compromise on this. Chiropractors must accept the tenets of their own reform movement (see Chapter 3), abide by them, and help enforce them. This will include changing the way they practice and promote themselves, and it may include lobbying in legislatures for reform measures and against self-serving chiropractic associations. It may also include testifying in court against fellow chiropractors involved in assorted fraud or malpractice. Unless chiropractors become part of the solution, they will remain part of the problem.

What Educators Can Do

"Our nation is at risk. Our once unchallenged preeminence in commerce, industry, science and technological innovation is being overtaken by competitors throughout the world. . . . We have, in effect, been committing an act of unthinking, unilateral educational disarmament." These alarming words are from *A Nation at Risk: The Imperative for Educational Reform,* a report prepared by the National Commission on Excellence in Education in 1983.

Since then there have been many more reports by such groups as the National Research Council, the National Science Foundation, and the National Science Board, all of which document a dismal state of affairs with little progress being made. Students from at least a dozen countries in Asia and Europe consistently out-perform American students in math and science. Experts estimate that only about 6 percent of Americans are scientifically literate. As we approach the twenty-first century, many times this number believe in astrology, creationism, telepathy, and other pseudosciences and myths. This not only affects our productivity as a nation, it also threatens our future as a democracy in a technological world facing major decisions about genetic engineering, the greenhouse effect, acid rain, nuclear power, and so on.

A democratic nation cannot make rational decisions if its citizens can't distinguish astronomy from astrology, chemistry from alchemy, and reality from fantasy. Science is not just a body of knowledge, but a way of thinking that is responsible for practically all the progress humans have made in improving our lives and understanding our world. Without it, individual decisions on health matters and policies regarding public health are inevitably irrational. The best weapon against quackery is a scientifically literate populace. Our educational system must develop ways to teach rational thinking.

Teachers of health, physical education, and home economics have ample opportunity to instill skepticism about dubious health products at an early age. All of these educators teach nutrition either formally or by giving advice to their students. Health classes could easily include material on bogus diets and phony cures in their nutrition sections. Students would not only learn about good nutrition, but would recognize bad nutrition when they encountered it. Home economics classes should help prepare students to make rational decisions in the health marketplace. They should include material on the vast array of nutritional supplements and other health-related products heavily promoted to the public.

Athletic coaches may be in the best position of all to help guide students away from quackery. Budding athletes these days waste millions of dollars on worthless supplements, especially amino acids, protein powders, glandulars, and vitamins. They have been taught to read, but they haven't been taught not to believe everything they read. They read the muscle magazines and have little reason to suspect that the articles and ads lie about products in order to sell them. Many young athletes, especially wrestlers and others who compete in weight categories, go on bizarre diets. They may even binge and purge like bulimics. Informed coaches should educate them on the dangers of these practices and the reality of sharks in the marketplace.

Academic writers, those who write textbooks for high-school and college students, should look at a publisher's entire catalog before signing a contract. All too often their good work is undone by mass-market titles from the same publisher, often under different imprints. This kind of publisher dispenses science-based and socially responsible texts out the front door while peddling pseudoscience out the back door.

Another way educators can combat quackery is to stop the teaching of health fraud and paranormal pornography on college campuses. In many areas, colleges are being used by quacks, scammers, and misguided zealots under the auspices of the continuing education divisions. The universities get some revenue from night room rentals for noncredit classes. The quacks get instant credibility by virtue of their association with the universities, including advertisements for themselves and their classes in official university publications. This arrangement has proven profitable to an assortment of astrologers, psychics, phony nutritionists, herbalists, naturopaths, and other fringe practitioners and con artists who sometimes make the rounds on local talk shows and represent themselves as university instructors who have scientific proof for their contentions.

I hate to pick on my alma mater, but the following episode illustrates how irresponsible continuing education programs can be. I once submitted to the University of Hawaii College of Continuing Education a detailed proposal for a noncredit class in nutrition quackery. It was to focus on the hazards and costs of the many quack diets, supplements, and remedies now so popular, including laetrile, the phony cancer cure. My proposal was rejected because the administrator in charge of choosing classes believed it would not draw well and money would be wasted publicizing the class and reserving me a room. I disagreed but had no right to appeal.

A few months later I came across an article in a local daily about a noncredit nutrition class at the university. It was a gullible piece about a real neat class on "alternative nutrition" taught by a real neat guy, a young pharmacist with lots of real neat ideas like curing cancer with laetrile and diet and using "vitamin B_{15}" (a fraud) to increase stamina. Aaarrrggghhh!!! They rejected a responsible, consumer-oriented class taught by a qualified nutritionist, but accepted a class promoting cult nutrition and cancer quackery taught by someone with no qualifications in the field. Fortunately, two real nutrition professors complained, and the course was not renewed.

There are two important lessons here: noncredit divisions may prostitute a university's integrity for the bottom line—or occasionally out of ignorance—and responsible critics in the university community probably can stop them.

What Accreditation Officials Should Do

The U. S. Office of Education (USOE) does not take scientific validity into account when it awards recognition to agencies that accredit our nation's schools. Nor does USOE investigate or pass judgment on either the truth or social utility of the material taught. Rather, it judges such factors as financial solvency, curriculum outlines, internal review processes, and legal recognition of graduates. So far, agencies have been recognized to accredit schools of chiropractic, naturopathy, and acupuncture. A USOE official actually has said that an accrediting agency for astrology schools could be recognized if it could meet the agency's other criteria. This enormous threat to consumer protection and the accrediting process should be changed. Perhaps a Congressional investigation should be the first step.

What Librarians Can Do

Librarians are special kinds of educators. In grade schools, colleges and communities their selections can deeply affect their users and influence their attitudes on major issues. Unfortunately, most librarians help perpetrate myths, hoaxes, and frauds by stocking their shelves with books that promote them.

The Hawaii State Library, for example, has about sixty books about astrology, all but two of which promote astrology as a *science*. The library's computer listing has twenty-six categories, such as Astrology and Diet, Astrology and Birth Control, and Astrology and Hygiene, which give no clue that the books are nonsensical. The two science-based books that debunk astrology as nonsense are categorized as "Astrology and Controversial Literature."

The book *In His Image: The Cloning of a Man* [Lippincott, 1978], by David M. Rorvik, claimed that a British multimillionaire had himself cloned and that this "offspring" was an identical twin the age of his grandson. A biologist mentioned in the book brought a lawsuit because he felt he had been defamed by being mentioned in a way that tended to promote fraudulent claims in the book. In 1982 the book was declared "a fraud and a hoax" by the judge at a pretrial hearing. Lippincott then apologized and settled out of court for a sizable sum.

Even though the publisher conceded the story was untrue, the book remains on nonfiction shelves in libraries all over the country. Librarians I have asked about it are surprised to hear the book is a hoax, but they don't know what to do about it. I suggest they do what others already have: add to the entry for the book in the card catalogue or computer listing, "Work declared a fraud and hoax by Philadelphia judge" and "Publisher acknowledged work is untrue in 1982"; add the subject headings "fraud in science" and "hoaxes"; and reclassify the book to 001.95, Deceptions and Hoaxes.

It is time for librarians to seriously consider greatly increasing the number of books classified 001.95. A book titled *The Third Eye,* by "Tibetan" Lobsang Rampa (really Cyril H. Hoskins of London), was exposed as a hoax by *Time* magazine in February 1958. Yet for the next thirty years, Ballantine, a subsidiary of Random House, published it as fact, and it remains on the nonfiction shelves of bookstores and libraries. The Don Juan books by Carlos Castaneda almost surely are hoaxes, as are many UFO titles, yet they are on nonfiction shelves. It's tempting to suspect that Shirley MacLaine's books are hoaxes, but they are more likely the products of delusion. Unfortunately, there is no practical way for libraries to classify books as "delusional."

What about the diet book hoaxes? It is too much to expect librarians to judge the validity of books on diet and health and to classify them accordingly. Committees of experts to classify books would be seen as censors, and their every act would cause an uproar. Clearly, routine classification of popular health books in this way would not be feasible. Yet, an occasional book of this sort could be placed in the Hoax category for the deceptive manner in which it has been promoted. For example, Warner Books sent Harvey and Marilyn Diamond on talk-show and lecture circuits allowing and encouraging the false belief that they are genuine experts on nutrition with real credentials in the field. The same publisher paraded another money-making team in its stable, Durk Pearson and Sandy Shaw, as leading authorities and experts in the field of aging, but they, too, have nothing close to expert credentials.

All the books by both of these couples are full of foolish assertions and potentially dangerous advice. Can librarians not find a way to separate these and similar books from legitimate and helpful books and identify them as such? Unfortunately, there is probably no practical way this can be done except in specific cases that have been adjudicated in court. For example, suppose a mother were to claim that she brought her child up according to the advice in one of the Diamonds' books and that the child consequently suffered grave injury. Suppose a court ruled in her favor and awarded damages from both the authors and the publisher, on the grounds that the claim the book was written by experts was false and misleading and the advice therein led to harm to the child. In that case it would be reasonable to either remove the book from the shelves or reclassify it to 001.95 and make a note in the catalogue entry for the book. A warning sticker stating the facts of the case could be placed on the inside front cover.

Enterprising librarians might also want to consider placing a warning label when an author dies of a disease after claiming that an "alternative" method has cured him. An example would be the books by Dr. Anthony Sattilaro, who died after suggesting that a macrobiotic diet had put his cancer of the prostate into permanent remission (see Chapter 1).

At the very least, libraries that carry popular diet and health books should also carry responsible critiques of them, such as those from *Consumer Reports,* Prometheus Books, the National Council Against Health Fraud, and *Nutrition Forum.* These materials should be prominently displayed or promoted in posters and flyers. Librarians asked about the latest best-seller diet book can say something like, "You might also want to read about it in *Nutrition Forum,* over in the corner."

Many librarians rely on book reviews in *Publishers Weekly* and *Library Journal* to help them decide what books to buy. Many reviews are done by nonexperts who cannot tell the difference between a fact and a piece of nonsense. Even when a reviewer knows that a health book is nonsensical, the published review will describe it as "controversial" and "likely to be something many patrons will want to read." The public might benefit considerably if book reviews in these magazines were written by experts or with the help of expert consultants. Unfortunately, this is unlikely because the magazines are not likely to publish negative reviews of the books published by their major advertisers.

When it comes to acquiring and retaining material, librarians should consider much more than short-term popularity, such as consumer advocacy and long-term value to society. If libraries simply reflected the public taste, the encyclopedias and important periodicals would be crowded out by tabloid papers; girlie, biker, and lurid detective magazines; pulp romance; comic books; and the like. Most libraries keep such trash out. They should start looking for ways to also keep out the quacky diets and other health pornography.

What Government Can Do

Health fraud is a dangerous form of white-collar crime. Of all the immoral and illegal ways people swindle each other, quackery is among the most dangerous and expensive for the victims and the safest for the perpetrators. Selling counterfeit stocks, phony gems, and diluted apple juice can bring heavy fines and jail terms, but diverting seriously ill patients from effective therapies with the lure of phony miracle cures carries little risk for the quack. This situation could be turned around by actions in the legislatures, administrations, and courts at the municipal, state, and national levels. A thorough review would take a large volume. A few examples here point to the kinds of reforms that are necessary.

Most states lack effective antiquackery laws. In some it is illegal to practice medicine without a license, but action is rarely taken unless a person falsely represents himself as a physician. In Hawaii, for example, a follower of Harvey and Marilyn Diamond and the Natural Hygiene cult, calling himself "Dr." on the basis of a mail-order diploma, runs a "health clinic." He has openly advertised his health consulting services and has given horrendous advice to seriously ill people, including cancer and AIDS patients. The state's Regulated Industries Complaints Office has warned him not to represent himself as a physician. Once he complied with the order, the agency backed off and refused my suggestion that they send a "patient" to the clinic to investigate. In another case, a chiropractor teamed up with a diploma-mill nutritionist to run a clinic in which iridology is used to diagnose illnesses, which are then treated with megavitamins, herbs, and other snake oils sold at the clinic. I could find no state or city office interested in investigating the operation.

The situation is similar in other states, as illustrated by an article in *Medical Economics* (December 18, 1989) titled, "No Medical Degree, No License? Come Practice Here." In North Carolina a man who had been an x-ray technician set himself up as a naturopath and "wholistic physician." For three years he diagnosed patients with a "bioelectromagnetics" machine and treated them with megavitamins, intravenous vitamins, herbs, and the like. He even ordered lab tests, electrocardiograms, and biopsies. The Board of Medical Examiners could do nothing because the "naturopath" had no license to revoke. The state attorney general said the activities constituted only a misdemeanor similar to cutting hair without a license and took no action. Even though there was evidence of Medicare fraud, no one investigated. Only after three years and two thousand patients did the State Bureau of Investigation charge him with practicing medicine without a license. He was fined $500 and given the maximum two-year sentence, which was suspended. Nothing was done to prevent him from plying his trade in another state.

While most states need stronger antiquackery laws and stronger enforcement, the trend is frequently the opposite. Nevada has nurtured the quackery industry as a tourist attraction. Its homeopaths, naturopaths, and peddlers of laetrile, Gerovitol, and other snake oils have been a disgrace to the state. Arizona, too, has a separate State Board of Homeopathy and has legalized the practices of homeopathy, acupuncture, chelation therapy, megavitamin therapy, and other unproven methods by medical and osteopathic physicians. Those licensed by this board are not accountable to the state's medical board. The president of the Arizona Homeopathic Medical Association is openly enthusiastic about diagnosis by hair analysis and electroacupuncture diagnosis, as well as remedies dreamed up by "psychic" Edgar Cayce in his slumbers.

Quacks in other states hope to legitimize their practices by emulating the strategy used in Arizona. If the legislators are as gullible and irresponsible as those in Arizona and Nevada, consumers across the country will have even less protection from quackery than they do now. Intelligent and courageous legislators must resist this trend and educate their constituents about the importance of quality health care and the dangers of quackery. Considering that most states already have chiropractic pseudoscience written into the laws and others have legitimized acupuncture and naturopathy, it is hard to be optimistic, but an effort must be made. The deceptive use of diploma-mill degrees in nutrition and other health-related fields should be outlawed in all states as it is in a few. On the federal level, the FDA must be strengthened, and that charlatan's dream known as the Proxmire Amendment to the Federal Food, Drug, and Cosmetic Act, which weakens FDA regulation of dietary supplements, should be revoked.

The judiciary is also guilty of being soft on quackery. Judges tend to treat health fraud about as seriously as jaywalking. Fringe practitioners who practice medicine without a license and kill people with bizarre and dangerous therapies are generally given little more than a slap on the wrist. In California, self-proclaimed healer Stanley Burroughs, who has no professional credentials, was convicted of second-degree murder, unlawfully selling cancer treatments, and practicing medicine without a license. His deep abdominal massages had caused a young woman with cancer to hemorrhage and die. The state Supreme Court reversed the murder conviction on the absurd grounds that practicing medicine without a license is "not inherently dangerous." Tell that to the victim. In another notorious case, Judge Luther Bohannon of the Western District Court of Oklahoma issued an injunction that allowed the peddling of laetrile to cancer patients in violation of federal law. His decision allowed the defrauding of some 25,000 cancer patients over eight years, the last four years in defiance of a unanimous U. S. Supreme Court ruling.

The FDA has great potential to slow the quackery industry, but so far it has lacked sufficient resources and will. In May 1985, *Consumer Reports* concluded that the FDA had "thrown in the towel" in the war on quackery. True, it has only a few million dollars a year budgeted to control an industry raking in billions, so it's not surprising that upholding the law has proven difficult. But sometimes I wonder whether its leaders really *want* to do the job. A few years ago I made an appointment with the head of the FDA office in a major city. I took an assortment of items I had purchased at a local "health food" store. They included purported remedies for cancer, arthritis, kidney disease, heart disease, and other serious ailments that were clearly illegally labelled and promoted.

The receptionist showed me to his large plush office and I entered. He was on the phone and signaled me to sit in the chair by the door. There I sat for ten full minutes while he bragged to his sister a few thousand miles away about his great view and the lovely weather. When he was finished, I had less than five minutes to ask him about the products. Were they legal? Not really. Was the FDA going to take action against them? No, they didn't have the resources to go to court. How about some warning letters? It's not worth the trouble. I walked out wondering what he gets paid for.

The tryptophan tragedy epitomizes the FDA's shabby effort against quackery. In 1972 the FDA banned the sale of isolated amino acids because of potential hazards that needed investigating. The ban was defied by the "health food" industry, however, and was not enforced by the FDA. In the late 1980s, more than 1,500 tryptophan users developed a painful and crippling disorder called eosinophilia-myalgia syndrome, with at least 28 deaths. The FDA finally announced a ban on tryptophan and enforced it. During the past ten years, I have wondered whether the public might be better served if the FDA used its entire antiquackery budget to warn people that it was not protecting them from quackery, that they must protect themselves. By pretending to do its job, the agency has lulled consumers into a false sense of security. Most people mistakenly believe that the products they buy must work as claimed and must be safe or the FDA would not allow them to be sold.

Having said this, however, I would like to express cautious optimism about recent developments. David Kessler, M.D., J.D., who was appointed Commissioner in 1990, has breathed new life into the FDA. Under his leadership, the agency has stepped up product seizures and proposed tough new food-labeling regulations, which, if they become final, will be of tremendous benefit to consumers. The FDA is also developing a cadre of criminal investigators and has announced plans to bring more criminal charges against violators of the Food, Drug, and Cosmetic Act. In fact, the "health food" industry is so frightened that, as we go to press, it has begun a massive advertising, letter-writing, and lobbying campaign to urge Congress to curb the FDA's powers.

What Attorneys Can Do

Attorneys can do many things to help fight quackery. While I agree with critics that Americans are too litigious and we should solve more problems out of court, there is too little litigation in some areas. Personal injury attorneys will find tremendous opportunities if they acquaint themselves with the quackery industry, which, so far, is getting away with murder and mayhem. Victims of health fraud deserve justice. If criminal law doesn't protect them, then the most must be made of civil law.

Thousands of people are being harmed by chiropractors, naturopaths, and other fringe practitioners; manufacturers of assorted snake oils, including vitamins and other supplements that don't carry warnings against overdose; wholesalers and retailers of the snake oils, especially "health food" stores whose unqualified employees presume to give medical and nutritional advice; multi-level operations whose officers conspire to defraud their salespeople and the public by lying about their products; publishers of books containing worthless or dangerous advice; publishers of newspapers and magazines that knowingly carry deceptive advertising; radio and television personalities and producers who deceptively or negligently promote quacks as genuine experts and allow them to run their scams without challenge; and the stations and networks that negligently allow the irresponsible activities.

What Journalists Can Do

Each "journalist" must decide whether he or she is a real professional dedicated to getting the story right or a charlatan in the business of lying for entertainment and profit. Is the journalist's job to enlighten the public with facts, or is this just a front, a pretense to help make a buck? Some people get college degrees in journalism, but end up with tabloids concocting wild stories about abductions by UFO, sightings of Elvis, and the like. They are not journalists, but hoaxers, prostitutes, and professional liars.

What about those who work for women's magazines and "health food" magazines and write "complementary copy" for their advertisers? This practice of publishing articles that are thinly disguised extensions of advertisements is a way of skirting the regulation of commercial language in order to deceive consumers. It has worked wonders for the quackery industry. Surely those who indulge in this sleazy business are not journalists.

Those cases are clear enough, but here's a harder one. What about the "journalist" who doesn't exactly make up stories and doesn't get paid under the table for plugging products, but does get rewarded for sensational stories that distort the facts. For example, he panders to irrational fears with misleading stories about the dangers of pertussis (whooping cough) vaccination and creates widespread fear that leads to a reduction of vaccination rates. This is followed by outbreaks of the disease, which causes death or brain damage in some children. Or he hypes an alleged cure for cancer or arthritis on the basis of sloppy research, gives the product unwarranted credibility, and increases the demand for it and therefore the harm it does. Is the person who makes a living writing such stories a journalist?

CBS-TV's "60 Minutes" occasionally indulges in the latter type of unprofessional and irresponsible "journalism." For example, in 1979 it did a story basically favorable to a remedy for arthritis and multiple sclerosis made from snake venom. It ignored the advice of experts that the product was bogus and dangerous and their warning that any story on it would create customers. The exoerts were right on both counts. Other "60 Minutes" programs have boosted cancer quackery and the "mercury amalgam toxicity" hoax.

Here are some suggestions for journalists (print and electronic) who cover health and medical subjects: get a college degree or at least a minor in a physical or biological science; always be skeptical; check the credentials of "experts"; if you give coverage to fringe ideas, give equal time or more to responsible experts who disagree; avoid excessive and overly positive coverage of medical "breakthroughs" and misleading headlines about them; cultivate expert contacts in the fields you want to write about; and resist the tempting evil twins, miracle mongering and paranoia peddling. And—perhaps most important of all—*criticize the shoddy work of others whose publications and broadcasts promote quack nonsense.*

What Feminists Can Do

In July 1987, I wrote the following letter to *Ms.* magazine:

> How do you people live with your hypocrisy? You supposedly stand for the rights and welfare of women, but you are deeply involved in two of the most lucrative and damaging ripoffs of women ever conceived. You have long made millions peddling cigarettes to women even though lung cancer rates in women are skyrocketing and smoking is the largest single cause of preventable death and disability among women. And now, with the two-page ad for "Spectrum 360," you have joined the diet hoax industry. Magical cleansing herbs wash out fat and shrink fat cells, and the product burns fat while you sleep. Sounds like the *National Enquirer*. If it's really so wonderful, why don't you run an article on it? Of course, we will never see articles or editorials in *Ms.* dealing with the hazards of smoking and phony diet aids. Is there anything you won't take money and limit your scope of investigation for? How are you any different from the other industries that exploit women for profits?

The letter was not published. *Ms.* went out of business for a few years, but has returned in a new format—with no ads. Maybe it will now start running articles on the hazards of smoking and the fraudulent nature of most weight-control products. In any case, the promotion by *Ms.* of nutritional quackery illustrates the depth of the problem. *It is time for feminists to realize that quackery is a women's issue because women are its main victims. The same is probably true of paranormal scams such as astrology, psychic readings, channeling, and all the New-Age humbug so popular these days.*

Sexual stereotyping (women are more intuitive and spiritual, men are more rational, etc.) tends to steer girls away from science and math. Women are often consoled with the notion that they are more intuitive than men. The consolation compounds the problem as some then decide that intuition is superior to science. Many a New-Age woman becomes seriously paranoid about everything and everyone scientific. She may pass this antiscience bias on to her children. Thus, sexual stereotyping helps create generations of easy prey for quacks and mystical flimflam artists.

Clearly, a major goal of both the feminist and antiquackery movements should be to greatly increase the scientific literacy of girls and women. It would also help if feminist leaders took an active role in combating pseudoscience and quackery.

A Final Comment

Health care in America is costly and sometimes incompetent. Its imperfections are legion and the subject of best-selling books, talk shows, and political rhetoric. Millions of concerned citizens are frustrated and angry about the situation. Unfortunately, a great many of them are being misled by the quackery industry, which has successfully used the terms "alternative medicine," "complementary medicine," and "wholistic healing" to peddle modern snake oils as well as ancient, recycled ones. The public has been deceived into believing that there is a cornucopia of marvelous antiaging and healing techniques, herbs, pills, powders and extracts of every kind that the "medical establishment" ignores and suppresses.

People interested in their own health and the health of their families must ignore all this nonsense and stick to the basics, the proven measures such as prenatal care, eating right, exercising, getting immunized, getting appropriate screening tests, and getting one's RDAs of love and laughter. This is the real wholistic, preventive medicine. Unlike the quacks' megavitamins, amino acids, algae, bee pollen, herbs, enemas, and crystals, these things are mostly free or inexpensive.

The quackery juggernaut has been gaining steam for several decades. Because the public is scientifically naive, the mass media hopelessly irresponsible, and the legislators ignorant and corrupt, it is hard to be optimistic about stopping it. Yet, the alternative is so dangerous and expensive that sooner or later, we must come to our senses. Eventually the pendulum must stop and begin to swing the other way. The obvious must become public policy: we cannot afford to continue to legitimize unproven and fraudulent healing methods. We need a lean, clean health-care system, not one that becomes more bloated.

The American health-care system will be improved by weeding out the incompetent and the greedy, those whose misdiagnoses, irrational prescribing, and unnecessary surgery cost fortunes and lives. It will not be improved by allowing ever-more quacks of every stripe to peddle their fraudulent nostrums freely and without accountability. The answer to poor science is better science, not nonsense.

Appendix

Reliable Sources of Health Information

The following publications can help you deepen and keep current your knowledge of health information and misinformation. Most of the books can be obtained from bookstores, either directly or by special order. For items not usually available through bookstores, we have provided the publisher's address. Out-of-print books not available at your local public library may be obtainable through an inter-library loan. The organizations listed at the end of this chapter may provide information and/or help with filing complaints.

Contemporary Quackery

Arthritis Foundation: *Unproven Remedies Resource Manual.* Atlanta, 1991, Arthritis Foundation.

S. Barrett (ed.): *The Health Robbers: How to Protect Your Money and Your Life.* Philadelphia, George F. Stickley Co., 1980. A comprehensive exposé of health frauds and quackery.

S. Barrett and the editors of Consumer Reports: *Health Schemes, Scams, and Frauds.* Yonkers, N.Y., Consumer Reports Books, 1990.

S. Barrett and B.R. Cassileth (eds.): *Dubious Cancer Treatment: A Report on "Alternative" Methods and the Practitioners Who Use Them.* Tampa, American Cancer Society, Florida Division, 1991.

A. Bender: Health or Hoax: *The Truth about Health Foods and Diets.* Buffalo, Prometheus Books, 1986. An analysis of the "health food" industry and many of its products.

L. Bennion: *Hypoglycemia: Fact or Fad?* New York, Crown Publishers, 1985. A lucid analysis of the fad diagnosis vs. the real disease.

R.J. Brenneman: *Deadly Blessings: Faith Healing on Trial*. Buffalo, Prometheus Books, 1990.

C.C. Cook-Fuller and S. Barrett (eds.): *Nutrition 92/93*. Guilford, Conn., Dushkin Publishing, 1992. A sourcebook containing more than sixty well-written articles from magazines, newsletters, and journals. Updated about once a year.

R.P. Doyle: *The Medical Wars*. Buffalo, Prometheus Books, 1985. A lucid analysis of the scientific method and its application to sixteen medical controversies.

H. Cornacchia and S. Barrett: *Consumer Health: A Guide to Intelligent Decisions*. St. Louis, Mosby Year Book, 1992. A referenced textbook covering all aspects of health care.

The Editors of Consumer Reports Books: *The New Medicine Show*. Yonkers, N.Y. Consumer Reports Books, 1989. A practical guide to common health problems and products.

F. Fernandez-Madrid: Treating *Arthritis: Medicine, Myth, and Magic*. New York, Plenum Press, 1989. Combines a fascinating history of arthritis quackery with insights about modern treatment.

K. Frazier (ed.): *The Hundredth Monkey and Other Paradigms of the Paranormal*. Buffalo, Prometheus Books, 1991. An updated anthology of articles originally published in the *Skeptical Inquirer*.

J. Fried: *Vitamin Politics*. Buffalo, Prometheus Books, 1984. The classic investigation of megavitamin therapy and its proponents.

M. Gauquelin: *Dreams and Illusions of Astrology*. Buffalo, Prometheus Books, 1979. A detailed account of the history and debunking of astrology.

H. Gelband et al.: *Unconventional Cancer Treatments*. Washington, D.C., U.S. Government Printing Office, 1990. A comprehensive report from the Office of Technology Assessment.

H. Gordon: *Channeling Through the New Age: The Teachings of Shirley MacLaine and Other Gurus*. Buffalo, Prometheus Books, 1988. A critical look at mysticism, yoga, reincarnation, psychological techniques for "increased awareness," and other components of the "New Age" movement.

V. Herbert and S. Barrett: *Vitamins and "Health" Foods: The Great American Hustle*. Philadelphia, George F. Stickley Co., 1981. An investigative exposé of the "health food" industry.

L.E. Jerome: *Crystal Power: The Ultimate Placebo Effect*. Buffalo, Prometheus Books, 1988. Historical and scientific perspectives on crystal mythology.

C. Marshall: *Vitamins and Minerals: Help or Harm?* Philadelphia, J.B. Lippincott Co., 1985. A comprehensive look at the sources, functions, benefits, dangers, and controversial aspects of vitamins and minerals.

G. Mirkin: *Getting Thin.* Boston, Little Brown, 1983. Weight-control facts and fads.

W. Nolen: *Healing: A Doctor in Search of a Miracle.* New York, Random House, 1974. A two-year study of prominent faith healers.

J.P. Payne et al.: *Alternative Therapy.* London, British Medical Association, 1986. A detailed report on "alternative" therapies and how they can be scientifically evaluated.

C. Pepper et al.: *Quackery, A $10 Billion Scandal.* Washington, D.C., U.S. Government Printing Office, May 31, 1984.

J. Randi: *The Faith Healers.* Buffalo, Prometheus Books, 1989. A devastating exposé of evangelistic faith healers and related subjects.

J. Raso: *Mystical Diets.* Buffalo, Prometheus Books, 1992. A fascinating exploration of food cults, their gurus, and offbeat nutrition practices.

D. Stalker and C. Glymour (eds.): *Examining Holistic Medicine.* Prometheus Books, 1985. A devastating exposé of "holistic" propaganda and practices.

F. Stare, V. Aronson, and S. Barrett: *Your Guide to Good Nutrition.* Buffalo, Prometheus Books, 1991. A discussion of dietary balance and avoidance of nutrition fads and frauds.

F. Stare and E. Whelan: *Panic in the Pantry.* Buffalo, Prometheus Books, 1992. An analysis of facts and fallacies related to the safety of America's food supply.

V. Tyler: *The New Honest Herbal.* Binghamton, N.Y., Haworth Press, 1992. A referenced evaluation of more than one hundred herbs and related substances.

J. Yetiv: *Popular Nutritional Practices: A Scientific Appraisal.* Toledo, Ohio, Popular Medicine Press, 1986. (Current address: P.O. Box 1212, San Carlos, CA 94070.) A referenced analysis of more than one hundred nutrition topics of current concern.

J.F. Zwicky, A.W. Hafner, S. Barrett, and W.T. Jarvis: *Reader's Guide to "Alternative" Health Methods.* Chicago, American Medical Association, 1992. An analysis of more than 1,000 reports on unproven, disproven, controversial, fraudulent, quack, and/or otherwise questionable approaches to solving health problems.

History of Quackery

R. Deutsch: *The New Nuts Among the Berries.* Palo Alto, Bull Publishing Co., 1977. How nutrition nonsense captured America.

B. McNamara: *Step Right Up.* New York, Doubleday & Co., 1975. An illustrated history of the American medicine show.

J. Roth: *Health Purifiers and Their Enemies.* New York, Prodist, 1977. An overview of the "natural health" movement and its critics.

R.L. Smith: *At Your Own Risk.* New York, Pocket Books, 1969. A critical look at the history and shortcomings of chiropractic. (Available for $4 from LVCAHF, P.O. Box 1747, Allentown, PA 18105.)

J.H. Young: *The Medical Messiahs.* Princeton, Princeton University Press, 1992. A social history of health quackery in twentieth-century America.

J.H. Young: *The Toadstool Millionaires.* Princeton, Princeton University Press, 1961. A social history of patent medicines in America before federal regulation.

Reference Books on Scientific Health Care

C.B. Clayman (ed.): *The American Medical Association Encyclopedia of Medicine.* New York, Random House, 1989. An 1,184-page guide to over 5,000 medical terms, including symptoms, diseases, drugs, and treatments.

K. Butler and L. Rayner: *The New Handbook of Health and Preventive Medicine.* Buffalo, Prometheus Books, 1990. A guide to preventing and treating common health disorders.

J.F. Fries: *Arthritis: A Comprehensive Guide to Understanding Your Arthritis.* Reading, Mass., Addison-Wesley, 1990. Facts about the causes and treatment of arthritis.

V. Herbert, G.J. Subak-Sharpe, and D. Hammock (eds.): *The Mt. Sinai School of Medicine Complete Book of Nutrition.* New York, St. Martin's Press, 1990. A comprehensive sourcebook by a nationwide team of experts.

D.E. Larson (ed.): *The Mayo Clinic Family Health Book.* New York, William Morrow and Co., 1990. A comprehensive guide to health and medical care.

R.S. Lawrence et al. (eds): *Guide to Clinical Preventive Services.* Baltimore, Williams and Wilkins, 1989. A detailed assessment by the U.S. Preventive Services Task Force of 169 strategies for preventing and detecting health problems.

D.R. Stutz, B. Feder, and the editors of Consumer Reports Books: *The Savvy Patient.* Yonkers, N.Y., Consumer Reports Books, 1990. How to be an active participant in your medical care.

United States Pharmacopeial Convention: *The Complete Drug Reference.* Consumer Reports Books, 1992. A comprehensive guide to more than 5,500 prescription and over-the-counter drugs. Updated annually.

D. Vickery and J.F. Fries: *Take Care of Yourself: Consumers' Guide to Medical Care.* Reading, Mass., Addison-Wesley, 1990. A practical manual with many flow sheets to help decide when medical care is needed.

Magazines

Consumer Reports, P.O. Box 53029, Boulder, CO 80322. Covers a moderate number of topics related to health and nutrition.

FDA Consumer, Superintendent of Documents, P.O. Box 371954, Pittsburgh, PA 15250. Covers nutrition, food safety, drugs, and other medical topics.

Health, P.O. Box 54218, Boulder, CO 80322. Features well-researched articles about health issues. Formerly called *Hippocrates* and *In Health*.

Living Well, P.O. Box 7550, Red Oak, IA 51591. Published by *Good Housekeeping* in cooperation with the American Medical Association. Outstanding coverage of a wide variety of health topics.

Priorities, American Council on Science and Health, 1995 Broadway, New York, NY 10023. Focuses on controversies involving life-style, environmental chemicals, and quackery.

Skeptical Inquirer, Box 703, Buffalo, NY 14226. Features critical analyses of paranormal claims.

Newsletters

Consumer Reports on Health, Box 36356, Boulder, CO 80322. Presents detailed reports on health strategies, with occasional reports on quackery.

Harvard Health Letter, P.O. Box 420300, Palm Coast, FL 32142. Features superb analyses of controversial issues, particularly those involving recently published research.

Johns Hopkins Medical Letter, Health after 50, P.O. Box 420179, Palm Coast, FL 32142. Solid information on basic health strategies.

Lahey Clinic Health Letter, P.O. Box 541, Burlington, MA 01805. Solid information on basic health strategies.

Lawrence Review of Natural Products, Facts and Comparisons, 111 West Port Plaza, Suite 423, St. Louis, MO 63146. Authoritative monthly monographs on herbs and other naturally occurring products.

NCAHF Newsletter, P.O. Box 1276, Loma Linda, CA 92354. Covers a wide variety of events related to quackery and health frauds.

Mayo Clinic Health Letter, P.O. Box 53889, Boulder, CO 80322. Solid, practical information with occasional reports on quackery.

Nutrition Forum, P.O. Box 1747, Allentown, PA 18105. Features in-depth reports and undercover investigations related to quackery and health frauds.

Tufts University Diet and Nutrition Letter, P.O. Box 57857, Boulder, CO 80322. Solid, practical information, with occasional reports related to quackery.

Antiquackery Organizations

American Council on Science and Health (ACSH), 1995 Broadway, New York, NY 10023. Telephone: (212) 362-7044.

Commitee for the Scientific Investigation of Claims of the Paranormal (CSICOP), P.O. Box 703, Amherst, NY 14226. Telephone: (716) 636-1425.

Consumer Health Information Research Institute, 3521 Broadway, Kansas City, MO 64111. Telephone: (816) 444-8615.

National Association for Chiropractic Medicine, P.O. Box 794, Middleton, WI 53562. [Provides referrals to scientifically oriented chiropractors]

National Council Against Health Fraud (NCAHF), P.O. Box 1747, Loma Linda, CA 92354. Telephone: (714) 824-4690.

Federal Enforcement Agencies

Federal Trade Commission, 6th and Pennsylvania, Washington, DC 20580.

U.S. Food and Drug Administration, 5600 Fishers Lane, Rockville, MD 20587.

U.S. Postal Service, 475 L'Enfant Plaza, Washington, DC 20260.

Index

Consumer Health Library® Order Form

A Consumer's Guide to "Alternative Medicine":
A Close Look at Homeopathy, Acupuncture,
Faith Healing, and Other Unconventional Treatments
    Kurt Butler, M.S.   Paper $17.95

Examining Holistic Medicine   Cloth $31.95
    Douglas Stalker, Ph.D., and Clark Glymour, Ph.D.   Paper $19.95

The Faith Healers
    James Randi   Paper $18.95

Follies & Fallacies in Medicine
    Petr Skrabanek, Ph.D., and James McCormick, M.D.   Cloth $21.95

The Harvard Square Diet
    Fredrick J. Stare, M.D., Ph.D., and
    Elizabeth M. Whelan, Sc.D., M.P.H.   Cloth $24.95

Health or Hoax? The Truth About Health Foods and Diets
    Arnold Bender   Cloth $24.95

Mystical Diets: Paranormal, Spiritual,
and Occult Nutrition Practices
    Jack Raso, M.S., R.D.   Cloth $23.95

The New Handbook of Health and Preventive Medicine
    Kurt Butler, M.S., and Lynn Rayner, M.D.   Paper $17.95

Panic in the Pantry: Facts & Fallacies about the Food You Buy
    Elizabeth M. Whelan, Sc.D., M.P.H.,
    and Fredrick J. Stare, M.D., Ph.D.   Paper $13.95

Consumer Health Library®
Series Editor: Stephen Barrett, M.D.
Technical Editor: Manfred Kroger, Ph.D.

Other titles in this series: